D1519145

The Art of Veterinary Practice

The Art of Veterinary Practice

A Guide to
Client Communication

Myrna M. Milani, D.V.M.

University of Pennsylvania Press

Philadelphia

Library of Congress Cataloging-in-Publication Data

Milani, Myrna M.
  The art of veterinary practice: a guide to client communication /
Myrna M. Milani.
        p.   cm.
  Includes bibliographical references (p.   ) and index.
  ISBN 0-8122-3260-7
  1. Veterinary medicine. 2. Veterinarian and client. 3. Human-
animal relationships. 4. Pet owners—Psychology. I. Title.
SF 745.M55   1995
636.089´0696—dc20   94-40919
                                                       CIP

To

D. Michael Rings, D.V.M., M.S.
Associate Professor of Food Animal Medicine and Surgery
The Ohio State University College of Veterinary Medicine,

for letting me bounce my real world ideas off his ivory
tower

Contents

Introduction

The hulking six-footer peered down at me semidefiantly as I peered up at him in total confusion while the golden retriever on the examination table between us grinned good-naturedly. I had just completed a text-book-perfect examination and diagnosis, which I concluded with what I considered the correspondingly perfect textbook recommendations for treatment. Consequently when my client calmly said, "No," I was flabbergasted.

"What do you mean, 'No'?" I asked, grabbing one of the veterinary bibles from the counter and opening it to the problem in question. "Look," I stabbed at the page. "Here's McDuff's problem and here's how we treat it. Now you're supposed to say, 'That's wonderful, Doctor. How much do I owe you?'"

I flashed him my most encouraging smile. He smiled back and flipped the book shut and closely examined its spine while the old dog thumped his tail and studied us both carefully.

"But this is the 'Working Husband with Rich Wife Home All Day to Take Care of the Dog' edition," my client announced solemnly. "We need the one for single, self-employed people working twelve-hour days just to make ends meet."

In such a way I first encountered a basic truth of veterinary practice I'd never even considered before: The most wonderful state-of-the-art medical science and technology has no value if it results in a treatment the owners find unacceptable for whatever reason.

That happened almost twenty years ago, and since then an awareness of that and other highly subjective truths has become even more critical for the successful practice of veterinary medicine. In addition to major life-style changes affecting both small and large animal owners, the relationships between humans and animals also have changed greatly.

Although we may argue that owners who view animals as fur-covered humanoids more likely will want the best possible veterinary care than those who treat their animals like so many bales of moldy hay, both kinds of relationships can complicate the treatment process enormously. Consequently, knowing how to deal most effectively with these relationships as well as objectively evaluating our own feelings about animals have become an increasingly important part of practice.

Similarly, human beliefs regarding the grossly unscientific emotions of guilt and love can sabotage even the most carefully orchestrated treatment regime, and successfully handling these responses requires more art than science. Sometimes we need to lean on Jake Hausmer a little to get him to pay closer attention to basic herd health or other preventive measures; lean too much, though, and getting him to do anything can turn into an uphill battle that benefits neither humans nor animal. By the same token, every practice can lay claim to clients who don't hesitate to use guilt to manipulate practitioner and staff alike: "I would have gotten her spayed before she got pregnant, but it's *so* expensive." And even practitioners who routinely use guilt themselves often resent such clients to the point that it undermines the working relationship.

The notion of love likewise evokes a wide range of client/clinician responses. Although some may choose to believe this emotion manifests only in the small animal arena, nothing could be further from the truth. Granted, those in large animal work might prefer a more neutral term such as "caring" when describing their own feelings or those of their clients, but the fact remains that all practitioners recognize what a critical role this feeling plays in the healing process. Unfortunately, what many of us also discover is that clients may not feel the same way about their animals as we do: We think the Carlins care too much and the Mayers not enough. Either way, unless we can find an equitable way to balance our own feelings with theirs, treating the animal will not be a rewarding experience for anyone.

It's been said that if you don't know where you're going any road will get you there, and a surprising number of practitioners have no idea how they relate to their clients, even though their clients often have very clear ideas on the subject. In general we tend to assume one of three roles in the treatment process—god, best friend, or facilitator—and once again no hard rules apply. Some clients want and need to be told what to do, whereas that same approach will alienate others. Similarly, that easygoing style that gains 100 percent compliance from the Browns may function as an open invitation to the Greens to call at any hour of the day or night with even the most minor concern. Most problems arise because we don't take the time to consider what kind of relationship we want with a particular client and patient. Instead we may assume one generic professional façade and stick with it whether it works or not, or wait for the client to do something and then react passively and often inconsistently. Once again we discover that the art of practice involves understanding our own orientations first, then we can change and adapt if necessary to best serve the needs of our clients and patients.

As veterinary medicine becomes more complex the art of knowing when, how, and to whom to refer a client will become an even more important part of practice. Although we traditionally think of referring when we reach our technical limits, there are other times when referral serves as a valuable option. Sometimes clients who give only halfhearted compliance to their regular practitioner will give 100 percent to a specialist. In terminal cases, referral may fulfill the client's unscientific but nonetheless very real desire to have the animal die under the very best care. Because the reasons for referral can be subjective as well as objective, practitioners must choose their specialists wisely, always bearing in mind that the client often sees the expert as an extension of the general practitioner. Consequently, and as we shall see in Chapter 12, we need to apply selection criteria to these experts that go beyond technical competency.

Integrating our own and our clients' views of alternative therapies also comprises a component of the art of veterinary practice. Although the scientific community may choose to take a slow and cautious approach to this subject, a growing number of people are considering alternatives for themselves and their animals right now. Furthermore, these people tend to be both educated and well-off—two qualities we prize in any client—and it would seem foolish to alienate them. Does this mean we need to do something we don't believe in or support something we don't condone? Not at all. It does mean we need to develop the skills necessary to communicate with this growing population in such a way that both their and our own needs can be met.

The book also considers those issues that cost practitioners the most sleep, including the issue of money. How can the Adlers put a dollar value on the treatment of a great horse like Saber? Why aren't the Barretts paying their bill after all the hard work you did for them? Because money often functions more as a potent symbol than as a simple medium of exchange, it behooves us to work through our feelings about payment as well as develop a sensitivity to those of our clients so we can free ourselves from this often very troublesome aspect of practice.

The emotional response evoked by the subject of money pales considerably when the subject of animal rights comes up. As we shall see again and again, the issue isn't the "rightness" or "wrongness" of a particular orientation so much as the need to work through our own beliefs and gain the self-confidence necessary to accept views that differ among our clients. Although food animal practitioners might consider themselves immune to an emotional issue like animal rights, nothing could be further from the truth. The current attitudes of both the animal rights movement and the food animal industry leave food animal practitioners in the much more vulnerable position. Those who don't work through their own beliefs about this emotionally charged issue could easily wind up wasting a lot of time and energy in unproductive them-against-us encounters.

The Art of Veterinary Practice devotes two chapters to the subjective aspects of terminal illness and euthanasia, topics we often dismiss as either irrelevant or too painful to discuss. Nonetheless, both issues remain realities of practice, and nowhere else can an awareness of the art of veterinary medicine so well serve both client and clinician. Not only can this awareness help to alleviate the devastating effects generated by these situations, it can enable us to see these situations as extraordinary opportunities to practice the highest quality medicine. Granted it requires that we develop a few new skills, but the rewards that come from seeing a client and patient through to the end in a dignified and caring manner make it more than worth the effort.

At the heart of the art of veterinary practice lies the human-animal bond, not as a warm, fuzzy public relations ploy or a scientific discipline, but as a dizzyingly variable, highly subjective, infinitely practical and reliable glue that binds patient, client, and clinician together in the treatment process. When practitioners and clients are asked what bothers them most about our profession, they rarely cite scientific or technological issues or incompetencies. Almost inevitably it boils down to the human factor: Practitioners complain that the animals are great; it's the owners who drive them mad. Clients complain that Dr. Wagner doesn't listen, or care, or understand how they and their animals feel.

It makes sense that practitioners feel somewhat at a loss when dealing with clients and that we consciously or subconsciously communicate this to them, because *Homo sapiens* has been meticulously dissected out of the veterinary educational process on two fronts. First, given the ever-increasing amount of scientific and technological data veterinary students and practitioners are expected to digest, adding something so highly variable as the client-patient relationship to the discussion of every medical problem would seem to necessitate cramming even more into a system already stretched to its limits. Second, just as the client has been dissected out of the educational process, so have the clinician and the student. Few faculty members have time to help the student or practitioner work through his or her own feelings about the objective aspects of a case, let alone the subjective ones.

Nonetheless, the costs of ignoring these aspects of the practice of veterinary medicine are high. Talk to those practitioners who have been sued because they failed to communicate effectively with the client; talk to those who have burned out; talk to those who drink a little too much, or rely on pills just a little too often to get to sleep at night. It's not not knowing the right treatment or surgical procedure that keeps these often very technologically competent and caring clinicians awake. It's the subjective and emotional aspects of practice that cause those in practice the most grief: the people who treat their animals like dirt or love them too much, the specialist who doesn't let us know what's going on, the critically ill patient whose owners just won't give up or want to give up too soon, the seemingly endless stream of unwanted animals to be euthanized, the burden of caring so much and wanting to save them all.

What follows is based on my own experience and discussions with thousands of veterinarians and animal owners over the years and is meant to serve as a guide rather than a definitive text as it delves into the most important of these subjective issues from the patient's, client's, and practitioner's viewpoints. The book utilizes composite anecdotes because much of the information that comprises the art of practice is anecdotal, even if some in the scientific community consider this form only slightly above trivial. However, reducing any animal-owner combination to a lowest common scientific denominator can only gain us a certain degree of accuracy in our treatment; it can never reveal all those subjective idiosyncrasies that enable us to precisely treat a particular problem of a particular animal which belongs to a particular person. That precision and all the benefits that go with it can only be achieved when we integrate the art with the science of veterinary medicine.

Finally, I would like to acknowledge the contributions of the following individuals: Patricia Smith at the University of Pennsylvania Press, who wholeheartedly supported this project from the beginning; Drs. Bonnie Beaver, Charles Neer, and James Wilson, whose valuable criticisms of the original proposal resulted in what I believe is a much better book; David Hollis at the Holstein-Fresian Association of America, for providing background information on the human-bovine relationship; spouse Brian Smith, for his insights into the business of veterinary practice and for keeping things running smoothly as I immersed myself in yet another book; and sons Jeremy and Daniel Milani, for never once in all these years asking me why I couldn't be like other mothers.

Without the help and support of all of them, I could not have written this book.

MYRNA M. MILANI, D.V.M.
Charlestown, New Hampshire

Chapter 1
The Bond and Behavior: The Core of the Art of Veterinary Practice

Years ago, Dr. D. O. Jones opened a senior lecture in Preventive Medicine at the Ohio State University College of Veterinary Medicine by noting that every profession consists of two parts: a science and an art. "The trouble with medicine," D. O. continued, "is that we've got too many scientists and not enough artists." A few research-oriented individuals and those headed for careers in large animal medicine smiled indulgently while the rest nodded respectfully, more out of habit than anything else. Today, however, it no longer suffices to practice only the science of veterinary medicine *or only* its art regardless what professional course we pursue: More and more the public demands that we do both. Nonetheless, developing the art of practice appears so maddeningly nonspecific and even inconsequential when compared to the burgeoning sea of medical science and technology that threatens to drown us that it's easy to ask, "Why bother?"

Two reasons immediately come to mind. First, we need only read texts such as James Wilson's *Law and Ethics of the Veterinary Profession* (1988) and the legal columns in various veterinary journals and animal-related publications to realize that miscommunication gets practitioners in far more trouble than medical incompetency: Bob Grant isn't nearly so upset that his cow died as he is that Dr. Brown didn't share her feelings about the severity of the problem and her doubts about the efficacy of the treatment from the beginning. Similarly, the equally troublesome problem of noncompliance frequently results from a breakdown in communication: By the time Dr. Brown realizes Mary McCormick's relationship to her setter makes medicating and bathing the dog impossible, the once-localized skin infection has spread over the animal's entire body.

Why do we experience these communications problems? As we shall see in the chapters ahead, many times problems arise because we haven't taken the time to work through our own beliefs and feelings about those more subjective aspects of practice that dwell within the province of its art. Lacking this awareness we may wind up projecting our own beliefs on the client: Ms. McCormick insists the setter growls and curls its lip ominously whenever she tries to do anything to it at home, but Dr. Brown loves all setters and dismisses Mary's remark as overreaction. Other times, we may find ourselves grappling with our beliefs for the first time in the owner's presence: The day the setter lunges and snaps at Dr. Brown, all of her thoughts focus on whether to freeze, fight, or run—reactions that contribute nothing to the diagnosis and treatment of the dog's skin condition let alone its behavioral problem. Third, and at the heart of the art of practice, many times we and our clients don't speak the same language: The veterinary educational system demands we speak the language of science and technology even as the majority of our clients communicate in terms of behavior and the human-animal bond. Because a surprising number of veterinarians consider the latter strictly small animal concepts, and many small animal clinicians see these as specialties, we can see why we must broaden our awareness of the bond and behavior if we wish to relate to and communicate with our clients and patients successfully.

The Science of Behavior

Like veterinary medicine itself, animal behavior and the human-animal bond each possesses science and art components, and we need to understand both to appreciate the whole picture. When most people think of the science of animal behavior, they think of Konrad Lorenz and his geese, Karl von Frisch's dancing honeybees, and the primate worlds revealed by the work of Jane Goodall and Dian Fossey. In the past those studying animal behavior adhered to the rules of science laid down by those in physics, astronomy, and chemistry, and these rules, in turn, relied on the supposition of objectivity—that is, on the assumption that the researcher could somehow separate him- or herself from the subject.

However, the very nature of animals and their relationship to humans made playing by these rules particularly difficult for those studying animal behavior, and gradually the science began to consider different standards. Perhaps no three books capture the essence of this evolution more than Edward O. Wilson's *The Diversity of Life* (1992) and Donald R. Griffin's *Animal Thinking* (1984) and *Animal Minds* (1992), which gained the attention of both the academic community and the general public. Wilson deliberately wrote his text in a lyric style to convey and blend the processes of scientific discovery and natural history, a blatant divergence from the scientific norm. Pioneer animal behaviorist Griffin continues his often highly controversial quest to convince his colleagues that animals must and do think in his presentation of numerous studies that offer compelling evidence for a less mechanistic view of animal behavior. Whether we agree with the approaches taken by these highly credentialed individuals or not, their work has found its way into the public conscience; and because the majority of our clients dwell in the public arena, it behooves us to recognize the reality of these orientations.

Within veterinary medicine, the science of animal behavior tends to view animals as displaying either normal or abnormal—that is, problem—behavior and an ever increasing number of texts describing both in large and small animals now exists (Beaver 1992; Campbell 1986 and 1992; Fraser and Broom 1990; B. Hart 1985b; Houpt and Wolski 1982; Price 1987). Although the veterinary profession as a whole still perceives behavioral problems as less important than medical ones, informal surveys of various segments of the public indicate that they do not share this view. Practically anyone intimately associated with an animal shelter will say that behavioral problems remain the number one killer of dogs and cats in this country. Nonetheless, practitioners who wouldn't hesitate to do something to help a dog which vomited three times in forty-eight hours will allow their clients to endure shredded furnishings for years because "everyone knows black Labs like to chew." However, this never-ending quality of behavioral problems—that they rarely either go away or kill the animal without treatment within a relatively short time, like many diseases—causes them to loom in their owners' minds far more clearly than that fractured femur or bout of colic. Ironically, the very fact that so many of these animals fit our deeply ingrained, albeit limited, definition of health as a strictly physiological phenomenon permits many practitioners to dismiss behavioral problems as inconsequential.

The Art of Behavior

As obvious as it seems that clinicians should pay attention to their patients' behavior from a scientific perspective for practical as well as moral reasons, an awareness of the subjective aspects of animal behavior plays an equally critical role in client communication. Consider the following list:

coughing
diarrhea
off-feed
limping
depressed

Every veterinarian immediately recognizes these as signs or symptoms that trigger an often precise sequence of diagnostic and treatment procedures. However, a day spent manning the phone in an average practice reveals that many clients don't share this view. To them, the cough or diarrhea isn't a sign of the problem: The abnormal behavior *is* the problem.

The failure to recognize the discrepancy between these two orientations leads to a common and very frustrating practice experience. The Smiths present their animal to Dr. McPherson because it's coughing; they want the veterinarian to stop the cough. However Dr. McPherson perceives stopping the cough as the final step in a process that begins with the question, "What is causing the cough?" To that end, he hospitalizes the animal and begins an extensive work-up. When the Smiths call for a progress report hours later, he confidently reports the available results and promises more by noon the next day.

"Is Tuffy still coughing so bad?" ask the Smiths, thereby giving Dr. McPherson his first inkling that he and his clients may be experiencing a communication problem.

At this point explaining that no attempts have been made to treat the animal pending the completion of the tests strikes Dr. McPherson as only slightly less dreadful than telling the owners that the work-up—which he now realizes they might not see as related to their animal's problem—is going to cost them several hundred dollars. Because the veterinarian didn't recognize that he and his clients started from quite different points relative to the definition of the animal's problem, he must now justify asking them to accept and pay for treating *his* version of the problem instead of theirs. A practitioner once described this challenge as akin to telling someone who thought he was in Philadelphia why you took him from your office in Denver to Los Angeles instead of to New York City, which is where he really wanted to go: It can be done, but it's not easy.

Theoretically one way to avoid this dilemma would be to educate clients to see these behaviors as signs the same way we do. However, this also can lead to miscommunication because each one of us assigns a wide range of meanings to these behaviors based on our education and experience, two data bases most of our clients do not share. Dr. McPherson examines a calf and diagnoses gastrointestinal parasitism based on the evaluation of numerous objective and subjective factors. However he only mentions the animal's watery diarrhea and listlessness as he explains the condition to the owner. Several months later the farmer stops in for medication for another calf displaying "the same signs as the one that bounced right back after worming" and Dr. McPherson dispenses the same medication. When he sees the now severely ill animal a week later, there's no doubt in his mind it suffers from coccidiosis.

In addition to lacking the time and wherewithal to teach clients to perceive their animals' behaviors as symptoms of disease on the same level we do, we also run the risk of imbuing our clients with our own diagnostic prejudices when we expect them to speak our language.

Perhaps the most glaring example in this category involves feline urinary problems. The client presents the cat with the complaint that it's not using the litter box, and the examination and work-up confirms a diagnosis of urinary tract disease. If the veterinarian then says to the client, "Not using the litter box is a major sign of this problem," the client links that behavior with that medical problem and we can wind up with a situation in which the client calls up and confidently announces "Socks has that urinary infection again," and requests medication every time the cat doesn't use the litter box. Because these problems do tend to recur in cats, few clinicians give dispensing medication without seeing the animal a second thought.

However, not using the litter box is also the number one behavioral problem of cats; but unless clinicians recognize the validity of the behavior in and of itself, they will continue to view it as strictly a sign of a medical problem. After treating Socks repeatedly and living with the cloud of impending urinary blockage hanging over herself and her cat for months, the owner reluctantly accepts Dr. McPherson's suggestion that he perform a perineal urethrostomy to eliminate at least that troubling aspect of the problem.

"Darn," says Socks's owner as the veterinarian carries the cat off to surgery. "I wish I'd never gotten that other cat. Socks never had any problems until then."

In this particular case the link between the behavioral and medical problems is so strong, it seems safest to assume the potential for both always exists. A "pure" case of in-house territorial marking in response to a new cat in the neighborhood becomes a cystitis and potential obstruction when the presence of the interloper sufficiently stresses Socks to the point that he no longer eats, drinks, or eliminates normally. His resistance goes down and he becomes a prime candidate for infection, at which time he begins leaving small puddles of urine in random locations throughout the house as well marking his usual spots. Conversely, Socks could begin urinating on the rug because of an infection but his territorial nature might compel him to continue doing so long after his medical problem is resolved. Treating only the behavioral or the medical component won't cure the cat because each one represents only half the problem.

Although this example may appear dramatic, virtually every problem seen in practice possesses a behavioral component. Once we recognize this, as well as that that behavior can serve as the greatest source of the owner's concern, we can more readily communicate with clients and expand the scope of our treatment to include this parameter.

The Science of the Bond

Of all the discoveries that have affected the veterinary profession, perhaps none has confused more than the studies of the human-animal bond. When we read Katcher and Beck's *New Perspectives on Our Lives with Companion Animals* (1983) or scan the increasing number of studies citing the positive benefits of animal companionship for the physically, mentally, and emotionally impaired, these simply add scientific credibility to something most of us knew intuitively: Being around animals makes many people feel better. However, the scientific validation of the bond now hangs over our heads like the sword of Damocles. On the one hand, we use it to justify treatments that rival those for humans in terms of sophistication and expense. On the other hand, if we err in our judgment or if the treatment fails, we can no longer quite so confidently hide behind that once inviolate protective legal shield that defined animals as chattel.

Here again large animal practitioners who feel tempted to heave a huge sigh of relief and exclaim, "Thank God I don't have to worry about *that!*" could find themselves in an increasingly vulnerable position in the years ahead. When we couple the positive answers to the scientific studies which currently seek to answer the question, "What can companion animals do to improve human physical, mental, and emotional well-being?" with the increased number of wildlife studies that take a less-than-chattel approach as indicated by Griffin's work, we can see that food animals exist in an artificial void between these two populations. As studies expand to include the multifaceted human-equine bond and the relationships between children and their 4-H projects, and as wildlife biologists wax ecstatic about the highly complex relationships that exist among wild ungulates and ruminants, it will become increasingly difficult for large animal clinicians to hang on to any strictly chattel attitudes. Even if the veterinary profession would support such an orientation, it seems highly unlikely that the vast majority of the population who live off the farm will allow it. Like Dr. Brown confronting her belief that all setters are lovable when the dog lunges at her, it would seem wiser to work out our beliefs about the food animal bond ourselves rather than have beliefs regarding it forced on us by others.

One scientific finding relative to the human-animal bond possesses such profound implications for the practice of veterinary medicine, it's difficult to believe that few even acknowledge its existence. The study, conducted in 1929 by W. Horsley Gantt, essentially reversed the roles of human-animal bond studies as we now know them. Gantt remotely monitored the heart rate of a dog at rest and then when an assistant entered the room and interacted with the animal. During this interval, the dog's heart rate went from a resting 100 beats per minute to 150, then gradually dropped to 40 BPM as the assistant stroked it. When the petting ended, the animal's heart rate returned to the resting level, all with no change in the animal's outward appearance following the initial greeting display (Lynch 1987, 16:16–21).

Or consider a study done at The Ohio State University College of Medicine by Frederick Cornhill, who fed rabbits a diet designed to create arterial plaque so he could test the efficacy of an anticholesterol drug. After a specific feeding period, Cornhill tested the animals' blood cholesterol levels and couldn't understand why some of the rabbits consistently exhibited 50 percent lower rates than the others. Eventually he discovered the culprit: The technician who cared for the animals liked these particular rabbits and spent time holding and stroking as well as feeding them each day (Padus 1992, 502).

So even as the scientific data convincingly argue that animals can make *us* feel better, other work offers compelling evidence that nothing more or less than our concerned presence and touch can make animals feel better, too. And because the goal of our profession is to use our knowledge and skills for the benefit of society as well as to relieve animal suffering, it seems only logical to incorporate this awareness of the bond into the practice of veterinary medicine.

Lewis Thomas, president emeritus of the Memorial Sloan-Kettering Cancer Center, noted that human medicine took a major step backward when the stethoscope replaced the physician pressing his ear against the patient's chest, an expression of mutual trust that seems practically suicidal in these litigious days in which the specter of real or imagined political incorrectness and sexual harassment lurks everywhere (Thomas 1983b, 57–58). However, veterinarians and their staffs still can legitimately and effectively make use of the healing touch in practice. Unfortunately, busy practitioners often claim they have no time for such displays as they rush from examination room to surgery to farm calls, a grave error on several counts. First, owners perceive the veterinarian's lack of intimate contact with the animal as not caring, an oversight far more unforgivable in their eyes than technical incompetency. Second, we deprive the animal of the benefits of that touch. And third, we deprive ourselves of the benefits that interaction with the animal confers upon us, too.

The Art of the Bond

To some extent the art of the bond, like the art of behavior, reflects our ability to go from the accurate answers of science relative to the general population to the precise ones that enable us to treat a specific animal owned by a particular person at a particular time in a particular place. The science of veterinary medicine teaches us the etiology, diagnosis, and treatment of the various autoimmune diseases, but the art of practice teaches us how to deal specifically with autoimmune problems in the Barnetts' sheep or cat.

An awareness of the art of the bond leads us to ask questions such as:

- How strong is the relationship between this person and this animal?
- What form does that relationship take?
- What kind of treatment is acceptable to these owners?
- What kind of financial commitment do these owners want to make?
- What kind of time commitment do they want to make?

Although we will discuss each of these parameters in more detail throughout the book, at this point we should note that, unlike an evaluation conducted from a scientific point of view, the answers to these questions are most variable and relative—that is, no "right" answer exists save the one that holds true for that owner and that animal at that particular time. Moreover, and the far greater challenge, the owner's "right" answer may not be the same as ours and we must find some way to make peace with that; otherwise we'll spend a lot of time trying to change the owner instead of treating the animal. For example, every practitioner sees patients which they consider to be in a deplorable state of neglect, either in terms of general husbandry or a particular problem. At such times, the urge to chastise the owner or herdsman looms as the most natural and caring response. However, the very fact that we stand in a stall or examination room with the owner tells us that this person does care in his or her own way—otherwise we wouldn't be there. Although we may tell ourselves that pointing out the owners' sins will insure they never make them again, in fact this usually alienates clients because we've taken what they viewed as a right and good response—getting professional help for the animal—and turned it into an attack on those very values. Consider the following clinician responses to the Smiths' admission that their pet has been coughing for more than a month:

- "How in the world could you let that poor animal suffer so long!"
- "I'm glad you brought Tuffy in. Let's see if we can help him get rid of that cough."

Although the first response may make the veterinarian feel better, it effectively dooms any chance for open communication with the client. The Smiths thought they did the right thing when they brought the dog in when they did; when Dr. McPherson condemns them, they feel confused and disoriented and this makes them defensive which, in turn, irritates Dr. McPherson even more. Compare this to the second response, in which Dr. McPherson commends the owners for bringing the animal in, then focuses all his energy on treating the animal with the owners' full cooperation.

An awareness of the bond also makes it very clear that to some extent all of our treatments function as placebos in that they won't work if the owners don't believe in their rightness for their animals and themselves at least enough to implement them as directed. Moreover, and one of those miracles of practice, if a solid bond exists between the owner and the animal and the practitioner and the owner and the animal, even the most rudimentary treatments can yield the most amazing results.

For example, surely every practice is blessed with at least one client like Bob Donahue and his family, who adore their pet but can barely keep food on the table, let alone afford anything extra for an animal. What makes Bob stand out as the perfect client in many ways is his relationship with his dog, Lady, and his honesty. During his first meeting with the practitioner, he introduced himself as "Call me Bob," and unashamedly admitted he was a little slow and would keep asking questions until he clearly understood exactly what the veterinarian wanted him to do. He also promised that he and his family would do anything they could for the dog in terms of home care, but he couldn't afford to spend much and wouldn't take charity.

When Bob brought Lady in with her hind leg smashed and solemnly announced a dollar limit that barely covered the cost of an examination and the most minimal medication, no acceptable course of action rushed to fill the void his words created in the veterinarian's scientifically trained mind. Nonetheless, the way the dog and her owners felt about each other and the way the clinician felt about them all made anything seem worth a try.

To make a long story short, the dog fully recovered on a primitive regime based on strict confinement, good nutrition (which meant family members upgraded the dog's diet with specific items from their own plates), meticulous care of the wounds and the dog's environment, some questionable antibiotic back-up, and lots of support from the family and everyone who knew them and the dog.

Throughout this process, the idea of formulating such an irresponsible regime in terms of her training never strayed far from the practitioner's mind. And yet when Bob would call or stop in with his children, the awareness of both the reality and the power of the bond would erase those doubts—at least momentarily. Although the clinician most certainly would never include this case on her scientific résumé, that outrageous nontreatment brought several new clients to the practice because everyone liked Bob and Lady, and Bob delivered beer and soda to practically every general store in the county. He could never say enough good about the veterinarian even though she did next to nothing and some of that was questionable. But she can never say enough good about Bob, either, because he taught her about the power of the bond in a way no text could.

This in no way means that an awareness of the bond serves like St. Jude, the patron saint of hopeless cases, to bail us out when clients won't allow us to practice our medical magic. In fact, cases such as this demand that we summon virtually every scrap of medical knowledge we possess as we take a meticulous history and conduct a scrupulous physical examination because there will be no blood tests, radiographs, or any other technological aids to fill in any details we might miss.

Conversely, an awareness of the bond plays an equally crucial role when clients place no limits on our technology. Dr. McPherson describes the work-up and treatment of a cow to Harry Simmons in terms of the animal's market or breeding value and the owner says, "I don't care what it costs. I want you to do everything you can to save her." Or the practitioner negotiates that mostly uncharted minefield known as the human-equine bond and tells Chip O'Brien, the animal's caretaker, that the ancient mare has multiple problems. "Frankly, I'd shoot her," says Chip, making no attempt to hide either his disgust for or dislike of the animal. "But my mother insists you do everything you can."

In these two situations, the practitioner's mind veers in three different directions simultaneously. One part immediately begins formulating a diagnostic protocol. Another (hopefully smaller) part notes that new tires for the truck just might be possible this month. A third part grapples with totally unscientific questions like "What's the deal with old 'Bottom-Line' Simmons? How come this cow means so much to him?" or "Am I going to spend days working up this mare only to have that O'Brien clown louse up the treatment?"

Although some may prefer to ignore the latter considerations, every practitioner soon learns that solid owner commitment to the animal and the treatment process makes the high of a sky's-the-limit case even higher. And few can deny the feeling of vulnerability that results from the awareness that the owner's commitment to the animal and the treatment process goes no further than his or her checkbook.

Most of us learn to incorporate bond factors into our treatment regime, but unfortunately often as the result of what happened in the past when we failed to do so rather than as a matter of choice. Before Dr. McPherson lays a hand on her animal, Ms. Fellows defiantly announces there's no way she's going to fight with her dog three times a day to shove pills into it like he made poor Ms. Dickinson do, and Dr. McPherson suddenly sees liquid amoxicillin in a whole new light. Similarly, we learn to recognize those clients for whom environmental concerns take precedence over efficacy when we prescribe products for external parasite control: Even though their animals always sport a flea or two, the Carmichaels tell their friends about their great veterinarian who cares about the planet as well as the animals.

For those who never have considered the ramifications of the bond, all this subjectivity can prove most disconcerting.

"Whatever happened to the good old days when you diagnosed a problem, prescribed the best treatment you knew, and the owner did whatever you said, no questions asked?" they ask wistfully.

Actually, we can recreate such good old days with certain clients, as we shall see in Chapter 9, but changes in human-animal relationships, owner life-style, the increasing cost and sophistication of medical technology, and the presence of alternatives make this only one of several approaches clinicians must use if they wish to meet the needs of their clients. Granted the idea of meeting the often highly subjective, sometimes bizarre needs of someone like Ms. Fellows, who feeds her Pomeranian from a spoon, strikes some as personally denigrating and a blatant attack on the values espoused by the profession. And most certainly practitioners who believe this should not subject themselves to the Ms. Fellowses of the world. However, unlike the case during the good old days, fewer and fewer veterinarians practice in areas where they offer the only game in town, and clients must play by the practitioner's rules—or at least pretend to—if they want veterinary care for their animals. Not only is it increasingly likely that some veterinarian down the road would be more than happy to see Ms. Fellows simply to generate income, it's also more likely that Ms. Fellows would go to someone in the next county if she believed that clinician more attuned to her relationship with her animal. Now the first practitioner could lose on two counts:

- He or she loses a client.
- Ms. Fellows could tell anyone who will listen that she quit going to the Valley Veterinary Hospital because "the doctor there doesn't care."

But what do you do if you find the relationship between the owner and the animal personally offensive for whatever reason? A quick rule of thumb reminds us that the only guaranteed change we can make is in ourselves; we might be able to change another, but it's hard work with no guarantees. So you look at Ms. Fellows and her dog and ask yourself, "Can I change my beliefs to the point I can accept this woman and her dog as they exist right now?" If the answer is "No," then do yourself and Ms. Fellows and her animal a favor and refer them to a colleague you believe would meet their needs better.

Although this seems like a no-win situation, in reality it can turn into a no-lose one. If Ms. Fellows does take your advice, she will view you as a caring person who put her and her animal's needs first. Such people not uncommonly say to their friends, "Baby and I go to the Hillcrest Veterinary Clinic because her problems require special handling, but I bet you and your animals would be very happy with that nice doctor in the valley who's much closer to you." If Ms. Fellows says she doesn't want to go anywhere else and asks why you don't want to treat Baby, this gives you a legitimate opportunity to share your feelings about her relationship with the animal. Many times just expressing those concerns in a professional manner—that is, "Treating Baby like a person can lead to all kinds of medical and behavioral problems and that bothers me," versus

"You must be sick to feed that dog with a spoon"—enables these people to see their relationship in a whole new light.

Point of View

The key to effectively and efficiently integrating behavior and the bond into practice rests upon the practitioner's ability to objectively evaluate these often highly subjective parameters as they affect the relationships between the owner and the animal, the owner and the practitioner, and the practitioner and the animal. Aside from noting that the idea of objectively evaluating subjective factors sounds like a New Age oxymoron, more than a few busy practitioners might also point out that there aren't enough hours in the day as it is without taking on this additional burden. However, many times it's our failure to summon the necessary objectivity that makes integrating these concepts time-consuming and emotionally draining.

For example, imagine Ms. Fellows revealing she spoon-feeds her dog. What kind of responses might this elicit?

- Ms. Fellows obviously lacks a few neurons.
- Ms. Fellows is definitely going to be a Problem Owner.
- People like Ms. Fellows shouldn't be allowed to own animals.

Although all of these might sound legitimate, all spring from an emotional rather than an objective evaluation of the relationship between Ms. Fellows and her dog and offer no viable solutions. Having defined the relationship between owner and animal as aberrant, then what? What usually happens is that every time that client's name shows up in the appointment book, the practitioner groans and prays he'll be called out for a large animal emergency that day—provided it's not to Farwell Farm because their herdsman is such a fussbudget about his Holsteins it can take all afternoon just to treat one case of mastitis there.

As we can see, such responses can generate a lot of negative emotion for the practitioner and take up a lot of time while doing nothing to resolve the problem. In fact, such evaluations only make the problem worse: Who wants to spend anything beyond the barest amount of time with people displaying the attributes ascribed to Ms. Fellows or the herdsman at Farwell Farm? It would seem we deserve a medal merely for tolerating them and not saying "I told you so" when their animals succumb to the negative effects of the relationship somewhere along the line.

However if we remove our emotions from the process and look at the owner's relationship with the animal as well as the resultant behavior objectively, this more likely will lead us to ask meaningful questions than pass judgment:

- Is this relationship acceptable to the owner?
- Is the relationship detrimental to the animal?
- How can I best maintain the animal's physical and behavioral health within the context of the relationship?

By seeing the problem as it affects the owner, the animal, and the clinician, the veterinarian positions him- or herself as a viable source of information and assistance to the client rather than as a judge, and in doing so leaves the door open for a mutually rewarding relationship.

As we shall see time and time again as we explore the many subjective factors that comprise the art of practice, this ability to view behavior and the human-animal bond objectively from the owner's and the animal's as well as our own point of view can do much to untangle some of the most complex issues encountered in practice.

Chapter 2
Common Human Orientations Toward Animals

As we noted in Chapter 1, one of the paradoxes of veterinary practice is that the individual client-patient relationships that make each interaction unique and exciting can also leave practitioners feeling disenchanted when they misread them. Dr. A. thought Mr. Chapman would be willing to plate Spot's leg because the terrier is such a great little dog; he's stunned when the owner refuses because Spot is, after all, just a dog. Dr. B. recommends culling a cow because of a nonresponsive condition and the normally objective farmer looks at her as if she recommended doing in his spouse: He could never do that to Emily, the only cow that survived when the old barn burned to the ground.

Adding to the confusion, human-animal relationships can be highly dynamic and variable. Owners who respond to their animals as little children one day may see those same animals as incomprehensible beasts the next. They also may respond differently to different animals in the same environment: Spot gets the same quality medical care as the kids whereas Fluff is left to fend for himself. Similarly, clinicians may respond differently to different individuals, breeds, or species or in response to the animal's condition based on their own beliefs and experience: Nip is wonderful, but Tuck is a jerk; retrievers are calmer than Yorkies; horses are more skittish than cows; terminally ill animals get more petting and reassuring murmurs than routine milk fevers or ovariohysterectomies.

Consequently, even though individual clients may form relationships with various animals that span the spectrum from what we might consider gross overindulgence to criminal neglect, recognizing the broad categories to which most human-animal interactions belong enables us to better understand what clients are thinking. And because the clinician always forms a triumvirate with the patient and the client in the treatment process, clinicians should also recognize their own orientations toward their patients, too. Above all, practitioners should acknowledge that no matter how aberrant a relationship may appear, it exists because the person maintaining it believes it works at that particular time.

The Anthropomorphic Orientation

As the name implies, people who view an animal anthropomorphically tend to assign it human qualities and this results in a relationship that carries the maximum emotional charge. Moreover, and as any practitioner can attest, what human qualities owners ascribe to an animal when is arbitrary at best. Although viewing an animal anthropomorphically is certainly a more common response of companion animal owners, owners of food animals kept as pets also often relate to these animals in this manner, as do seemingly detached farmers and herdsmen who may form such relationships with one particular animal in the herd or flock or with a family pet or barn cat with whom they closely identify for some reason. Similarly, owners who would never think to relate to a healthy animal anthropomorphically may do exactly that when the animal becomes ill.

A common stereotype portrays anthropomorphically oriented owners relating to their animals as somewhat dimwitted children, but these people may also attribute very sophisticated and complex responses to their charges. Thus Mary Stevens may babble baby talk to her poodle in the waiting room, but then place the dog on the examination table and declare with certainty, "Muffin says he has a headache."

Before denigrating the owner's view as well as her remark, bear in mind that all human attitudes toward animals reflect anthropomorphic views to some extent for the simple reason that that's the only way we can view members of a different species. What makes the anthropomorphic orientation different lies in these people's willingness to see animals, or perhaps just that one particular animal, as animate extensions of themselves, a view best summed up in the old saying, "Love me, love my dog." To do this requires an emotional investment on the owner's part which further colors the quality of the relationship. Mary Stevens does not assign general human species' qualities to Muffin. She sees the dog as possessing a very specific set of attributes that can reflect some of her most intimate beliefs about herself.

Is this good or bad? As we shall see repeatedly as we study the art of veterinary practice, it isn't so much a question of good or bad or right or wrong as whether it works for the person and the animal in that particular situation.

Advantages of the Anthropomorphic Orientation

One obvious advantage enjoyed by anthropomorphically oriented owners is that they always believe they know what their animals are experiencing because it's what they themselves would experience under similar circumstances. However, if we don't recognize where these clients are coming from, miscommunication can result. For example, the human symptom "headache," translated into veterinary terms, logically could point the clinician toward a presumptive diagnosis of head trauma or a central nervous system problem, but in Muffin's case it could mean something entirely different. Further adding to the problem, sometimes these owners' overly solicitous manner and delivery may irritate us to the point that we discount what they're saying. However, they do tend to pay very close attention to their animals and with a little effort it's possible to separate their self-projections from meaningful information about the animal. When asked how she knows Muffin has a headache, Ms. Stevens answers that the dog rubs the side of his face "just like I do when I have a headache," a statement that leads us to shift our focus from CNS toward eye, ear, teeth, or skin problems.

The second advantage of this orientation is that these clients often will embrace everything that science and technology have to offer if they want and expect the same for themselves. Ms. Stevens gets her teeth cleaned twice a year; so does Muffin. Her physician routinely orders blood work when Ms. Stevens feels under the weather; naturally she wants the same for her dog. Even the farmer who never would consider any treatment whose cost exceeds market value for those animals in his flock or herd in general may willingly go to extraordinary lengths for one particular animal who carries a particularly strong emotional charge.

A third advantage is that anthropomorphically oriented clients often listen very attentively, as long as we bear in mind that they respond better to analogy than linear fact: They want to know what they would be experiencing if they had the same problem as the animal. Consequently statements that begin with phrases such as "It's a lot like when you [twist your ankle, catch a cold, eat something that disagrees with you]" appeal to them more than specific references to the animal's anatomy and physiology.

Disadvantages of the Anthropomorphic Orientation

A major disadvantage of this orientation results from the uncontestable fact that animals aren't human. Even as the media and convention champion treating an animal as a person as the very highest state an animal could hope to achieve, in reality doing so represents the state of least human knowledge. We needn't know anything about dogs or cats or horses or cows to treat them like humans: We only need to know ourselves. The ramifications of this are familiar to all practitioners:

- Anthropomorphically oriented owners feed the animal what they eat instead of a balanced diet because they think what they eat looks and tastes so much better.
- They apply remedies that work for them to their animals, unmindful that these remedies may be problematic.
- They attribute their own feelings—and especially their fears—to the animal.

Similarly, just as these owners will go to extremes to treat their animals if they believe the treatment right for themselves, they often just as adamantly will refuse any treatment they see as detrimental to themselves for any reason: No matter how beneficial steroids might be for his horse, John Griffin can't get beyond his own negative experiences with the drug to allow treatment of his animal with it.

Another drawback of this orientation is that these owners can serve as the source of great emotional stress for the clinician because telling them their animals have a problem often amounts to saying the owners have one too. Recall that standard media event, the pet look-alike contest, during which owners boast of their similarities to their animals. We laugh at the saggy jowled owner with the saggy jowled bulldog; we don't laugh when the obese owner waddles into the examination room with the obese old English sheepdog in tow. Because these owners perceive the animal as an extension of themselves, they are much more likely to take anything the clinician says about their animals personally and that usually means emotionally. Because of this, it works better to listen carefully to their view of the problem and then respond to them in that same context.

Consider these two postexamination clinician responses to Muffin and her owner:

- "Muffin doesn't have a headache. He has an infected tooth."
- "No wonder Muffin's head was bothering him! He has an infected tooth."

The second response may seem like a non sequitur in the traditional medical sequence which equates head pain with head trauma or a CNS problem, but it acknowledges the client's unique relationship with her pet rather than dismissing it. Not only that, it makes the owner feel good because it recognizes that she knows her pet well enough to notice a problem and seek treatment for it. Compare that to the first response, which dismisses Ms. Stevens's headache definition as wrong, then goes on to imply that the owner missed Muffin's tooth problem. Which response more likely will leave the client feeling good about herself, her dog, and her veterinarian?

A third critical disadvantage of this orientation will be discussed in more detail in subsequent chapters: Because anthropomorphic relationships can be intimate to the point that these owners see the animal as four-legged, fur-covered mirrors of themselves, not only are they more likely to fall prey to some of the more troublesome human-animal conditions, such as codependencies and separation anxiety, they also can create nightmare scenarios for the practitioner when faced with the terminal illness or death of the animal, to say nothing of its euthanasia. To some extent, the latter conditions can prove even more traumatic for these owners than facing similar circumstances involving a human loved one because medical insurance and the sheer complexity of the human treatment process often make it possible for family members to take themselves out of the treatment loop if they so desire. However, the very nature of veterinary practice demands the inclusion of the owner in the process, and both the economics of terminal conditions and the euthanasia option make timely owner involvement crucial. Although some clinicians may feel sorely tempted to avoid the often highly emotional encounters with these clients, the veterinarian may serve as the only reliable objective reference at such times. Barring his or her reassuring presence and guidance, these people may give in to their fears as well as feelings of abandonment, both of which can feed a belief that has precipitated more than one legal action: "That Dr. Stoneheart didn't care what Muffin and I were going through!"

Recalling that miscommunication with our clients often results from our failure to speak to them in their own language, we see that a more beneficial approach involves recognizing the owner's orientation and then responding in a manner that complements it. This in no way means we must play peek-a-boo with Muffin if we're not a peek-a-boo kind of person. It does mean acknowledging the validity of that orientation if it works for the animal and the owner.

What if the anthropomorphic orientation doesn't work? In this situation, the practitioner's ability to relate to these clients in a manner that doesn't denigrate either them or their relationship with the animal becomes even more critical. For example, every practitioner knows the medical consequences awaiting animals fed strictly table food, but imagine an anthropomorphically oriented owner's response to the clinician who berates her for this practice and predicts dire consequences for the animal every chance he gets, versus her response toward someone who suggests various table foods the animal might enjoy that would also enhance its plane of nutrition: Which clinician would such an owner more readily turn to for help when problems do arise?

The Anthropomorphically Oriented Veterinarian

Although practitioners, just like anyone else, can become involved in anthropomorphic relationships with particular animals, some clinicians do assume this as their primary orientation toward their patients. Some might feel tempted to attribute this approach primarily to the women in the profession because it is a more emotional, parental response and women tend to experience fewer inhibitions about expressing such feelings. However, men also adopt this orientation, and they do it for the same reason their distaff colleagues and their clients do: It works for them.

Maintaining a generalized anthropomorphic orientation toward all patients carries all the advantages and disadvantages for the clinician that it does for the owner—plus a few extra. An obvious advantage relates to the principle of like begets like: If the clinician practices in an area with a sufficient population of those who view their animals anthropomorphically, these owners will naturally gravitate toward a practitioner who shares that view. When anthropomorphically oriented Dr. Sheldon opened her practice a mile down the road from Dr. Stoneheart, Mary Stevens and Muffin were among her first clients and soon Mary's friends made up half of Dr. Sheldon's client base. In this case the orientation became a valuable practice builder.

On the negative side, however, even though veterinary education and training enable clinicians to easily avoid the anthropomorphic assumptions that could lead to medical or surgical errors, when these practitioners get into areas such as bond or behavioral problems where the training is not nearly so rigorous, they can find themselves in trouble. For example, Dr. Sheldon labels a client's cat which breaks its housetraining but shows no clinical evidence of urinary problems as "spiteful," and another client's biting horse as "naturally mean." In these cases the clinician's anthropomorphic response creates two problems. First, these labels don't recognize the problems as remediable let alone do anything to resolve them: The only logical treatment for a spiteful or mean animal suggests some sort of as yet unavailable veterinary psychiatric counseling for the miscreant. Second, such anthropomorphic veterinary pronouncements leave the owner in the awkward position of owning a spiteful or mean animal, not a positive feeling under the best of circumstances and certainly not one that will enhance the human-animal relationship as these people daily clean up the mess or treat their wounds. One practical result of this is that owners who don't feel good about their animals feel less inclined to seek out veterinary care for them. Consequently, an anthropomorphic evaluation of such problems can result in lost revenues to the practice.

A second disadvantage that befalls those who assume a uniformly anthropomorphic attitude is that those clients who don't share this view often find it irritating and unprofessional. Such owners may consider the anthropomorphically oriented practitioner's response as silly and lightweight and automatically assume the same holds true for that person's grasp of medicine and surgery. Mary Stevens's husband hates to take Muffin to see Dr. Sheldon because "she acts as silly around Muffin as Mary." Sensing his antagonism, the clinician feels obligated to justify rather than explain virtually everything she does to the animal, a time-consuming and emotionally draining process that contributes nothing to the treatment process.

Another disadvantage of the generalized anthropomorphic view is that these clinicians may identify so closely with their patients that they lose their objectivity; like the anthropomorphically oriented owner, they take everything that happens to their patients personally. Dr. Sheldon literally winces every time Muffin winces during the examination. Aside from the tremendous emotional burden this can place on the clinician, it also can interfere with the relationship between the owner and the animal if the veterinarian cares more than or in a way different from the client. When Mr. Stevens brings Muffin in for treatment, Dr. Sheldon can't believe he refuses to cuddle the animal following its vaccination; he, on the other hand, wishes she would stop babying Muffin whenever the dog overreacts.

The Chattel Orientation

Unlike those who relate to animals anthropomorphically and see the animal's condition and its treatment as a direct reflection on and of themselves, people who adopt the chattel orientation perceive the animal as an inanimate possession. Although people who maintain strong anthropomorphic views may accuse practically anyone who doesn't share their views of treating animals like inanimate objects, in reality the true chattel orientation rarely occurs among individuals who experience routine one-to-one contact with the animal. Nor do those who dislike a particular animal or species usually ascribe to this view. Because the primary distinguishing characteristic of this orientation is the *lack* of an emotional tie with the animal, those who experience negative feelings about an animal share more in common with anthropomorphically oriented owners than those who adopt the chattel view.

The chattel orientation most commonly occurs among absentee owners: the purebred animal owner whose animal is trained and handled by someone else; the part-owner of a thoroughbred bought for investment purposes; the gentleman farmer or agribusinessman who rarely sets foot in a barn. However, people lacking sufficient training in the subjective aspects of the human-animal bond may also adopt this orientation when placed in situations where the sheer number of animals and/or the emotional components of human-animal interaction could otherwise overwhelm them. Previously anthropomorphically inclined, overworked, underpaid animal welfare workers may take the chattel approach in an effort to protect themselves from the never-ending stream of abandoned and abused animals. Very busy practitioners may seek to free themselves of the time-consuming, energy-draining emotional aspects of practice by embracing this orientation.

Advantages of the Chattel Orientation

The primary advantage of the chattel orientation is that it disavows the existence of the human-animal bond and in so doing comes about as close to creating the illusion of objectivity as possible in the real world. Furthermore, because market value and utility serve as the foundation of the chattel orientation, people who ascribe to this view often maintain very clear ideas regarding what they will and won't do for the animal. Ted Belanger never treats a cow unless Dr. Walsh can guarantee the animal will recover completely. Jane Forsythe wouldn't consider repairing a broken leg on a racing greyhound with a mediocre track record.

A second advantage of chattel-oriented owners lies in their willingness to accept the language of science and technology spoken by many practitioners. Whereas owners who view animals as animate often see the animal's condition in terms of what it means to them personally and may ask questions which require the clinician possess knowledge of the person's relationship with the animal as well as of the animal itself, owners who view animals as chattel seldom voice such concerns.

The lack of emotional attachment that characterizes the chattel approach also spares the clinician the often idiosyncratic responses displayed by owners who view their animals as animate. Dr. Walsh makes his diagnosis and describes the proposed treatment, its cost, and the prognosis; Ted Belanger weighs that information against the animal's production and/or breeding record and makes a decision. Although the farmer may cringe a little if the sick or injured animal is one of his top producers, his decision to treat it or not depends solely on whether the cost of the proposed veterinary care will exceed the monetary value he places on the animal. Compare this approach to that of his neighbor who will spend far more to treat his wife's three favorite Jerseys and his daughter's 4-H heifer than any other animal in his herd.

Disadvantages of the Chattel Orientation

What we gain in objectivity from the chattel-oriented owner, we may lose in commitment to the animal's welfare. This poses little problem if the orientation is embraced by an absentee owner who makes the decision to treat, but it falls upon a more involved herdsman or handler to actually call the veterinarian and carry out any treatment. However, when chattel-oriented owners also serve as the animal's primary caregivers, their emotional detachment can be detrimental.

For example, consider the case of David Bennet, who always wanted to be an engineer but inherited a farm and dairy herd from his father-in-law; as far as he's concerned, cows are hay- and grain-eating milk-producing machines. Because of this definition, this herdsman misses many of the early signs—the slight depression, decrease in appetite, or reluctance to move—a more involved owner might notice immediately. Furthermore, because he recognizes no emotional link to the animals, he sees treating their ailments as just one more thing to take up his time. Interestingly, animals suffering from relatively mild problems may fare worse than the seriously ill because this client's commitment increases directly in proportion to what he could lose financially if he didn't carry out the treatment. Consequently, he takes a lax approach to basic husbandry and routine preventive care but will treat a good producer down with milk fever very conscientiously.

A second disadvantage of this orientation centers around client communication. Although practitioners tired of dealing with emotional owners may welcome the chattel-oriented client's willingness to accept all our scientific jargon, it behooves us to make sure this acceptance reflects true understanding rather than disinterest. When Dr. Walsh gives a textbook-perfect description of the problem afflicting one of the animals which includes drug withdrawal times, possible complications, and public health significance, the farmer nods distractedly as he simultaneously scans the instructions on the medication in his hand, convinced they tell him everything he needs to know. If they do, no problems will arise; if they don't, both the animal and the veterinarian could be in trouble, the latter for taking his client's lack of response as indicative of his understanding.

A third disadvantage of this orientation springs directly from a paradox that underlies veterinary education: Even as many of our texts routinely ignore the existence of any owner, they often simultaneously assume that person possesses maximum emotional commitment to the animal as well as the treatment process. Consequently, when practitioners encounter owners who express less than this ideal, they feel disoriented. And although most of us can learn to accept variations in financial and time commitment and even in the different kinds of emotional commitment owners make, most find the lack of emotion that characterizes the chattel approach incomprehensible and extremely frustrating.

This lack of owner emotion can prove a very emotional experience for the veterinarian, enough so that it can undermine both the client-clinician relationship and the treatment process. Suffice it to say that clinicians who believe they can *make* a client care about an animal can waste a great deal of time and energy. As we noted with the anthropomorphic response, we can save ourselves a lot of mental anguish if we can nonjudgmentally accept the orientation as normal for that particular person and that particular animal at that particular time, and focus all our energy on providing the best possible care within the limits of that relationship.

The Chattel-Oriented Veterinarian

Veterinarians who assume a generalized chattel orientation commonly adopt it as a protective mechanism. For those in food and laboratory animal practice, the sheer number of animals may preclude the opportunity to relate to them in any but the most superficial way. The fact that many of these animals are destined for slaughter further negates the desirability of any emotional involvement. Similarly, those who work in shelters or economically depressed areas may find that this orientation enables them to perform their duties under circumstances that would be incapacitating were they to allow themselves to become emotionally involved with their charges. Third, practitioners stressed by personal problems and/or overwork may adopt this orientation in an effort to eliminate all the variables that the human-animal bond introduces into the treatment process. As noted in Chapter 1, while this theoretically should simplify things, in fact it makes them worse because these clinicians cut themselves off from the positive effects of the bond that far outweigh the negative.

Much more commonly, most of us assume the chattel orientation on a per case basis even though we may not realize this. We all periodically encounter those animals who, for whatever reason, simply do not evoke an emotional response. One practitioner may feel no affinity toward birds whatsoever; normally animal-loving Dr. Walsh finds the Bennets' Appaloosa the dullest animal he ever worked on. It's not that we don't like these animals; we just don't feel any emotional tie to them.

Other times, we may deliberately sever the tie because it interferes with our ability to relate to the client and treat the patient. Dr. Sheldon, who routinely gushes over her patients, knows from (sad) experience to adopt an almost mechanical demeanor when she examines Colonel McIntyre's pit bull because the colonel considers anything the least bit emotional to be frivolous. As any practitioner who has treated his or her own animal can attest, sometimes we assume the chattel orientation when faced with a critical emergency involving a patient for whom our feelings are so great we must sever all emotional ties in order to perform efficiently.

Finally, we may manifest this orientation at the end of a day filled with emotionally draining emergencies and hysterical owners. We examine and vaccinate the placid black Lab as though he were a sack of potatoes; we don't feel anything for the dog because we're too tired to feel anything at all.

In all of these situations the chattel orientation serves as a safety valve to protect us. Whether it becomes problematic depends on how often we use it and whether our clients accept it.

The Integrated Orientation

People who maintain an integrated approach relate to animals neither as people nor as objects, but rather as separate, animate beings who become incomprehensible beyond a certain limit. The good news is that this orientation recognizes the animal as a unique and separate animate creature; the bad news is that these owners may place what we consider detrimental limits on the animal and its needs. Because this relationship appears much less emotional than that in which the owner treats the animal as a fur-covered humanoid yet more caring than that which reduces the animal to an object, a strong temptation exists to perceive these liaisons as more realistic. However, this orientation can rest on human beliefs and prejudices rather than on knowledge of the animal and its needs every bit as much as the anthropomorphic and chattel approaches do. While the hypochondriacal anthropomorphically oriented owner who insists on immediate attention every time his cat sneezes confounds us as much as the farmer who wouldn't spend a dime to treat a barn cat, the owner who ignores his cat's obvious respiratory distress because he believes that cats can take care of themselves leaves us feeling equally troubled.

Unlike anthropomorphically oriented owners who don't distinguish their own feelings and responses from their animals' and those who sever all emotional ties with the animal as in the chattel approach, those who take the integrated approach establish a mental barrier that defines the limits of their relationship with and responsibility to the animal. When the animal crosses that barrier, these owners see the animal as independent of their influence. This, in turn, may lead them to emotionally and/or physically abandon the animal to fend for itself, or it may lead to the evocation of a completely different set of rules.

For example, every practitioner is familiar with owners who create a barrier that sets a dollar value on the relationship: Denise Bottomly acts like an ideal clear-thinking client involved in a stable, affectionate relationship with her dog when seen annually for routine examination and vaccinations. However, when the dog succumbs to a readily treatable liver problem, the owner adds up the costs and opts for euthanasia because she doesn't want to put that much money into him.

Other owners may maintain very strong definitions regarding what constitutes unacceptable behavior which can prove particularly problematic for practitioners who lack knowledge in this area. Whereas anthropomorphically oriented owners routinely blame all hostile displays on outside factors beyond the animal's control—"Muffin was abused when he was young," "Those pills you gave Sequin make her grouchy"—those owners who take the integrated approach may hold the animal totally responsible for any behavior that violates their definition of normal or good. The frightened gelding with the badly lacerated cornea strikes out when George Labrie grabs the halter right below the injury to steady the horse's head for examination, and the normally placid owner beats the animal unmercifully: "No horse is going to kick me!"

Advantages of the Integrated Orientation

Although integrated relationships can carry very potent emotional charges when situations arise that challenge the limits of owner commitment, within those limits these clients often share very solid relationships with their animals. Had Ms. Bottomly's dog never developed that liver problem, the staff at Sunnydale Veterinary Hospital would have considered her one of their most conscientious clients. During discussions of the animal's minor problems she always listened attentively, asked intelligent questions, and followed instructions as directed. Unlike anthropomorphically oriented Mary Stevens, Ms. Bottomly didn't cringe and rub her own ears gingerly when the veterinarian showed her how to medicate her pet's ears. Similarly, George Labrie impressed everyone as one of the most savvy and concerned horsemen in the area until he attacked the injured gelding.

Another advantage of the integrated relationships is that the limits set by these owners tend to be relatively well defined. Whereas Ms. Stevens might maintain all sorts of definitions regarding Muffin based on her own skin, dental, and ear problems, positive or negative reactions to various drugs and diets, and a host of other often inconsequential human experiences, Ms. Bottomly only maintains one: the cost of the treatment. Once the clinician recognizes the nature and magnitude of that limit, he or she can work to keep the animal medically and behaviorally healthy within it as much as possible.

But how do practitioners identity those limits? Although the increasingly symbolic relationship between humans and animals can lead even the most intelligent, seemingly rational clients to establish parameters that only a psychotherapist could comprehend, most people who maintain an integrated orientation set limits affecting veterinary care that fall into one of six general categories:

- financial
- time
- emotional
- physical

- behavioral
- public health

To be sure, anthropomorphically oriented owners do the same thing, but whereas they will seek ways to surmount these barriers—and often see doing so as evidence of their great feelings about the animal—those who take the integrated approach see these factors as creating a protective barrier beyond which the owner will not pass. Ms. Bottomly sees veterinary care as just another item in her budget, not an expression of love for her dog or a projection of her feelings about her own medical care. Another owner knows he can only spend about two hours more a day with his sheep and still fulfill the obligations of his full-time job; whether he will treat a sick animal depends on how much time it will take. Yet another owner will only treat problems that "don't make me crazy," while others will balk at treatments that would create physical inconveniences as varied as threatening the owner's bad back or resulting in a physically imperfect animal. Still others maintain strong ideas regarding what they consider intolerable behaviors that run the gamut from submission to aggression and everything between, while others draw the line at treating those conditions that could be transmitted to people or other animals. Using such awareness as a guideline, we can determine the exact nature of the limits set by a particular client.

Why bother? It's the difference between accuracy and precision again. The more we understand the specific relationship between the owner and the animal, the more we can tailor a treatment regime to meet their needs; the more it meets their needs, the greater the chance of compliance.

Although careful observation and listening often will reveal any limits set by anthropomorphically and chattel oriented owners, that may not hold true for those maintaining the integrated view. Because of this, sometimes a more direct approach becomes necessary to avoid at least the shock, if not the owner confrontations, that may occur when we inadvertently blunder across the line. This often can be accomplished via the question "Does this sound like something you would want to do?" following a description of the animal's problem and any proposed work-up and/or treatment. This purposefully owner-directed question gives clients the opportunity to express a wide range of concerns, and solidly positions them in the treatment loop rather than automatically assuming they will agree with the clinician's approach.

For example, consider the case in which the clinician diagnoses a parasitic skin condition and recommends dipping the animal at specific intervals. In response to the question, the owners may counter with questions of their own, such as:

- "How much time will this take?"
- "Is this dip safe?"
- "Where am I supposed to do this?"
- "Can I [the kids, the other pets, the rest of the herd] catch this?"
- "How will the animal respond to this?"
- "What's this going to cost me?"

These questions sound perfectly normal, and yet all of them relate much more to how the problem and its treatment will affect the relationship between the owner and the animal than to a desire for more scientific information. Moreover, owners usually list their concerns in order of importance to them, which also provides valuable clues to the nature of the relationship. Were the clinician to focus only on the process of diagnosing and treating the condition, he or she could miss these often very revealing indications of the nature of any owner limits that could affect the treatment process.

In spite of the extra effort necessary to determine the owner limits, practitioners who recognize them can greatly enhance their ability to treat their patients effectively. Once Dr. Walsh knows Ms. Bottomly will spend only so much and that another client's relationship with his cows reflects his very strong environmental concerns, he can strive to maintain the health of their animals within those definitions. Although some practitioners may view doing anything but the textbook best as practicing less than quality medicine, many enjoy the challenges offered by these clients and the opportunity to broaden their treatment regimes in an effort to fill these owners' needs.

Disadvantages of the Integrated Orientation

The major disadvantage of the integrated approach is that practitioners may not agree with the limits set by these owners which, in turn, undermines the client-clinician relationship. How can Denise Bottomly place a dollar value on such a great dog? Doesn't that farmer realize all the effective dips are potent insecticides? Granted those owners who treat their animals like furry humanoids or pieces of furniture also can hold their animals hostage to what we consider detrimental beliefs, but most of us consider these views sufficiently different from our own that they threaten us less than the more intellectual approach taken by those maintaining an integrated view. As Ms. Stevens goes on and on about her own infected tooth and how she knows exactly what poor Muffin is feeling, her approach so differs from Dr. Walsh's educationally groomed professional one, he sees her as an irritant at worst and an interesting example of the human-animal bond at best. However, when Denise Bottomly calmly looks him squarely in the eye and announces she doesn't want to put that kind of money into her dog, the idea that she could so coolly and objectively deliver a comment that violates the very core of his professional credo makes him defensive.

The second disadvantage of this orientation arises directly from the first: When these owners set limits with which we don't agree, a very strong temptation exists to define them as wrong and uncaring. Just as labeling an animal's perceived negative behavior as spiteful or mean leads to a dead end, so do such evaluations of human-animal relationships. Whether we agree with these owners' orientation or not, the fact remains it exists because it works for them and it reflects a magnitude and quality of caring they find acceptable. Practitioners who learn to accept and work within the boundaries of a particular human-animal relationship not only stand a better chance of insuring the animal's health within those limits, they can function as valuable sources of information when and if these owners seek to expand those limits in a more positive direction.

The Integrated Veterinarian

The integrated orientation is probably the most common generalized approach taken by practitioners because it appears both more objective and less emotional than the anthropomorphic approach, but more caring than the chattel orientation. The key to its success, however, lies in the flexibility of the individual practitioner, and that depends on the nature of the limits he or she sets on the relationship with animals in general and any patient in particular. For example, new veterinary graduates not uncommonly feel that the only right way to treat an animal means doing everything medically and surgically possible for as long as possible. Whether these people will find happiness practicing in the Los Angeles ghetto or Appalachian backwater community will depend a lot more on their ability to establish new limits than any knowledge of veterinary medicine.

For those veterinarians who recognize their own limits, the advantage of the integrated orientation is obvious: Like clients who adopt this orientation, they possess a clear idea of what they will and won't do. As long as their clients agree with them or they don't need those who don't, they experience no problems. Dr. Walsh can adhere to his belief that declawing is cruel because he only gets about two requests for the service a year and the majority of his clients share his view. In this environment Dr. Walsh's limits complement those of his clientele and serve as a practice builder.

The disadvantage occurs when our limits differ significantly from those of our clients and we view those limits as inviolate matters of principle rather than as choices we make that reflect our personal beliefs. Dr. Walsh refuses to euthanize healthy animals but knows nothing about behavioral problems. Because behavioral problems are an extremely common reason for euthanasia and most animals with behavioral problems appear physically healthy, Dr. Walsh's limits ignore the reality in which many of his clients live. While he might consider the owner who euthanizes a physically healthy animal as the epitome of uncaring irresponsibility, that owner may view him in exactly the same light for failing to take the animal's behavioral problems seriously and offer help. In this situation, Dr. Walsh's orientation undermines his professional credibility rather than enhancing it.

Of the three human orientations toward animals, the integrated one offers practitioners the most leeway because it enables us to strike a balance between the emotional and practical when relating to clients and patients. By the same token, however, it also challenges us with the greatest array of variables. Because of that, we need to consider some of the limiting factors that can influence the client-patient-practitioner relationship and thus the treatment process.

Chapter 3
The Art of Discussing Money

Of all the factors that may affect the treatment process, few confound practitioners more than money. However, we can rightfully claim this confusion for several reasons. First, a very large gap exists between our training, which often assumes money is no object, and the real world of our clients, where money can be a very big object indeed. Second, even as the cost of our technology soars, we live in a time when fewer people can claim financial security with certainty; upper level managers, investment bankers, and engineers are just as apt to find themselves unemployed as blue collar workers are. Owners of once thriving herds see their income swallowed up by raging floods or their inability to compete with increasingly large and powerful agribusinesses. Third, and most troubling, many people—practitioners and owners alike—may attach very potent and symbolic meanings to money which directly or indirectly may influence the treatment process.

Surely all veterinarians know the old saw that claims there are two kinds of veterinarians: those with time and no money, and those with money and no time. As ingrained as that particular sentiment might be within the profession, few veterinary business consultants share that view. Moreover, one of these, David Gallagher, cites two economic studies conducted by economist Dr. R. K. House that prove just the opposite. In both the large and small animal practices surveyed, veterinarians who charged the highest fees not only enjoyed the highest incomes, they also worked the fewest hours (Gallagher 1993, 7:1). Although this would seem to make a sound case for a "Damn the financial considerations, full speed ahead!" approach, many practitioners working long hours for low wages find it difficult to do this. Whether this results from an actual or an imaginary gap that the subject of money creates between them and their clients, its effect remains very real.

Communicate, Communicate, Communicate

Some business experts claim the three most important components of a successful business are location, location, and location. However, how happily a practitioner conducts his or her business in that location surely depends on that person's ability to communicate, communicate, and communicate some more. With the advent of computers, we can now calculate the cost of a certain procedure down to the penny and this amount generally reflects an objective evaluation. However, whether practitioners succeed in getting that price depends on two factors:

- Whether they ask their clients for it.
- Whether their clients are willing and able to pay it.

And both of these factors depend solely on the clinician's ability to discuss money matters openly with the client.

Although asking for payment would seem as natural an act as performing a particular service, many practitioners find this the most difficult part of practice, to the point that some will even foist it off on their office staffs or, worse, their computers. Ms. Evans stares stunned at the bottom line of the totally accurate, precisely itemized, neatly printed bill in her hands; Dr. Connor shrugs apologetically and says, "It's all done by computer," then scurries off to see his next patient. In this situation, Ms. Evans's shock—and perhaps her subsequent irate letter to the board of veterinary examiners—might not result from the fact that she doesn't believe her animal or Dr. Connor's work merit that amount, but rather that he didn't *tell* her how much the procedure was going to cost.

Which brings us back to communication again. Why do so many of us find it so difficult to talk about money? First, veterinary education often deals with the subject tangentially at best. Although computerization permits faculty members to keep running tabs on their cases, they may or may not share these with students, and any discussions with the client regarding cost and payment may occur in private. Other times those who bring an animal to a veterinary school do so with the idea that they'll do whatever the experts there recommend regardless of the cost, further separating students from the financial implications of the treatment process.

Second, as a profession we always have promoted and reinforced the public image that we became veterinarians because we love animals, even though few consider "people loving" or "teeth loving" a prime pre-requisite for physicians or dentists. This is not to say our orientation is wrong but rather that it, coupled with our training, easily if irrationally leads to the belief that a clinician who truly cares about animals doesn't care about money.

This belief, in turn, makes us reluctant to discuss money for fear our clients will think us uncaring, and that approach gives rise to a very neg-ative and counterproductive paradox. Because we find it so difficult to discuss money, we hesitate to bring up the subject before we commence treatment. However, the less we discuss money beforehand, the more likely we'll run into problems related to it afterward. At that time, the owners' reluctance to pay makes us feel abused because we did, after all, respond to the animal in what we considered a caring manner. The fact that the owners accuse us of being *uncaring* money-grubbers strikes us as totally opposite the truth. However, as we saw with Ms. Evans, these clients aren't accusing us of not caring about their animals; they're accusing us of not caring about *them.* And because our clients, not our patients, pay the bills, it behooves us to consider their needs, too.

Communicating Before the Fact

Unfortunately many practitioners think of communicating as some sort of touchy-feely client interaction which they reject because it either makes them feel personally uncomfortable or because it violates their definition of professionalism. However, the type of communication rec-ommended here shares little in common with small talk. Practitioners who excel at happy chatter may fail miserably in terms of imparting use-ful knowledge to their clients. And as we know from sources as diverse as the Bible (Proverbs 24:4 and 25:12), Francis Bacon (1597), and Samuel Johnson (1759), knowledge is power. The more people know, the more they feel in control of the situation. Moreover, John F. Kennedy expanded that notion in a manner of particular importance to practitioners when he noted, "In a time of turbulence and change, it is more true than ever that knowledge is power" (Kennedy 1962). Un-fortunately, it is at such times of turbulence—when faced with the fam-ily pet hit by the car, the near comatose horse, the down cow—that most of us focus on summoning as much medical knowledge as we can to treat the animal while letting the owners fend for themselves.

Because consistency, and only consistency, of response leads to last-ing change, it makes sense to formulate a practice policy that integrates information about both the animal *and* the costs involved in its treatment from the every beginning. For example, compare these two scenarios.

1. Mr. Croteau arrives at the Happy Valley Veterinary Hospital for his first appointment and sees a large sign announcing, "All services must be paid for at the time they are rendered!"—his first exposure to Happy Valley's payment policy. He curses and slaps his pocket in hopes his checkbook will magically appear there.

2. When Mr. Croteau calls Happy Valley for his first appointment, the receptionist tells him how much the examination and vaccinations he requests will cost. She then notes that clients are expected to pay for services at that time unless other arrangements have been made with one of the doctors in advance. When he arrives for his appointment, he sees this same policy on a small sign next to one which invites clients to ask staff members for any assistance they may need. The same payment policy also appears at the bottom of the information form the receptionist asks him to complete.

Even though we may rationalize that people don't go into a supermarket and expect credit, the fact remains that few people consider veterinary practices on a par with supermarkets and we've worked long and hard to create an image that doesn't support the view that they are. Furthermore, a lot of people do go to physicians, dentists, lawyers, accountants, and other professionals who do not expect immediate payment for one reason or another. When clients first become aware of Happy Valley's credit policy via a sign that allows them no gracious way out of what could be an innocent oversight, payment takes on a negative emotional charge that may interfere with the treatment process. When the client in the first scenario realizes he left his checkbook at home, his embarrassment and dread about admitting this cause him to miss much Dr. Connor tells him about his animal.

Once we actually see the client, another old adage that directly relates to communication comes into play: Most people really do believe they get what they pay for. But how can our clients know what they're paying for unless we tell them? This certainly doesn't mean informing the client of the dollar value of every syringe and cottonball used in the process of examining and treating the animal. However, pertinent financial facts may be integrated into the information we share with the client relative to those aspects of the case that will add to the estimate mentioned when the appointment was made. For example, consider these phrases for use when seeing routine cases.

- "Because of the nature of this infection, I think we should use one of the newer, more potent drugs to treat it. It will cost about X dollars to treat Snuffy, but I think it will give us much faster results."
- "The nice thing about this drug is that it's very effective in cases like this and you only need to give it once a day, but it does cost three times more than the other treatment available."
- "These tests cost Y dollars but I think it's money well spent because they'll tell us more about Snuffy's thyroid [adrenal gland function, immune response]."

In addition to supplying the owner with information regarding the animal's condition and the possible costs of treating it, these responses all keep the owner firmly in the treatment loop. The clinician does not say, "This is what we're going to do and this is what it's going to cost you," or, worse, "This is what we're going to do. Period."

When we combine this approach with a clearly stated and reinforced payment policy that permits clients to make alternate arrangements in advance, we gain several advantages. In the first situation, the client may agree that the price of the drug is very steep, but he wants to show the animal soon and opts for the more expensive treatment to get the infection under control as quickly as possible. In case two, the fixed-income owner home all day with the easy-to-medicate animal may opt for one of the less expensive treatments, while the client in the third case may agree to the tests only if she can spread the cost out over several payments. Regardless what approach the clients may take, the practitioner involves them in the financial aspects of it from the beginning.

In addition to removing the element of surprise, another advantage of this approach is that it severs that problematic link between money and caring. The practitioner responses in no way insinuate that a client who opts for another route doesn't care for his or her animal. Similarly, because these responses allow clients to make the final choice regarding both the treatment process and the method of paying for it, they can hardly accuse the clinician of being insensitive to their needs. When we add the fact that the financial data is shared in the context of solid information about the animal, the clinician comes across as caring about both the animal and its owner.

A third advantage of this approach is that it doesn't assume what an owner will or won't spend. Dr. Connor sees a shabby old farmer and his equally bedraggled terrier suffering from one of those sky's-the-limit nonspecific skin problems. He feels sorry for the owner and dispenses some equally nonspecific medicated shampoo. The client then proceeds to peel a fifty dollar bill off a roll of fifty dollar bills bigger than Dr. Connor's car, then takes the dog to one of Dr. Connor's colleagues who ultimately finds the cause of the dog's problem somewhere in the medical and economic stratosphere. As if that weren't bad enough, the client tells Dr. Connor's colleague that Dr. Connor obviously doesn't know what he's doing.

In this case, Dr. Connor erred on two counts: He judged the owner's ability to pay based on his physical appearance, and he grossly underestimated the owner's relationship with the animal. Ironically, however, the converse also may hold true: The town's most ostentatiously wealthy citizen may balk at spending an extra cent on his animals and harshly— and publicly—criticize the practitioner who treats his animals as if money were no object.

Finally, integrating financial and medical information from the beginning helps neutralize the emotional charge many people place on money, and this makes it easier for both the client and the practitioner to discuss the case more objectively and honestly. Furthermore it seems safe to say that the less people know about what's going on, the more critical they are about the cost—especially when things go wrong.

Estimate, Estimate, Estimate

Of all the tools that simplify talking to clients about money, the prepared estimate surely ranks as the most helpful. For example, the clinicians at Happy Valley have designed simplified estimate sheets for each of their most commonly seen small and large animal problems— blocked cats, pyometras, milk fevers, colics—a set of which is kept in the appropriate examination rooms or vehicles. Each form includes a statement of Happy Valley's payment policy and a brief description of the disease or condition. It then lists diagnostic and treatment options with their unit costs as well as a space in which the clinician may either check off or estimate the total cost for that part of the procedure.

Unlike the standard inventory-linked, computer-generated estimates which may list every gauze sponge, these forms contain composite totals for broader categories such as examination, anesthesia, fluid therapy, catheterization, removal of obstruction, surgery, medication, hospitalization, dietary management. At the bottom of the page is a space for the clinician to write in any special financial arrangements or additional information for the client.

The various items appear in the order in which the clinician would normally perform them, which confers several benefits. First, this enables the clinician to educate the owner regarding the nature of the animal's problem and its treatment as well as the anticipated costs in an organized fashion rather than jumping all over the page. Second, the order serves as a systematic reminder for busy or frazzled clinicians regarding possible aspects of the problem they might otherwise overlook. Third, it makes it possible for the clinician to go over the material even as he or she examines the animal. This third benefit is particularly useful in dealing with cases of acute illness or injury where talking about money while the animal suffers obvious distress surely strikes everyone as uncaring.

Although we will discuss the often highly emotional aspects that may complicate the treatment of seriously ill or injured animals in Chapter 15, at this point note that a "Buy Time" estimate can prove especially helpful in such cases. As the name implies, this estimate describes the nature and cost of the treatment necessary to stabilize an animal and make it comfortable, usually for six to twelve hours depending on its condition. By breaking down the treatment in this manner, owners who become so overwhelmed when the crisis occurs that they may agree to anything gain some time to evaluate the situation more objectively. Similarly, sometimes practitioners faced with a crisis may want nothing more than to get rid of the client so they can get to work. Such estimate sheets enable clinicians to describe the preliminary treatment and its cost as they examine the animal. They then note a specific time on the bottom of the sheet for the owner to come in or call to discuss the case in more detail.

Practitioners who find the idea of talking to clients about money or preparing estimates too difficult and time-consuming might want to run a quick reality check: Add up the dollar value of all past due accounts, those turned over to collection agencies, and those classified as "uncollectible" for the past year and divide that sum by what you consider a fair hourly wage for your time. Next add up the number of hours spent worrying about or pursuing these accounts and add it to the preceding sum. That total represents hours spent working for nothing. As long as you're not getting paid for it, why not spend the time developing estimate forms that will increase your odds of getting paid for the work you do in the future?

Payment Options

Offering payment options to clients takes advantage of the business premise that maintains a cost consists of two components: the price and the terms. The price refers to the dollar value set and the terms refer to how that amount will be paid. How services may be paid for is limited only by the creativity of the clinician and the client, assuming both are honest and we needn't worry about any legal implications. The more any option strikes the client as both fair and achievable, the more likely the clinician will receive full payment. The key here, however, remains that any option must result from an open and honest discussion between the clinician and the client with the conclusions of that discussion included in the patient record, the estimate, and the bill presented to the client.

What are some of the options available? Certainly in our time-payment society, the monthly payment first comes to mind. Because people are used to paying for services in this manner, many find it a simple matter to incorporate payment for veterinary services into such a schedule. This approach works best when the client and clinician agree on a specific monthly payment rather than the practitioner's dismissing the subject with a casual, "Oh, just pay me whatever you can." If Dr. Connor really doesn't care if he gets paid, fine; but he shouldn't make such remarks and then complain to his staff or criticize clients when he doesn't see a cent from them for months.

Consider this alternate scenario: Dr. Connor looks at the total cost of treatment and suggests payments of so much a month; the Hancocks hesitate and note that that amount would put quite a strain on their budget, but they'll try to do the best they can. At this point, Dr. Connor can accept that or continue negotiating.

Continued negotiation offers three advantages: It increases clients' input regarding a problem whose solution depends solely on their compliance; second, it decreases the probability that the clients will be unable to make the payments, which can lead to embarrassment and fear, the latter being the most common source of defensive or flight responses; and third, it positions the clinician as a caring, flexible person. If Dr. Connor suggests that the Hancocks make smaller monthly payments with the idea they can pay more if circumstances allow, or even asks them how much they feel they can reasonably pay per month, this once again puts the responsibility in the owner's domain while expressing the clinician's genuine desire to help animal and owner alike.

Whether this type of payment schedule succeeds goes back to the basics discussed previously:

- Clients must possess a clear understanding of what they're getting for their money.

- Cost and payment must be discussed with clients *before* the treatment begins.
- Any payment policy must take the client's needs into consideration and actively involve the client in the formulation of any alternate payment plans.

Another form of monthly payment involves offering clients a fixed rate for services conducted over a period of time. Some clinicians offer new animal packages that include all routine vaccinations, fecals, worming, and neutering during the first year for which owners pay a fixed amount each month. In addition to insuring payment, this approach confers a definite medical advantage because it offers an alternative to those owners who might otherwise delay these procedures for lack of funds, thereby increasing the probability that the animal will succumb to some avoidable condition. Although we may or may not accept cost as the real reason people don't neuter their animals, offering them the opportunity to do this as part of an easy-payment plan does much to address this issue. Other packages may address common problems such as treatment for heartworm disease, mange, or fractures. Similar programs designed to meet the needs of horses and food animals also make it easier for clients to incorporate routine veterinary care into their budgets.

Regardless of the species, this approach benefits the animal, the client, and the practitioner. Those designed for young animals give the animal a good start, and the special programs insure it gets care it otherwise might not receive. Clients gain an awareness of veterinary care as an ongoing, financially feasible concern. Finally, practitioners not only establish veterinary care as an essential element of responsible animal ownership, they get paid for what they do in an unemotional, timely fashion.

Another option involves the payment of half the cost before treatment begins and the other half at its conclusion. Obviously, whether this plan succeeds depends on whether the client has the initially requested amount and will have the other half when the treatment ends. The good news here is that the practitioner always gets at least half the amount no matter what happens. The bad news is that this approach gives owners who don't have the money to pay the second installment a very compelling reason to keep the problem going. The bone heals, the pin comes out, but the client complains the animal isn't using the leg normally yet. Dr. Connor finds no evidence of any problems and tries to dismiss the owner's concerns, but the client persists until the veterinarian suggests a recheck in another week. Even as Dr. Connor mentally reviews every step of the treatment and evokes any one of a number of medical problem scenarios, the client's only real concern is that she'll have the wherewithal to make the final payment the next time she sees him. If not, the animal's "problem" may persist. Once again we see a breakdown in communication: The practitioner puts himself through needless hours of worry regarding the medical aspects of the case when it's really a money issue.

At this point, it bears noting that yet another paradox may come into play in terms of what payment options we offer to which clients. Sometimes practitioners who fear that a client can't pay place even more stringent financial restrictions on that person than those placed on clients for whom payment poses no problem. Dr. Connor demands payment in full or two payments two weeks apart from the owner of the small farm that barely gets by while accepting monthly payments on a catch-as-catch-can, "Oh, they're good for it" basis from the owner of the plush spread a mile down the road. As the physician breezes past Dr. Connor's front office staff, he tosses out a casual, "Put it on my tab" for all those in the waiting room to hear, including the college students who search their pockets for loose change in hopes of coming up with enough to get the stray cat examined. In someone's book this may amount to sound fiscal management, but it certainly doesn't communicate either a consistent or a caring image to the public.

Another payment form requests payment in full for medication, outside laboratory work, and other fixed fees, and negotiates the cost of the clinician's time and expertise. On the one hand, this allows clinicians to project the reason for the request for money away from themselves, thereby dissociating them from any negative client feelings the subject may precipitate. On the other hand, practitioners who consider their service the most critical part of the process may feel this approach puts the emphasis in the wrong place.

Clients Who Don't Pay

Although treating medical and surgical cases can present us with some pretty dreadful scenarios, nothing can quite match the array of thoughts and feelings that assail us when the business manager or an employer presents us with a list of "no pays" and asks us what we intend to do about them. We immediately summon any memories of the case which almost invariably focus on the animal, the problem, and how we treated it. More often than not, we don't summon any memories of how we treated the payment aspect of the case because such a discussion most likely didn't occur in the first place.

At this point, many of us respond fearfully but, of course, we don't see it that way at all. We accept the list and promise to get to it "as soon as possible," and it sits in a pile with the other no-pay lists on the edge of the desk for months—a perfect example of a *freeze* fear response. *Flight* fear responses lead us to say things like, "I'm too busy to handle this. You take care of it (or send them into collections)." And surely every practitioner who has faced such a situation recognizes this common *fight* fear response: "Those rotten crumbs! After all the work I did for them!"

Even though the litigious climate of our society appears to champion replacing Hippocrates's implied "Above all do no wrong" with "Above all admit no wrong," the fact remains that the majority of bad pays represent a breakdown—or complete lack—of communication regarding the financial aspects of the case, whether we admit this to the client or not. Dr. Connor originally avoided mentioning money because he found it awkward or distasteful, and now he faces a money-related matter potentially ten times more awkward and distasteful than the one he tried to evade in the first place.

However, once we realize our own contribution to the problem, we can act decisively as a matter of choice rather than allowing these situations and our emotions to manipulate us. Within a week of the first missed payment, call the client and ask if there's some problem. Why so soon? The longer we delay making that first call, the less we can legitimately claim concern about the animal and the client as our primary concern, and the more it will appear that we care only about the money. Unlike sending a series of progressively stronger worded invoices which may invoke the same fear responses in the client that the clinician experiences when confronted with the unpaid account, this approach gives clients an opportunity to express their concerns directly to the clinician in a timely fashion. Although a staff member can make this call, it only complicates the process if the client raises issues that that person can't address.

Suppose the client says that his animal isn't responding as expected. Further discussion may reveal that an unforeseen problem has arisen; or perhaps the animal is responding normally, but the practitioner initially failed to describe the nature of the recovery period in a manner the client understood. In these situations, the practitioner may arrange a time to examine the animal or provide the client with the necessary information.

Similarly, if the animal is doing well but the client has fallen on hard times, the practitioner immediately can work out an equitable solution that becomes part of the record and is confirmed in writing to the client. This spares the client the embarrassment of dunning and once again positions the practitioner as a caring individual.

What about the client who comes right out and says, "I never would have done it if I'd known how much it was going to cost," a statement that carries a particularly negative charge if the animal doesn't survive? Although bottom-line-oriented clinicians surely will disagree, some practitioners not only place a value on their time, but also on their mental health—with estimates for the latter running as high as $1,000 a minute. In other words, they don't become involved in emotional exchanges with clients. Instead, they recognize that a breakdown in communication occurred, and explain in detail why they did what they did and the charges for those services. They then ask the client to pay what he or she thinks is a fair amount and consider the case closed. Most clients do deduct something from the total, but most clinicians who use this approach believe that they receive more than they would have from a collection agency and that they learned a valuable lesson about communication. Sometimes they even keep these people as clients.

Disengaging the Symbolic Connection

Unless we take a strictly bottom-line orientation and refuse to provide service unless clients produce irrefutable proof of their ability to pay—that is, cash on the barrel head in advance—we will encounter those clients who don't pay no matter how hard we try to avoid this situation. When this occurs, any symbolism we attach to money will wield far greater influence on our response than any logic or reason. For example, a clinician who makes $50,000 a year who considers himself half the veterinarian compared to one who makes $100,000 and vice versa (the practitioner who earns a $100,000 who sees herself as twice the veterinarian as the colleague who earns $50,000) probably will react much more negatively to no-pays because they see themselves in terms of money. Anything that decreases their incomes diminishes them as a person in their eyes.

Informal surveys reveal another subjective aspect of the money connection: Those who make the most working the least hours also enjoy their work the most. Although some might retort, "Who *wouldn't* under those circumstances?" they miss the point. These practitioners don't enjoy the work because it generates money; they simply enjoy the work, and all the positive effects of that enjoyment—including increased efficiency which reduces hours—lead clients to seek them out and pay their price.

Another aspect of this issue is that people who enjoy their work may feel comfortable with incomes that those dissatisfied with their work would find inadequate. Compare the practitioner who relaxes by reading journals and considers a veterinary meeting the best vacation a person could want to the colleague who sees veterinary medicine as a job made tolerable by a full social life and regular vacations to exotic places. Obviously the work will need to generate more income to fulfill the second person's needs. Put another way, there are two ways to have everything we want: We can make a great deal of money, or we can want less.

The last way to look at payment is that each client-patient potentially offers three different kinds of payment. First, there is the traditional dollar amount. Second, each case provides us with an opportunity to collect a knowledge payment by increasing our knowledge in an infinite number of ways: We encounter a new symptom or response to treatment in a patient with feline immunodeficiency virus or bovine viral diarrhea; a breeder shares information about a rare breed or new variety; we try a new procedure for the first time; the case leads us to establish a relationship with a new specialist. Third, each case provides the opportunity to collect a positive emotional payment: the sight of healthy calves romping following a serious outbreak of pneumonia; the goofy pup that makes us laugh just looking at him; the owners who give their heartfelt thanks even when we think we should or could have done more.

Practitioners who see a case only in terms of time and money naturally feel cheated and angry when clients don't pay. These clinicians can rightfully claim, "What a waste!" because they did spend their time and, by their definition, do have nothing to show for it. However, for those who appreciate all the levels of payment, it's possible to collect a minimum two-thirds on every single case. Every case offers an opportunity to increase our knowledge; and anyone who can't find something emotionally gratifying in every interaction with a patient or a client probably could make a lot more money and be a lot happier in some other line of work.

When we view the dollar amount as only one of the three forms of payment we receive from each case, the idea of writing off bad pays doesn't seem like such a frivolous idea. Some clinicians do this as a gift to themselves because they don't like the negative feelings these situations generate. Others do it as a gift to these clients, even going so far as to send them cards notifying them of the fact. True, some of these people may be deadbeats, but every so often a person is genuinely touched by the gesture. As one clinician noted, "What have I got to lose? I wasn't going to get paid anyhow, so I'd rather do something positive and end the agony for both of us."

For practitioners who choose to use dunning letters, collection agencies, or the civil courts, success depends on the ability to view the process objectively. If it rankles, if the practitioner loses sleep over it or dreads meeting the client in public, then it would seem that whatever the amount ultimately collected, it won't cover the emotional cost of collecting it.

Another advantage of not pursuing bad pays emotionally lies in the fact that even as some practitioners attach all kinds of symbolism to money, some clients do the same thing. When this occurs, we may find ourselves involved in situations in which even though it superficially appears that the subject is money, the client views it as something else entirely. Dr. Connor wants Ms. Evans to pay for the treatment he gave to the best of his ability; Ms. Evans believes she doesn't owe him a cent because his insensitivity so upset her she forgot an appointment with a very important customer, got chewed out by her superior, almost lost her job, and screamed at her mother, who hasn't spoken to her since.

As always prevention proves the best bargain. However, just as students anxious to try their hand at surgery often find preventive medicine boring, so practitioners faced with putting together estimate sheets and developing a comfortable manner in which to talk to clients about money often can think of many other things they'd rather do. Unfortunately, just as none of us can escape the sick feeling that occurs when an animal needlessly suffers or dies because we forgot the dull, boring basics of medicine, so practitioners who find themselves embroiled in time-consuming, highly emotional confrontations with clients over charges and payments often wish they'd paid more attention to preventing the problem.

Because money does tend to serve as the practical as well as emotional bottom line for many people, failure to understand the client's as well as the animal's needs in many areas ultimately may be reduced to this lowest common denominator. Consequently, we may wind up haggling over money with clients because we see this as the *cause* of the problem rather than the *effect* of our failure to consider the role other client limits may exert on the treatment process. Because of this, it makes sense to recognize the other limits so we can avoid this troublesome problem.

Chapter 4
Life-style and the Treatment Process

Because little in our training addresses life-style as it may affect the veterinary process, this chapter surveys an increasingly complex world where people work, go to school, and participate in a wide range of activities outside a wide variety of homes. Although we could argue that if they really cared about their animals owners would find the time to do what we ask, trying to force compliance by preying on owner emotion may complicate rather than simplify the treatment process. Because of that, it seems more realistic to recognize what comprises normal life for our clients and then seek to establish and maintain the health of their animals within those limits.

Consistent Inconsistency

Inconsistency looms as the hallmark of contemporary life even as consistency remains the crux of effective medical and behavioral therapy, and very few segments of the animal-owning population can claim immunity to its effects. We tell ourselves that owners of food animals surely will find some way to muster the necessary consistency to do what we ask because their livelihood depends on it, then discover that 70 percent of the beef herds in the country consist of less than fifty animals often kept in poorly managed herds by owners who sandwich their care between other activities or work off the farm (Herrick 1993, 203:501–2). Or we convince ourselves that the strong emotional ties between owners and companion animals certainly will guarantee 100 percent compliance, only to discover the parents who make up the bulk of this group may spend very few hours at home on any given day. Meanwhile childless couples and singles often pursue equally busy lives. Younger couples may work long hours in hopes of someday owning their own homes and starting a family; older ones may take full advantage of their child-free status and travel or immerse themselves in community activities. Singles of all ages may maintain a very full social life in addition to any other obligations.

Similarly, the rise of the two-income household as a matter of choice or necessity also introduces inconsistency into the human-animal relationship. In urban and suburban settings this may mean that no one is home from seven in the morning until six at night to care for the animal. On the farm, we may see this same phenomenon as well as a new variation: the farmer or herdsman who interrupts his chores to meet the school bus, take the kids to the pediatrician, or put dinner in the oven because he's a single parent or his spouse works a full-time job away from the home.

The Time Factor

Although many considerations may pop into owners' heads when their animals appear ill, time follows close on the heels of money. However, many texts read as if clients live in a timeless state in a manner delightfully summed up by the tale of the efficiency expert who roars down a country lane and passes the old Vermont farmer holding a pig up to the branches of an apple tree. The sight of the animal contentedly munching the fruit so astounds the expert, he comes to a screeching halt and demands, "Do you have any idea how much time that wastes?"

The old Vermonter ponders this a while then very seriously replies, "What's time to a pig?"

We probably never will know what time is to a pig, but an awareness of contemporary client time can do much to enhance the treatment process. Is it reasonable to expect clients to take off from work to bring an animal in for examination or wait for us to arrive at the farm? Can we realistically expect them to do whatever we tell them no matter how long it takes and whether or not it fits into their schedules?

It depends. Practitioners lucky enough to claim a captive clientele probably can do whatever they want. However, for those who must meet the needs of their clients in an increasingly competitive environment, it makes sense to recognize that for many people time *is* money. Connie Wharton works from 8:00 A.M. to 5:00 P.M.: if Dr. Morgan can't see her until 10:00 A.M., she must add any lost wages to the cost of veterinary care. Is it any wonder she may wait until her cat shows signs of serious illness before she calls for an appointment?

Furthermore, no matter how we and the owners may feel about the importance of animal health, employers who balk at allowing time off to care for sick humans let alone animals can add another negative quantity to that equation. Connie Wharton's supervisor has expressed his dislike of cats almost as frequently as he has stressed the importance of regular attendance. Should she take a sick day and pray he never finds out she used it to take her cat to the veterinarian? Or should she only take off the time necessary to have her cat seen and hope she can sneak into work without her superior noticing? Either way, she must deal with these obstacles created by her life-style before she even sets foot in the veterinary hospital.

Owner attempts to compensate for time incompatibilities with their veterinarians lead to two opposite approaches to veterinary care. As noted, for some all the juggling necessary to obtain veterinary care proves so troublesome that they postpone the visit as long as possible, often until a crisis occurs. Ms. Wharton decides to give the cat another day to see if he gets better on his own. However, a cat with a urinary blockage rarely gets better on his own and by the time the owner gets home that evening, the animal's condition has greatly deteriorated. Now she no longer needs to worry about all the implications of taking time off from work; instead she must deal with all the emotional and financial implications of taking a critically ill animal in for treatment after hours. We can only hope Dr. Morgan doesn't add to her burden by demanding indignantly, "Why did you wait so long!"

Following that nightmare experience, this owner might adopt the other orientation common to those who cannot synchronize their time with their veterinarian's: She focuses all her attention on preventive measures. She asks Dr. Morgan what signs her cat might display when problems occur, and he explains these and shows her how to take her pet's temperature, check the color of its mucous membranes, and keep track of its food and water consumption, urination, and defecation. Few would argue the validity of this approach for animal and owner alike. However it works much better when a strong sense of keeping the animal healthy—as opposed to the fear of a recurring problem—serves as the focus of the client-clinician relationship from the beginning.

Suppose Dr. Morgan never mentions these procedures or dismisses his client's concerns regarding ways to reduce the probability of the animal experiencing the same problem. She could reasonably feel she's on her own when it comes to preventive care. In this case and not unlike other owners who feel abandoned by their veterinarians following a bad experience, she becomes a fanatic. She scours books and magazines and canvasses coworkers and friends for information about how to prevent urinary problems. In these situations the animal not uncommonly winds up on a wide variety of often counterproductive remedies and supplements. Additionally, the owner's overly attentive attitude may jeopardize the relationship and undermine the animal's behavior as well as its health.

What's Time to a Veterinarian?

The clinician's concept of time plays as important a role in the treatment process as the client's. Although scientific acceptance of cyclic behavior in animals is long-standing, only recently have studies revealed that humans possess a biological "clock" in the superchiasmatic nucleus (SCN) of the hypothalamus. Among its activities, the SCN regulates the light-mediated output of melatonin by the pineal gland. Because melatonin affects mating, eating, and sleeping patterns in other animals, it seems likely similar effects will be found in people. We do know that many people experience seasonal mood changes directly related to the amount of light. Others classify themselves as day or night people; some feel at their best in the morning whereas others can't get moving until midafternoon or later (Marieb 1991, 254–55).

Although solo practitioners might feel their time sense a moot point, it can and should be taken into consideration along with clients' time-related needs. It does no good for Dr. Morgan to offer morning office hours if he can barely drag himself out of bed and he acts dull and grouchy when he does. The same holds true at the other end of the time spectrum: The morning person whose efficiency drops precipitously in the late afternoon may find him- or herself involved in an endurance test rather than any meaningful interaction with the animal and owner. Even though common sense tells us people should schedule their activities so they do their most challenging work at their peak hours, a surprising number of practices maintain schedules that meet neither the clients' nor the practitioner's needs. Just because the schedule worked when Dr. Morgan's predecessor founded the practice twenty-five years ago in no way means it works for Dr. Morgan and his clients today.

Another aspect of time concerns how long it takes an individual practitioner to do a job right. Some clinicians always need more than fifteen minutes to examine an animal, and scheduling appointments every fifteen minutes for that person only leads to back-ups. Although a colleague might envy that crowded waiting room, clients entering it are much more apt to groan in despair. Remember, some of them took time off from work to bring the animal in; others need to pick up children at the sitters or be home in time to meet the school bus. Nor do such waits do much for the patients who may become increasingly apprehensive and unruly, neither of which enhances either the clinician's image as caring, nor the treatment process.

If it takes twenty minutes to examine a patient, schedule it; don't hope to steal it from another client. If it only takes more time to examine young or new animals, exotics, or large animals seen on the premises, only schedule extra time for those clients. Similarly, if a large animal client always comes up with ten more things for you to do "as long as you're here," allow extra time for him so the next client who rushes home from work to meet you in the barn doesn't wind up waiting for hours cursing your insensitivity.

Although time-is-money thinking says the more people seen, the more money made, in reality successful practitioners know that they can make just as much money seeing fewer clients to whom they can devote their full attention. Add the negative feelings generated when busy people must wait, and trying to see more clients could cost the practitioner more in the long run.

Synchronizing Client and Clinician Time

As noted previously, whether alternative scheduling designed to meet client needs works or not depends on whether it meets the clinician's needs as well. Even as clients who feel manipulated by their veterinarians may undermine the treatment process, so may veterinarians who feel manipulated by their clients. For example, when we think of meeting the time needs of working clients, offering evening office hours comes to mind as the most logical solution to the problem. Interestingly, these may prove no more pleasing to the client than they are to the clinician. Just as few practitioners like to work all day, grab a quick dinner, and face two or three hours of clients, so few clients like to spend the evening in a veterinary hospital after a long day's work. Weary practitioners as well as clients may forget to ask necessary questions and share important information.

Although it would seem that the presentation of an acutely ill animal at such times creates the major headache, in fact the ones presented with relatively mild, nonspecific, or chronic symptoms—just a little off-feed, a little depressed, an occasional bout of vomiting or diarrhea—may pose the greater dilemma. Dr. Morgan knows he must treat the critically ill animal regardless of the time and how tired he is; and, in fact, the very nature of the situation may result in a revitalizing surge of adrenalin. However, as he weighs doing a work-up versus symptomatic treatment of the animal displaying mild, nonspecific, or chronic symptoms, time rather than the owner or animal may loom as the primary consideration. It's almost 9:00 P.M.; the animal isn't that sick; who wants to start a work-up now? Even practitioners enthusiastic to do the work-up may find themselves assisted by a weary technician or even working alone—that is, working under less than optimal conditions.

Suppose Dr. Morgan wants to do the work-up first thing the next day. He should tell the owners this and give them the option of leaving the animal that night or bringing it back the next morning. Under no circumstances should he leave the owners with the impression that he will do something to the hospitalized animal that night if he doesn't intend to do so.

Several factors may influence the client's response to the problem at this point. One owner may decide to leave the animal because he doesn't have time to drop it off the next morning. Another may opt to return with the animal the next morning rather than have it spend the night in a cage. A third voices a not uncommon working owner's dilemma that leaves more than a few practitioners feeling uneasy: "I really hate to pay for hospitalization since you're not going to do anything, but you don't open until eight and I can't afford to be late for work, either."

Upon hearing this, some practitioners may shrug and think if not say, "The way it is, is the way it is." Or they might consider offering some alternatives to meet the client's needs better. Some don't charge for keeping the animal overnight, believing the goodwill generated more than offsets any cost involved. Others offer early drop-off service on a routine or special basis depending on the needs of their clients. Whether the practitioner or a staff member admits the animal at that time, the success of this approach hinges on quality communication once again. In the case of the animal seen the evening before, this may mean doing little more than verifying a phone number where the owner can be reached the next day or setting up a specific time for the owner to call or stop in if his or her access to a phone is limited.

Increasing numbers of clients prefer to leave their animals for the day for routine preventive care as well as treatment of problem conditions. In this situation, some reliable method of sharing the necessary information must exist; and this most certainly holds true for those large animals examined in the owner's absence, too. Once again, preprinted forms can serve as a valuable adjunct to quality practice. Following the basic form of the estimate sheets (Chapter 3), these describe routine services and their costs, provide a checklist of the most common owner complaints (coughing, vomiting, diarrhea, itching, etc.), pose pertinent questions regarding the history of the problem, and furnish space for any special owner concerns. These may be completed by the person admitting the animal, or clients who use the service routinely may be given the forms to fill out in advance. For those practitioners who must examine large animals in the owner's absence, finding such a form (and the animal) in a prearranged, safe place offers many advantages over those scribbled notes taped to the stall door or impaled on a nail driven into a wall somewhere. However, regardless of how routine the services requested by the client appear, the importance of including some means whereby the veterinarian can contact the absentee owner cannot be overemphasized.

Naturally the more routine the desired treatment, the more readily clinicians can achieve it in the owner's absence, and many practitioners find this approach actually saves them time in the long run. Granted those making large animal calls must accept that there won't be any help available. However, at least they know this in advance, which many find preferable to spending half an hour waiting for the farmer to help them or, worse, discovering their "help" with the unpredictable gelding consists of a latchkey ten-year-old.

Timely Treatment Options

In addition to changing life-styles necessitating changes in scheduling, alternative treatment approaches also may be needed. We noted previously how busy owners may place a higher premium on preventive care than clients of the past because they simply can't afford to have their animals get sick. In addition, these clients may not have, or may not want to spend, as much time to treat their animals as we would like. The prescription says to medicate the eye or give the pills three times a day, bathe the animal every other day, or soak the foot for twenty minutes daily: In reality, the client administers the ointment or pills three times one day and once the next, bathes the animal only twice a week, or soaks the foot for ten minutes every other day at most. Or maybe the animal gets the pills three times a day, but at six, eight, and ten at night because the owner forgot the morning and noon doses and wants to get them all in before he falls asleep. Or maybe the owner gives the whole day's treatment at one time. (Practitioners tempted to accuse these owners of not caring should pause and imagine what they would do if one of their animals fell ill and they couldn't bring it to work to monitor and medicate it.)

Sometimes owners and clinicians with the very best intentions can create a cycle of miscommunication that greatly prolongs the treatment process. Dr. Morgan dispenses medication for Connie Wharton to give her cat every eight hours for ten days and requests a progress report at the end of that time. The owner can only medicate the cat as directed on the weekend, but she does manage to get three random doses into him four other days; of the remaining five days, the cat gets the pills twice on three, once on one, and misses one day completely.

At the end of the ten days, Ms. Wharton calls Dr. Morgan and reports that the cat is improving, but not completely back to normal. Fearing he will think badly of her, she doesn't tell him about the erratic treatment. Believing she has followed his directions to the letter, Dr. Morgan dispenses another week's worth of the same medication and the same erratic cycle begins again. In this case, the problem isn't the medication's efficacy; it's the fact that the owner's life-style doesn't permit her it administer it in the manner necessary for it to be effective. Unless the owner volunteers this information or the clinician anticipates it in the treatment process, not only can this lack of awareness needlessly prolong the animal's condition, the haphazard administration of drugs may contribute to the presence of resistant pathogens. In food animals such resistant microorganisms can pose public health problems in addition to impeding the animal's recovery. Consequently, it pays to verify that someone will be present to administer any medication as directed before prescribing it.

Another variation of the treatment theme can generate a fair amount of negative clinician emotion, especially for companion animal practitioners schooled in a tradition that calls for exhausting all alternatives before opting for salvage procedures. We do not enucleate eyes with recurrent ulcers until we try every medication and surgical treatment; we do not amputate mangled legs until we first try to pin, screw, wire, and plate them. Consequently, when an owner requests what we consider a salvage procedure prematurely or even as a first choice, we may feel more than a little disoriented as our scientific principles fall under siege yet again.

The worst thing practitioners can do is treat an animal in a manner with which they do not agree, and those who believe a specific set of requirements must be satisfied to warrant enucleation, peroneal urethrostomy, or amputation should not violate that rule simply because a client requests it. On the other hand, it does pay to evaluate the matter in terms of the bond and behavior. If the treatment process undermines the relationship between the animal and the owner in any way, those people more likely will consider options that will resolve the problem once and for all.

Consider the owner who spends frustrating hours trying to medicate the unruly animal's eye: That person may opt for enucleation for what the veterinarian considers a treatable condition. In this situation, behavioral as well as bond factors come into play. It is rather amazing how many clinicians don't realize that owners who stare in awe as the clinician medicates the animal and murmur, "Wow, how do you do that?" might be saying they don't know how to do that rather than praising the practitioner's mystical way with animals. Obviously, if clients can't accomplish the treatment because they can't handle the animal, the treatment will be no more effective than if it's not given because the owners aren't there to give it. It is far better to address behavioral problems immediately and separately when they arise than try to deal with them when they undermine the medical treatment process. Trying to teach a rowdy mare not to kick while simultaneously medicating her for an uncomfortable eye condition would challenge anyone, let alone the single parent with two young children who works an eight-hour day.

The Space Factor

Contemporary owners also may experience space problems that undermine the treatment process. Obviously if Dr. Morgan prescribes medicated baths for Ms. Baily's spaniel and she only has a shower stall, her complicated life suddenly becomes much more complicated. However, other space-related problems may also arise. Consider the not uncommon case of the owner of multiple animals who notices a patch of diarrhea on the rug or in the pen, but all the animals look essentially normal.

"Keep an eye on them for the next twenty-four hours so you can see who's doing what," confidently commands Dr. Morgan.

"But there are seven of them and I work all day," counters the owner.

"Well, then separate them so you can see who's doing what," suggests Dr. Morgan, a bit less confidently as the owner's situation becomes more clear.

Then the client asks the Dr. Morgan the Dreaded Question: "How?"

Companion animal owners will fare much better under these circumstances if clinicians have had the foresight to recommend crate training for young pups and kittens. In this situation, crate training refers to accustoming an animal to a fiberglass kennel or other secure enclosure as a safe space. Aside from preventing some of the more common territorial problems that may occur as the animal matures, animals so trained offer several advantages to their owners. Because they consider the crate a haven, whenever the animal goes anywhere in the crate, a piece of "home" goes with it. Compare an animal so trained to the one involved in a much more typical pre-veterinary visit scenario: The owner drags the carrier out of the back of the closet, the animal sees it and takes off. The owner chases it around the house several times before grabbing it and stuffing it into the crate. By the time the animal arrives at the clinic, its heart pounds, its pulse races, it pants, its pupils are dilated, perhaps it even vomited or defecated. The owner complaint? "She's been a little off the past day or two."

Granted, lugging retrievers around in crates presents problems, but many owners find that even the biggest dogs appreciate their own private space where they may retreat when they feel pressured by other animals or various circumstances in the household. Note that the goal of this form of training is not to restrain or punish the animals, but to provide them with an always accessible private space in a world of increasingly numerous territorial violations. Second, and of vital importance, clinicians should *never* recommend this technique for any reason unless they and their clients fully understand and accept the rationale behind it. The very concept of crate-training violates some people's personal beliefs about freedom; if these are not addressed, the technique will fail as miserably in their hands as if they used the improper procedure.

Companion animal and large animal owners lacking crating capacity are faced with the task of setting up a makeshift isolation facility to determine which animal is doing what. If space allows, owners may put each animal in a separate room or stall. If space does not allow, a single area may be set aside for this purpose and one animal placed in it for a twenty-four-hour period of observation. Obviously, the more animals, the more time it will take to put all of them through this process. However if they appear healthy to the owner, the options are limited. At such times, those owners whose veterinarians taught them to take temperatures and evaluate other vital signs will fare much better than those who have no idea what a normal animal—let alone a mildly sick one—looks like.

If owners can't accomplish this, then three options remain:

- The owner can wait and hope that the condition resolves itself or that the animal with it becomes ill enough to show obvious signs.

- The veterinarian can examine all the animals in hopes of detecting the one with the problem.
- The veterinarian can treat all the animals symptomatically.

None of these options fits the definition of what most practitioners would consider optimal. However, such frustrating experiences do tend to make those who felt they lacked the time to educate their clients in basic husbandry and preventive measures see this aspect of practice in a whole new light. When owners lack both the time and the space to accomplish what we consider the most basic procedures, even the simplest problem can become very complex.

The Art of Hospitalization

When we think of hospitalization, we tend to think of it in terms of the patient and our own needs: the animal requires a work-up that will take time to accomplish; it requires treatment that we only can give in-house. However, sometimes it is necessary to consider hospitalization in terms of the owner's needs, too. We already mentioned offering drop-off service for working clients. Similarly, contemporary owners face other situations that make hospitalization a viable option for them even though the clinician may not place their animals in that medically defined category.

For example, in the multiple animal household the owner might intuitively feel a particular animal is the most likely source of the problem and request hospitalization to confirm this suspicion. Other people may request hospitalization for an animal with mild gastroenteritis because their landlord would throw a fit if he saw vomit or diarrhea on the rug. Still others may see hospitalizing the animal as the only way to insure proper treatment because they cannot accomplish this at home for one of several reasons. First, as noted earlier, concurrent behavioral problems may make it difficult or impossible for the owner to medicate the animal. Second, some owners have aversions to medicating certain anatomical parts; the eyes and genitalia most frequently fall in this category. Third, some owners cannot stand the sight of blood, pus, vomit, or anything that looks or smells unpleasant to them—be it an exudate or the medication itself. In these situations, it is far better to hospitalize the animal now for what we might consider an idiot-simple treatment than later for more extraordinary care when the animal fails to respond to erratic treatment at home. Although the latter condition may strike us as a more justifiable reason for hospitalization than the former, it would seem more caring to do everything possible to insure that the animal never reaches that critical state in which no one would question the need for hospitalization.

Finally, sometimes owners will request—or welcome the offer of—hospitalization as a means to buy them some time away from the animal so they can evaluate a problem more objectively. This service can prove especially valuable to those owners who feel their absence contributed to a serious medical or behavioral problem. When faced with the prospect of expensive, long-term, and/or time-consuming treatment options, these owners can become paralyzed by their own emotions or make commitments they can't fulfill because of "the way Samantha keeps looking at me."

Another form of hospitalization whose day has come in many areas is the concept of day care. Connie Wharton leaves her cat with Dr. Morgan from eight to five to insure that the animal gets its midday medication Monday through Friday; another animal comes in Tuesdays and Thursdays for a medicated bath and spends the day. Owners of new pups and those with behavioral problems may request day care to prevent destruction or other negative behaviors at home in their absence.

Although there would seem to be no place for day care in the large animal realm, that might be because no one has considered it. Perhaps some of those persistent conditions as well as those infections that become resistant to antibiotic therapy result more from the inconsistencies inherent in the owner's life-style than from a problem with the animal's physiology.

Dynamic Life-styles

In addition to contemporary owners and clinicians' experiencing much more varied life-styles than in the past, life for many is also much more dynamic. People move, marry, have children, get divorced, take new jobs, get new animals; and each one of these changes may affect their relationship with their animals and/or the treatment process. Once robust animals may develop all kinds of nonspecific ailments when their owners begin working the night shift. A flock once optimally tended by a couple may become overindulged or ignored by the one who keeps it when the couple separates.

However, maintaining an awareness of the ever-changing nature of an owner's life-style in no way means practitioners must delve into their clients' private lives. Simply concluding the discussion of any proposed treatment with the question "Can you do this?" may lead clients to express their concerns about the time involved, any space limitations, handling the animal, and so on.

Because some clients will agree to anything, clinicians who doubt an owner's ability to carry out the recommendations should address the issue more directly, but in an unaccusing manner:

- "It's important that the animal gets this particular treatment three times a day, so if that doesn't fit into your schedule we can use something else."
- "This colt's become quite a handful since I last saw him. Is there someone here to help you medicate him?"

To some extent, we may say that the bond determines what owners *want* to do for their animals, but their life-style determines what they *can*. Rather than deny clients willing to juggle money, time, and space to maintain a stable relationship with a well-behaved, healthy animal that opportunity, it seems more sensible and caring to make it as easy for them to do this as possible.

Chapter 5
Special Human Needs

When veterinarians think of people with special needs, most maintain mental categories—senior citizens, children, the physically, mentally, or emotionally impaired, the immunocompromised—and treat those who fall into these groups in a particular way. Unfortunately, senior citizens might receive a 10 percent discount, children might get a coloring book, those impaired in one way or another might receive more solicitous care. Why unfortunately? Three reasons affecting the art of practice and the treatment process make this so. First, all our clients deserve the best care, not just those we consider special for one reason or another. Second, we live in an age in which many people in categories defined as special needs increasingly blend into the mainstream: Senior citizens may be more physically fit than parents in their twenties; the immunocompromised may appear physically healthy. Third, people's lives continually change: Last year's recipient of the Future Farmers of America Scholarship may be two months' pregnant or HIV-positive when Dr. Tobin asks her to hold the sheep with diarrhea a year later; the best herdsman in the county can become the worst when his wife leaves him.

This chapter proposes three broad areas—defined in the familiar trinity of body, mind, and spirit or, if preferred, the physical, mental, and emotional realms—for practitioners to consider during every client interaction. By responding to all clients in this manner, practitioners needn't summon a special protocol when someone with special needs appears in the barn or examination room. This not only simplifies the process, it reduces the chance that practitioners will fail to address the needs of these people because they appear capable. Also note that although this chapter will focus on the client and the clinician, the same limitations may affect staff members as well.

Physical Needs

Regardless of the species of the patient involved, human strength and flexibility loom as primary factors in the success or failure of the treatment process. Unfortunately, we tend to view strength as that physical parameter which enables *us* to restrain an animal long enough to do whatever needs to be done, and flexibility as that which enables *us* to achieve the procedure and get out of the way if necessary. Concurrent with this, we see (or should see) educating clients to use these same principles when treating their animals as a primary responsibility. When dealing with a well-behaved animal, however, we may accomplish the treatment so effortlessly that the idea of specifically addressing the issue of strength and flexibility with the owner may never cross our minds.

Not doing so poses two major problems. First, it assumes others possess the same physical capability as the practitioner, which may not be true for several reasons. Many clinicians do not realize that the very act of working with animals over a period of time imbues them with an ease and grace of motion that has a calming effect on many animals. If we compare this to the typically faster and jerkier motions of children, we can see how animals lacking experience with this segment of the population could feel threatened by a child no matter how easily the veterinarian handled the animal or how willing and mentally able that child may be to care for it.

Other owners, especially those with new animals or those confronting a condition in the animal that they consider threatening in any way, also may lack this ease of movement. A frail senior citizen reaches out tentatively to medicate the new kitten in a manner more likely to stimulate the animal's motion-sensitive predatory response than effectively restrain it; immunosuppressed individuals may treat animals with diarrhea much more tentatively than those displaying symptoms they consider less threatening to their own health. Many animals pick up on this hesitation and resist such handling even though it may be most minimal.

This leads to the second problem associated with making assumptions about the owner's physical capability: It denies the behavioral implications of every problem. Given the very strong position taken by the American Veterinary Medical Association Professional Liability Insurance Trust, which instructs practitioners to make every attempt not to have the owner assist during the examination and treatment process, practitioners conceivably might never see client-animal interactions and thus have virtually no idea whether their clients can handle their animals (Holgrieve 1992, 201:1681–82). This recommendation also negates any meaningful demonstration of treatment procedures to the client: What practical value does the single, elderly client with arthritis in both hands gain from Dr. Tobin's eye-medicating demonstration when a technician restrains the rambunctious miniature dachshund? Thus we face a frustrating Catch-22: Logic tells us that the only way we can insure that owners can properly treat their animals is by asking them to demonstrate this, which means they must handle their animals in our presence, which they're not supposed to do.

Given these restrictions, we may either hope to impart all our physical skills verbally to owners of ill-behaved animals or dispense a skilled technician along with any treatment; or we may focus on creating and maintaining animals whose behavior makes them safe and easy for their owners to handle. Once again, food animal practitioners tempted to dismiss this as a companion animal problem may need to reevaluate their beliefs in terms of a population whose individuals with special needs increasingly exist within—and many times are superficially indistinguishable from—the mainstream. To anesthetize a fractious animal for diagnosis and treatment, then tell the owner or herdsman to "keep an eye on it," or "take that bandage off in four days" would challenge even the most physically capable client, let alone one with any limitations.

By the same token, we also can see how those who lack the physical wherewithal to treat an animal would be willing to pay for someone to do this for them. In addition to offering full-time and day-care hospitalization options, some practitioners make daily treatment calls for large animals whose owners can't medicate them, while others send skilled technicians to provide this service following the initial visit.

The Bond and Physical Handling

Although often overlooked, the bond between owners and their animals also plays a critical role in the animal's behavior and the client's ability to physically handle it. People who do not trust or like an animal respond to it differently from those who do; in addition to the previously noted hesitant movements, we also may see excessively rough handling and heavy-handed displays. Because all domestic animals except the cat are social or pack animals, an observation made by William Campbell regarding dogs carries meaning for human interaction with all social species. Campbell notes that whenever a dog relates to a person, the question that will be answered is whether the dog is a four-legged member of the person's two-legged pack or the person is a two-legged member of the dog's four-legged pack (Campbell 1992, 49–75). In general, unless specific training and handling occur to teach the animal otherwise, dogs not uncommonly see adult human males as leaders of the pack (simply by virtue of the man's size, voice, and other sex-related characteristics), themselves as number two, and women and children below them. Hence the common female owner complaint that her husband, brother, or father can do anything he wants to the animal, but it always gives her a hard time. However, increasingly we now also see more men whose self-defined kinder, gentler natures may communicate submission to the animal.

When an animal perceives its owner or handler as submissive, certain dominant actions that person may consider neutral or even positive as well as necessary to administer treatment—establishing eye contact, placing the hands on the animal's shoulder or neck, holding it down—may cause the animal to respond aggressively. Moreover, animals who normally tolerate such dominant gestures may find them intolerable when compromised by illness or injury. Not surprisingly, food animals with whom the owner has had little contact not unnaturally play by animal rules. If the owner displays what the animal considers sufficiently dominant characteristics to warrant submission, handling and treatment pose few problems. However, if the animal perceives itself as dominant, then anyone involved with its care must seek to dominate it in some way, either by force or behavior. While always a consideration, this becomes particularly important if the animal belongs to a child, a not uncommon situation in rural communities with active 4-H or pony clubs. Unfortunately, if we don't observe owners interacting with the animal and don't ask questions regarding how, when, or even if they interact with it, we easily could assume they relate to the animal the same way we do.

Although numerous behavioral problems may be traced directly to the failure of the person to assume dominance, it is possible for some of these people to handle and treat dominant animals easily. A common scenario stars the woman practitioner who gains a reputation for her wonderful way with animals which menace her male colleagues. Before claiming any Dr. Doolittle awards, those in this position should recognize that these animals may *allow* the treatment because they don't consider it and the clinician a threat; that is, they feel perfectly confident in their ability to "discipline" her if she gets out of line. Second, many times clients and/or technicians may pay more attention to restraining an animal for a 110-pound woman than for a 180-pound male clinician.

In terms of accomplishing the goal—examining and treating the animal with as little human and animal stress as possible—it makes no difference whether the animal considers the clinician a leader or tolerable underling as long as the job gets done. However, just as brawny, physically fit Dr. Tobin shouldn't assume all clients can strong-arm dominant animals into submission, so those women clinicians whose patients allow treatment shouldn't assume the animal will accept this from the teenaged boy who owns the animal.

Mental Limits

When practitioners think of clients with mental limits, they may summon the image of the client with the Keeshond who lives in the sheltered home, or that of the farmer's slow nephew who helps out in the barn. Once we learn to communicate with them, these people rarely prove problematic, for two reasons. First, they tend to be very consistent—which we already noted is critical for effective treatment—and second, they tend to have more time than other clients. The Keeshond never misses his multiple medications for heart problems because administering these is the high point of his owner's day; any cow with mastitis tended by the farmer's nephew will be stripped religiously.

A good rule of thumb relative to clients' comprehension of the nature and treatment of their animals' condition is: Never assume anything. This in no way means treating all clients like the farmer's nephew; it means developing a manner of communicating with clients that insures they receive and understand the information necessary to properly treat their animals. If clients don't understand the value of the treatment and how to administer it properly, the chance of compliance plummets regardless of their—and the practitioner's—intelligence. The client looks at the medication labeled "Give one tablet three times daily," and then at the Abyssinian bouncing off the walls, and decides the animal can't be that sick.

An excellent way for clinicians to determine what, if any, mental requirements they impose on their clients is to speak to target groups such as:

- children
- senior citizens
- those from sheltered environments

Ideally, giving a presentation to each group in the group's own setting as well as a guided tour through the veterinary facility provides the most useful information about different client needs. Naturally, the more numerous and varied the groups, the more the clinician will learn. Teenagers think differently from preschoolers; seniors who meet at the community center express concerns different from those who meet at the country club; children in sheltered environments differ from adults in those same settings.

Those clinicians terrified by the idea of interacting with any group may gain some benefit by making conscious efforts to interact with single individuals from each group. However, groups provide a wider range of responses. Moreover, the reason many practitioners dread such encounters often may be traced to their first forced or voluntary forays into public relations during which they confidently presented a textbook-perfect description of a disease experienced by animals in the community only to have the audience stare dumbly at them as if they had two heads. For every clinician who experienced this at a 4-H or Cub Scout meeting, another exists who got the same treatment from the local Rotary Club or Business and Professional Women's Association. Nonetheless, the worse the experience, the greater the need for the clinician to repeat it until he or she can communicate effectively with these people in their own language.

Speaking to people in a classroom setting in many ways duplicates many examination room encounters, and very quickly practitioners learn that people respond to information given in one of two ways: linearly or analogically. The linear approach favored by science takes people from the known to the unknown following a progression they consider orderly. The key to comprehension here is that the progression must appear logical and orderly to the person to whom the information is directed.

Compare "Symptoms like Spot's are often caused by liver problems, so I'm going to take a blood sample from his front leg and do some tests to help me pin down the exact cause of the problem" with "Spot's icteric so I need to run a profile." Although the latter statement may result from a formidable mental process on Dr. Tobin's part, this statement tells the client nothing. Not surprisingly, it may leave the owner with the impression that the practitioner knows nothing about the animal's problem and expects the work-up to provide the necessary answers. When linearly attuned owners take this to its logical conclusion in these days of increasingly numerous and costly diagnostic procedures, they conceivably could envision themselves embarking on a very long and expensive process, even though Dr. Tobin may have no such thing in mind. Conversely, and barring that knowledge of medical technology, they might imagine a progression that involves just one test that will provide a definitive answer to the animal's problem while Dr. Tobin sees it as a preliminary first step in a longer and more complex process.

As noted in the discussion of anthropomorphically oriented clients, some people find it much easier to assimilate information presented analogically rather than linearly. Blank looks in response to a step-by-step linear explanation should stimulate practitioners to offer that same information analogically. This usually means describing the animal's condition in terms of similar human ailments, and the workings of various organs in terms of pumps, hinges, computers, or whatever best fits the situation.

Practitioners who speak to various groups quickly discover that automatically providing information both linearly and analogically rather than adopting one orientation and then trying to rephrase the information in terms of the other on the spot in response to confused looks is the most efficient way to insure comprehension. Moreover, just as the same person may manifest anthropomorphic or chattel orientations depending on the animal involved, so normally linear or analogical thinkers may assume the opposite approach in certain situations. The accountant who always accepts Dr. Tobin's linear scientific explanation suddenly can't comprehend it when he learns his animal suffers from the same serious condition he does; the anthropomorphically oriented horse owner becomes coldly linear and logical about treating a problem that may affect her ability to show the animal. By offering his clients information in both forms, Dr. Tobin needn't worry about these idiosyncrasies.

Group discussions also reveal that most people want the answers to two questions—"Why?" and "How?"—answered in a way that makes sense to them. Because science traditionally banishes the more subjective "Why?" to the realm of philosophy, some practitioners see answering it as immaterial, whereas others may give an answer that amounts to "Because I said so." However, when we ask clients to do things that require that they juggle money, time, and space limitations as well as challenge them physically and emotionally, it would seem reasonable to do this in a way that makes sense to them. In other words, the goal of communication should not be to tell clients what the animal's condition and its treatment means to us, but to describe it in a way that enables them to understand what it means to *them*. And not only that, to do this in their own language, be it that of a four-year-old or a senior citizen, the individual with Down's syndrome or the dean of the local college.

Offering guided tours through the veterinary facility provides additional valuable information along this line. Something so simple as going through the basics of a physical examination will elicit a host of "Why do you do that?" and "How does that work?" questions for those clinicians who don't routinely provide this information in their client presentation. As Dr. Tobin takes a group of Girl Scouts into his lab area, the group's interest wanes: Even his most sophisticated equipment looks like so many boxes with so many buttons and knobs to them. However when he sets up a fecal, then shows them a slide covered with *Toxocara* ova and the bottle of preserved specimens as well as a picture of an animal suffering from severe parasitic infestation, few of his visitors fail to react.

As the tour through his facility continues, Dr. Tobin gains an increasingly clearer idea of what people in a particular group consider important. Surely more than one practitioner has boasted proudly about various sophisticated pieces of equipment in treatment or surgery rooms only to discover that many children and grown-ups alike consider the foot-controlled faucets at the scrub sink the most memorable feature.

For those who despair over ever finding some common ground that will serve as the starting point of a communication process that seems filled with an infinite number of variables, ending the tour with a walk through the wards inevitably points out the identity of the most potent and universally understood starting point: the animals, not the clinician and his or her technology.

Special Emotional Considerations

Human emotional responses make up such a large proportion of the art of veterinary practice, we will discuss these in one way or another throughout the entire book. However, in general the emotional problems encountered in practice fall into one of two broad categories. We see clients with specifically defined chronic problems such as depression or alcoholism; and we see normally stable clients who respond in what we consider an uncharacteristic or aberrant way in a particular situation. Because animals often act as valued stabilizing influences in the lives of those with chronic conditions, veterinarians seem to be spared many of the problems that other professionals encounter when dealing with these people. Where others complain of missed appointments, veterinarians more commonly wonder how clients in such confused mental or emotional states mustered the wherewithal to bring the animal in. The alcoholic who arrived by motorcycle during a snowstorm with his dog stuffed in his jacket rather than miss his appointment for the animal's annual vaccinations comes to mind here.

Although all clients benefit from written descriptions of the animal's problem and treatment, these can be particularly helpful for those clients whose concentration may be impaired during the examination. Computerized invoices with space for the clinician to enter such comments make this a simple process. Similarly, supplying these owners with the absentee owner forms (Chapter 4) to complete prior to the examination may help those who find it easier to concentrate at home, during certain times of the day, or when alone. Finally, a request for a progress report serves as an invaluable aid to help assess owners' understanding of the problem as well as their desire and ability to carry out the treatment. Many times practitioners don't request such reports thinking they take up too much time. However, in reality they can save time because they enable clinicians to deal with problems as they occur rather than when a simple condition blows up because the client misunderstood or blanked out the instructions. Once again, food animal clients deserve the same consideration as those owning companion animals.

More commonly practitioners must deal with clients who, from the practitioner's view, respond excessively or aberrantly to a particular situation. Clinicians periodically see patients and owners during times of emotional crisis under circumstances that may border on the bizarre: the cat who gets hit by a car or the sheep mauled by dogs the day after the owner's spouse dies; the dog diagnosed with malignant lymphoma the same week as the owner. Some owners may use animals as symbols of other people no longer present in their lives. Empty-nesters may have very strong feelings about the departed offspring's dog or final 4-H project. When people whom others emotionally link to an animal die, the animals can carry a tremendous emotional charge: John gave Mary the toy poodle for her birthday six months before he died in an accident; she considers the dog her last link with her husband.

Additionally, owners may respond negatively to animals they see as reflecting their own inadequacy. A primary example of this takes us back to behavior again. The owner tries to strong-arm the horse or cow to medicate it and the animal knocks him flat. This so enrages the owner that he chases the animal around the stall and beats it until he's exhausted. At that point, he may forcibly medicate the animal "to show him who's boss" or he may decide to let it suffer for exactly the same reason. Others who lack the strength to vent their frustration on the animal physically under similar circumstances may ignore the animal. Consequently, what the clinician sees as a simple medical problem becomes a major source of emotional trauma for owner and animal alike because the ability of the owner to handle and treat the animal was not ascertained beforehand.

Other owners may place what we consider an excessive emotional charge on only one aspect of the animal or its treatment. Owners of purebred animals may be obsessed by the desire to breed an animal no matter how reproductively unsound; food animal producers may care only about function or forgo what some practitioners consider the most basic humane care for financial reasons. Others will treat an animal only if the clinician can guarantee a complete cure, something all but the most optimistic and skilled practitioners find difficult to do, while other clients will do whatever the veterinarian asks as long as it doesn't require anesthesia or hospitalization.

Patient Stress and Owner Emotions

A final form of emotional involvement that warrants consideration involves that collection of looks and behaviors to which people—owners and veterinarians alike—assign emotional definitions. Obviously Dr. Tobin won't fault the owner of the tail-wagging dog or nuzzling horse for exclaiming, "Oh, Doctor, he's so happy to see you!" However, he feels quite differently when the owner gives that same response to the animal which pins him against the wall. In such cases, it's beneficial for all concerned to help these owners establish more workable emotional-behavioral links. For some clients, simply telling them the behavior communicates dominance rather than affection to people who are unprepared for such a display may lead them to stop reinforcing it and substitute less problematic behaviors.

One practitioner routinely evokes a visit from mythological favorite Great-Aunt Harriet in these situations. Great-Aunt Harriet is eighty-two, weighs a hundred pounds, and this visit will determine whether she changes her will and leaves the client all her millions: What will she do when that Great Dane or horse squashes her against the wall?

In such a way this practitioner humorously makes the point that just because the owner knows what the animal will do under certain circum-stances doesn't mean everyone else does or will agree with any positive emotional meaning the owner assigns to the behavior. Nor can we ignore the image of Great-Aunt Harriet getting assaulted yet again by all those food animals and horses who have been cheerfully smacked on the rump to speed them on their way into or out of the stall or pen. The unsuspecting person who happens to be standing nearby or, worse, leading such an animal when it gives that spastic leap as it passes through the barrier associated with the blow may be in for quite a painful surprise. If that person happens to be impaired in any way, the implications of this seemingly innocuous human behavior can become enormous.

Animal and human emotions also create problems when clients or practitioners justify what everyone considers negative behavior. Dr. Tobin reaches out to stroke an animal only to barely escape its teeth or hooves. The owner's explanation? "You must have frightened [hurt, surprised] him." Although the idea of veterinarians condoning such negative behavior seems ludicrous, in fact a surprising number do primarily because they don't know how to correct it. Moreover, the opposite scenario also plays itself out in barns and examination rooms. As the clinician examines the perfectly behaved animal, the client complains about it kicking the kids or snapping at the grandchildren and the veterinarian says they must have done something to antagonize it. Unfortunately, the fear and lack of knowledge that keep both clients and clinicians from dealing with such problems when they arise almost inevitably lead to a crisis situation: A person gets badly hurt; a sick animal can't be treated because the owner is afraid of it.

If we think of the human-animal bond as a highly specialized emotional link, we also can appreciate why some animals respond better in their owner's presence while others behave worse. We know that humans and animals can affect each other's pulse and heart rate: Does it seem so unreasonable that Tippy becomes upset when he can see his beloved owner standing in the corner wringing her hands in distress while some technician holds him in a death grip on a stainless steel table three feet off the ground? If the dog sees himself as dominant he may resist handling, struggle to reach her, or even attempt to bite, all of which will distress his owner even more. If he considers her dominant, her distress will compound his own and may lead to the familiar freeze, flight, or fight fear response. Meanwhile, the probability of Dr. Tobin performing a thorough physical on this animal under normal physiological conditions decreases in proportion to the increase in its and its owner's stress.

In these cases, separating the animal and the owner may relieve the tension on everyone. Dr. Tobin first meets with the client and discusses the animal's history while merely observing the patient; the animal remains alone in the stall, its carrier, or on a leash which the owner holds during this time. Once the practitioner describes what he intends to do to the animal and the client agrees, Dr. Tobin then takes the animal into another room to accomplish the treatment or waits until the owner leaves the barn to begin his work. Some owners will stay for everything but the needles; others want no part of the process whatsoever. Considering the negative effects these people can have on the animal, it does no good to insist that they remain if they don't want to be there.

What about the opposite case—the animal and owner who go to pieces when separated? These pose a major client relations dilemma, and pointing to the poster claiming the staff will restrain the animal for the owner's safety more often incites than calms these clients. It's far better to take the time in the beginning to introduce these owners to the technician who will hold the animal and demonstrate exactly what that person and the veterinarian will do. Remember, knowledge is power. More than anything the fear of the unknown—What if they hurt Baby? What if Baby bites them?—makes these people feel impotent. By providing them with knowledge, we decrease their apprehension; because these animals take their cues from the owners, calming the owner helps calm the animal, too.

Calming the animal also can help calm the owner. Sometimes dispensing tranquilizers for pre-visit administration works wonders in these situations. Depending on the owner, this may mean giving a dose that makes the animal appear "normal"—not drugged, but not apprehensive or practically asleep. However, owners who take this approach must be made aware that it may take time to establish an optimum dosage for the animal.

Interestingly, some owners find the idea that their animals require such drugs spurs them to undertake the necessary training to eliminate the problem. In these situations, they may request the tranquilizers for use "just in case," but never actually use them. Rather, the drug serves as a reminder of what lies ahead for the animal if they don't alter the behavior. Naturally, however, these clients may not realize such animals do respond to behavioral therapy if the practitioner doesn't mention it.

What about the owner who insists on holding the animal, or the one the clinician considers a capable and beneficial handler? Each clinician must make his or her own peace with that, knowing all responsibility for anything that happens to the client most likely will fall on the veterinarian. Some companion animal practitioners pose the AVMA Professional Liability Insurance Trust recommendation as law: They will not treat any animal held by a client. Period. However, those treating large animals often depend on the owner to restrain the animal and may see taking a trained technician to calls where willing and able help is available as an added expense that takes veterinary care beyond the reach of many clients. Like so many aspects of the client-patient-clinician relationship, it boils down to trust in an era whose laws imply the existence of such cannot be trusted; and whether or not that trust exists depends on good communication.

The Clinician Response

In all these situations, the owner's response possesses the potential to trigger an equally strong emotional response from the practitioner. Dr. Tobin inwardly seethes every time he does sperm counts on the obnoxious, bow-legged husky who should be castrated, not bred; he cringes as he turns the sheep loose without further treatment even though he knows the eye will rupture; his stomach flips any time he feels forced to treat animals under what he considers less than optimal conditions.

Unfortunately, once practitioners respond emotionally, an already emotional problem becomes even more so. Because of this and in order to successfully deal with these clients, practitioners must deal with their own emotions first. Ideally, this means objectively considering all sides of these emotionally charged issues *before* they occur, rather than ignoring them and hoping they never happen. This offers several advantages over trying to accomplish this in the client's presence:

- It gives clinicians the time to consider aspects of the issue and treatment options that might escape them in the midst of an emotional client encounter.
- It enables them to formulate their own philosophies regarding these issues, which are then easier to articulate unemotionally to clients at such times.
- The less emotionally practitioners present their positions, the less threatened clients will feel and the more likely they will listen.

In no way does this mean practitioners should rationalize to the extent they talk themselves into doing something they believe wrong. In fact, this approach will help insure that they *don't* do that in the heat of the moment when a normally reasonable client surprises them with such a demand. It also will help insure that clinicians present their positions professionally rather than as some heated harangue against the client. Compare Dr. Tobin's calmly delivered "I can't do that because it violates my standards of sound [safe, humane] treatment," to his shouted "That's a stupid [cruel, rotten] thing to do and I won't do it!"

Although the second sentiment may sound like the most passionately caring, the first one conveys the clinician's thoughtful consideration of the problem rather than a spur-of-the-moment emotional response to it. Where the latter assumes an adversarial stance toward the client, the former makes a simple statement of fact with which the client may do what he or she chooses.

All practitioners know their emotional hot spots as well as the most common owner emotional danger zones, so no reason exists for not working these out beforehand. Failing to do this, or if caught by an unanticipated negative emotional response, do not treat the animal until these issues are resolved to your own and the owner's satisfaction. Time and time again we come back to the same theme: Veterinarians do not get themselves in trouble because they use the wrong drug or charge too much nearly as often as because their behaviors express a lack of caring to the owner, and this includes a disregard for the owner's needs as well as the animal's.

Furthermore, it seems safe to say that insuring total comprehension and verifying the client's physical, mental, and emotional wherewithal to treat the animal as directed will become an increasingly important part of food animal practice for several reasons:

- The public is becoming increasingly concerned about the improper use and/or excessive level of drugs and other chemicals in the food supply.
- The presence of a growing immunocompromised population mandates strict control of zoonotic organisms in the food supply which will lead to even greater scrutiny of their sources.
- The increased presence of the immunocompromised in the workforce means the practitioner must educate his or her staff and the farmer/herdsman in proper handling and husbandry procedures that will ensure their own safety as well as the health of the animals.

Although a strong temptation might exist to see the human needs considered in this chapter as just one more thing to worry about in a day already lacking enough hours, clinicians may easily address these issues in the course of normal quality client communication. Not only will developing these skills benefit the typical client, it will help insure that we don't inadvertently overlook those with special needs.

Chapter 6
Problematic Owner-Animal Relationships

As animals become increasingly potent symbols in our society, we may reasonably assume that their relationships with their owners will become more complex as they reflect this changing orientation. This chapter discusses several problematic owner-animal relationships that can be particularly trying to the practitioner for several reasons. First, in all of these relationships the feelings and beliefs of the owners become inextricably tied up in the welfare of the animal. Although this is true to some extent in virtually every case we see, in these situations the animals may function as animate manifestations of the owners' beliefs rather than as four-legged, fur-covered mirrors reflecting them; in other words, the animal becomes the belief rather than just a symbol of it. Compare the owner who talks baby talk to the dog to the one who consciously or subconsciously creates and reinforces dependency in the animal until it is incapable of functioning on its own. In the former situation the owner sees the animal in a manner that complements his or her own beliefs while still maintaining the animal's separate identity; in the latter, both the animal and the owner need each other to complete their identities.

A second reason for considering these problems is the fact that, although they are relatively rare, informal discussions with practitioners indicate they may be becoming more frequent. Currently what little information exists tends to be primarily anecdotal and confined to the companion animal arena. However, because these owner-animal relationships can carry such a tremendous emotional charge for owner and practitioner alike, once again it would seem better for clinicians to work through their thoughts and feelings about these situations beforehand rather than when they discover themselves in the middle of such a relationship while they're trying to treat a seriously ill animal.

Third, in these situations above all others, practitioners must deal with any illusions they may harbor that they can treat any animal separate from its owner or primary human caregiver. Although dividing up the medical turf such that the physicians get all the *Homo sapiens* and we get everything else possesses a certain linear logic, it denies reality. However, much as those of us who say we got into veterinary medicine because we wanted to help animals (and even may believe animals warrant our help more than people) may chafe at finding ourselves agonizing more over the human than veterinary aspects of the problem, such constitutes the real world of veterinary practice. Those tempted to evade the issue by claiming we are, after all, veterinarians trained to treat animals, not people, inevitably will discover that attempting to treat only the animal in most of these situations may actually make the animal's problem worse, even to the point of jeopardizing its life.

Codependencies

Although the term codependency may carry a highly specific meaning within a particular human behavioral science, we will use it to refer to those animals and owners who share similar medical and/or behavioral problems. Surely every small animal practitioner can recall at least one diabetic pet-owner combination or overweight miniature poodle with congestive heart failure whose overweight owner shares the same fate. And who can be in practice more than a week and not notice how many uptight animals belong to uptight people?

Even though the idea of a pathologically dependent animal superficially may appear bizarre, it follows naturally from a process of domestication that views animals as animate quantities we genetically manipulate to reflect human beliefs, among them our desire to make animals dependent upon us for their most basic needs. The more an animal depends on us, the more likely it will stay around giving milk, laying eggs, or hunting with us rather than taking off on its own.

Furthermore, veterinary medicine is inextricably bound up in this process. A breeder's comment that he gives no vaccines or medical treatment to any pup until it reaches six months of age because he believes the animal should possess sufficient vigor to survive that long on its own elicited more than a few gasps of horror and remarks about animal abuse among the veterinarians present. These clinicians obviously did not share the breeder's view that medically intervening to sustain animals who lacked sufficient wherewithal to survive without that help constitutes the perpetuation of an unnatural dependency. Because domestication, by definition, creates a state of neediness in animals even as it fulfills certain human needs, we can appreciate that problematic codependencies reflect little more than an extension of the norm rather than an unrelated aberration.

Many studies of the human-animal bond position animals as indicators of the soundness of the intimate human physical and psychological environment, just as miners of old took canaries into the mine to monitor air quality and marine biologists and limnologists use certain target species as indicators of water quality (Allen and Blascovich 1990; Ascione 1991; Beck and Katcher 1983; Bergler 1992; Friedman 1990; McCullough 1989; Ruth 1992; Sykora 1992). Logic tells us that an animal which maintains a close relationship with an owner will share that person's life-style, and that may include eating the same high-salt, high-fat foods, and other unhealthy practices that may undermine the animal's health. Moreover, because the animal is smaller and of shorter lifespan, related health problems will show up sooner in the animal. However, as yet few clear correlations consistently exist between medically codependent owners and animals and their environments. Although some of these owners do maintain highly anthropomorphic relationships with their pets, others may share perfectly stable or even detached relationships with their animals.

That an animal's behavior intimately would reflect its owner's to the point of creating negative behavioral codependecies also finds a basis in fact. Allelomimetic behavior in social animals such as dogs leads them to mimic what other members in their group or pack are doing (Campbell 1992, 32–34). When humans become incorporated into the animal pack or serve as the pack's only other member of any significance, it seems reasonable that our animals could pick up our bad habits as well as our good ones. Similarly, the cat's solitary and maternal/sexual nature, which leads kittens to relate to people as queens, lends credence to the idea that animals also can serve as very intimate mirrors of their owners' psyche as well as physical being. Just as people may knowingly or unknowingly respond to an animal's physical needs in such a way that the animal's health reflects the owner's poor eating or exercise habits, so owners may knowingly or unknowingly reinforce those animal behaviors that reflect human needs rather than benefit the animal. Consequently, to attempt to treat these animals' problems separate from the owner amounts to trying to change the mirror because we don't like what we see in it.

Once we accept the possibility that some animals can and do interact with their owners this way—whether the owner chooses that particular animal because they consciously or subconsciously recognize it as "like me" or create it via their own habits and attitudes—we can see why we can't dissect the owner out of the treatment process in these cases above all others.

Medical Codependencies

In their most positive form, medical codependencies can be a boon to the treatment process for several reasons. Dr. Russo diagnoses the animal's problem and dispenses the medication and Ms. Hepner exclaims, "Those are the same drugs I'm taking for that same problem!" Because she wants to stay healthy, she faithfully takes her medication and easily incorporates the animal's treatment into her own medication schedule with the result that compliance can be very high even when the treatment regime is complex. Second, if these owners understand the nature of their own illnesses, the practitioner more easily can expand this knowledge base to include the similarities and differences between the owner's condition and the animal's. Dr. Russo commonly spends at least an hour discussing the ramifications of diabetes with a client before he commences treatment to insure compliance; he and Ms. Hepner complete this discussion in a fraction of the time because she already knows much of this from her own experience. Third, owners sharing chronic problems with their animals may maintain a more realistic view of the dynamic nature of these ailments. Ms. Hepner expects her animal to experience ups and downs because it happens to her. Finally, these people not uncommonly will go the extra mile for their animals. This may occur because they see the animal's problem as their own or because they've been preconditioned by a human medical process that gives them little or no choice in the matter.

Medical codependencies most commonly become problematic when a breakdown in communication occurs between the *physician* and the patient. In this situation, the owner turns to the veterinarian as a source of information for him- or herself as well as the animal. Nothing can quite compare to the sinking feeling experienced by practitioners confidently discussing an animal's treatment and prognosis when they realize the owners are asking all those questions in an attempt to better understand their own condition rather than the animal's. Nor does it take any great insight to imagine what the lawyers would say about veterinarians dispensing such information!

At such times the temptation to backpedal furiously may seem overwhelming, but this only will complicate the problem. If the information given is accurate, trying to downplay the severity of the animal's condition and/or prognosis to keep the owner from drawing conclusions about his or her own problem amounts to lying. Moreover, it could cause these owners to take a less conscientious approach to the animal's treatment which, in turn, could lead to a crisis situation that could increase owner anxiety regarding their own health even more. After all, if it happened to the dog and they were doing everything they were told to do to treat it, why couldn't it happen to them?

Regardless of the owners' relationships with their animals, most seem intrigued by the idea that they and their animals share the same problem, and few practitioners experience any difficulty learning the name of the owner's physician in normal conversation about the phenomenon. Nor do practitioners appear to experience difficulty explaining to these owners that they will tell them whatever they want to know about the animal, but any information about their own medical problems must come from their physicians. If clients say they cannot talk to their physicians, the practitioner can suggest these people contact a patient advocate provided by some hospitals and insurance companies to act as an intermediary in such situations. If this service is not available, advise the patient to contact a medical social worker or other member of the hospital counseling staff for assistance. In such a way, practitioners can show concern for the owner's problem as well as firmly establish themselves as the animal's and not the owner's clinician.

Sometimes problems arise when practitioners attempt to share the information about the animal with the client's physician. Then why bother? Good physicians want to know about anything that could affect the health of their patients, especially those with chronic and serious problems, and informing them about a medically codependent situation amounts to good medical practice as well as basic professional courtesy. However, physicians, and particularly specialists whose training may be highly linear, often view animals strictly as carriers of pathogens and allergens and have little or no concept of the human-animal bond, all of which can complicate the communication process. Consequently, veterinarians in these situations may need to summon all their communication skills to speak to these physicians in their own language. Practitioners should clearly state their willingness to discuss the animal's condition with the client, but place the full responsibility for discussing the client's health on the physician.

Territorial Codependency and Separation Anxiety

Although different kinds of behavioral codependencies exist, separation anxieties tend to create the most common detrimental effects in the medical treatment process. All practitioners recognize the dilemma posed by the animal who refuses to eat when hospitalized under the very best of conditions, let alone when ill. On the one hand we know it won't eat on its own, yet on the other we don't want to send it home until it does—especially to a household where it might be alone all day. Even more frustrating, and sometimes frightening, is the Siamese cat or Afghan who comes in for some common procedure (OHE, simple mid-shaft femoral fracture repair) and then proceeds to just give up and fade away following surgery unless we initiate extensive nursing care.

In these situations, the animal's sense of territory may lie at the heart of the problem. All animals are territorial and establishing and protecting the territory remain a primary species concern, often taking precedence over eating, mating, and all other activities. However, as domestication, genetic manipulation, and human-animal relationships blur basic species instincts, we see animals displaying more and more territorial variations. Some animals become more territorial and defensive in an examination room or cage, whereas others will make no attempt to claim territory under those circumstances and behave much more docilely at the veterinary hospital than at home. An animal's territorial nature becomes detrimental to the treatment process when the animal's definitions of enough or the right kind of territory cannot be fulfilled in the treatment setting. For example, those animals who feel so threatened by the veterinary clinic that they resist handling or experience fear responses (hypersalivation, increased heart rate, respiration, and temperature, hypermotility of the gut) may respond much more calmly to practitioners who make house calls.

Separation anxieties commonly reflect the two primary kinds of territoriality seen in domestic animals: place and person. Animals with a strong sense of spacial territory feel uncomfortable out of that physical setting, whereas those who define a person as their territory feel uncomfortable away from that person. How uncomfortable? Some realtors recognize what they call yo-yo pets, those animals whose owners move and take the animal with them only to have it return to the old home again and again because that's where it feels secure. For some animals the instinct to remain in that physical space may prove so strong, the owners wind up selling the pet along with the house. Other times the owner moves and leaves the animal, only to have it show up weeks or months later. These and other so-called "incredible journey" stories give us glimpses into the magnitude of the bond that exists when a particular place or person functions as the animal's primary territory.

Regardless what causes these phenomena, when we remove these animals from their territories they may feel so threatened that they refuse to eat or drink, and only sleep when exhaustion overtakes them. Some may even refuse to urinate or defecate because they see this as a form of territorial marking that they don't want to risk in what they consider a hostile environment. Obviously none of these behaviors enhances the recovery of the animal. If sufficiently overwhelmed by the situation, some will just give up and treating them for even the most simple condition can become problematic.

Even as some animals' territorial nature may undermine their recovery in a hospital setting, another space-related territorial assault may await hospitalized animals when they return home. Consider the case of Rosie, the ten-year-old Brittany spaniel hospitalized with acute pancreatitis complicated by renal problems. The day she was released three weeks later was such a joyous occasion for owners and practitioner alike, nobody considered not inviting the owners' other dog, Muffin, to join in the festivities. When the practitioner led Rosie into the examination room for the reunion, Muffin took one look at his former playmate, snarled, lunged, and pinned her to the floor, much to everyone's horror. Similarly, in multiple cat households the hospitalization of one animal for even a day may lead the others to attack or keep it from eating, drinking, or using the litter box when it returns home.

In some cases the strange scents carried by the hospitalized animal may lead others to treat it as an intruder, and spraying both the hospitalized and stay-at-home animals with a scented flea product or coat conditioner before reuniting them may help neutralize this affect. In situations where the animal is hospitalized for a noninfectious problem for more than a day, having the owners bring bedding from home and taking the hospitalized animal's bedding home for laundering can help maintain the scent link between the animals.

In other situations, the territorial peace evidently is maintained so tenuously in the household (too many animals in too little space, for example), the disappearance of one animal causes the remaining animal(s) to claim the departed animal's space. When it returns the others treat it like an intruder and attempt to drive it out, hardly a situation that bodes well for full recovery. Although still a relatively rare occurrence, the cat's solitary, territorial nature coupled with the increasing cat population and numbers of multiple cat households could make this a more common problem for members of this species and their owners in the future.

How can we work around these animals' basic nature? Training animals to accept a crate as a safe haven can help remove the territorial pressure during hospitalization because the crate can be placed in the cage with the frightened animal if necessary. Barring this, placing towels over cage doors or providing cats with paper bags or inverted boxes to hide in may help decrease their apprehension. In multiple animal households, crate training not only can reduce the individual space requirement per animal and thus decrease the possibility that any hospitalized animal will be ostracized when it returns, it also provides the latter with a safe space for recovery where the owner can easily monitor it as well. Compare the cat recovering from a urinary blockage in the owner's bedroom in a crate big enough for it, food and water, a favorite blanket, and a litter box, to that same animal hiding under the couch until it feels well enough to reestablish its territory. Again, bear in mind that the crate training advocated here means accustoming the animal to the crate as a private space it can use as it pleases, not as a source of confinement.

Animals who experience space-related territorial problems may share normal, stable relationships with their owners. However, the animal's behavior during or following hospitalization may greatly undermine that relationship as well as that between the client and the clinician. When the owner of the blocked cat calls an hour after the animal's discharge screaming, "My God, the other cat is trying to kill him! What did you do to him!" is not the best time to discuss this possible side-effect of hospitalization. Far better to discuss the nature of the relationships between the animal and other animals and humans in the household before hospitalization so owners may take precautions to avoid or limit these problems as much as possible.

Wise practitioners recognize that animals may not eat, drink, urinate, or defecate for behavioral as well as medical reasons and keeping them hospitalized until they do may hinder rather than hasten their recovery. If the animal does not respond even though medical science says it should, involve the owners in the process, first by keeping them informed about the animal's attitude as well as its medical parameters. Ask them to visit the animal and don't snicker when they bring an old sweater for the animal to sleep on or some of its favorite food or toys. Thank them. If all else fails, send the animal home on a trial basis to see if it responds better there.

Owner-Related Territorial Codependencies

When animals claim the owners as their territory, we not only see all the negative effects previously described, we also may need to deal with a distraught person because these owners may be as attached to the animal as it is to them. Just as we noted that sometimes we must hospitalize animals for normally at-home treatments because of owner limitations, so we may need to treat animals suffering from conditions for which we would normally recommend hospitalization on an out-patient basis when these animals belong to codependent owners.

How come? Two basic reasons make this a valid option.

- These animals won't respond away from the owners.
- These owners will disrupt the clinician and staff with constant inquires about the animal's condition.

Even if we can supply these often highly anthropomorphically oriented owners with what we consider irrefutable proof that our technology can benefit the animal far more than their loving presence, they won't believe it. Worse, many times their animals' failure to respond will support their view, which leaves practitioners in the awkward position of either admitting they made a mistake or trying to overcome a bond problem medically. In short, these owners can represent a major communications and public relations nightmare for the unsuspecting clinician. On the one hand, they're the last people any practitioner wants hanging around the wards and, on the other, that's exactly where they should be unless they take the animal home.

The true codependent owner often turns out to do an excellent job caring for the animal given enough support from the practitioner and veterinary staff. Because these owners' own sense of well-being is so strongly linked to the animal's, they are very conscientious about treating the animal as directed because they can't feel good until the animal does.

Those practitioners who cannot send these animals home or allow their owners free access to them because it violates either their definitions of good medical practice or their own sense of territory should refer these clients to a colleague who does not maintain such beliefs. To these owners, isolation from their animals communicates a blatant lack of caring for animal and owner alike, regardless of the medical and technological skill and best intentions of the practitioner who requires this. Once that feeling takes root, client and clinician become adversaries rather than partners in the treatment process and the animal gets caught between them.

Although many practitioners view these typically highly anthropomorphically oriented owners as attentive to the point of excess relative to their animals' care, in reality such owners pose fewer problems than the pseudo-codependents. Pseudo-codependent owners attempt to divest themselves of their furry creation when the animal develops problems. They enjoy boasting to their friends that "Muffy would die without me!" as long as Muffy stays healthy. However, when Muffy becomes ill and it becomes quite clear that the animal would, in fact, die without the owner's constant attention, they feel abused. When we add the guilt that often accompanies such ambivalent feelings, these owners' behavior may vacillate wildly between suffocating attention and total neglect.

The Preventive Practitioner Response

Once again good communication preferably before rather than during or after any crisis functions as the most important ingredient in the success of the treatment process. Practitioners should gently but firmly remind clients who encourage dependent behavior that they must assume full responsibility for any negative consequences this may cause the animal. Ideally such information should be imparted during that first examination when the owner overreacts to the process then cuddles and babies the animal following it, thereby reinforcing rather than neutralizing its fears. (Veterinarians who offer the animal food treats and sympathy rather than good-natured support under these circumstances also help perpetuate rather than alleviate the animal's fears.) Explaining that these often submissive animals take their cues from their owners and that owners who sympathize can magnify rather than reduce the animal's fears may induce even the most hesitant clients to put on a show of bravado for the animal's sake. Additionally, telling the owners exactly what will be done to the animal as well as any possible negative reaction on the animal's part before commencing the procedure can help alleviate owner apprehension.

Dependent social animals can gain confidence from training, particularly in groups where they are exposed to other animals and people. Many times owners see training as a mechanism whereby young animals learn certain basic commands or as a remedy for specific behavioral problems. However, the interaction with other animals and people and exposure to novel stimuli can do much to alleviate these animals' fears; the less fear, the less dependency on the owner. By the same token, those owners who would encourage dependent behavior as a result of their own lack of confidence also can benefit from training programs, especially those in which they handle other animals as well as their own. The latter approach does much to neutralize the "one-man dog, one-dog man" dependent mentality that results when owners and animals reinforce each others' fears.

Preventing dependent human-feline relationships proves more difficult because the cat's relatively recent arrival on the domestic scene coupled with its solitary and maternal/sexual nature may lead it to form very close ties to its owners, particularly when taken away from the queen too soon. Unfortunately "too soon" is an extremely relative term. Some breeds like the Siamese and Persians and their derivatives seem to need longer (at least twelve weeks) with the queen to develop a sense of "catness," although some individuals within those breeds may develop this earlier and others never do. However, the more a cat recognizes its cat nature, the less likely it is to become detrimentally dependent on its owners. Good breeders know the developmental curves of their animals and knowing such people to whom to refer interested clients seeking kittens can help prevent dependency problems. Granted most practices can claim thousands of cats among their clientele who were purchased or adopted at eight weeks or even younger with nary a problem. However, trying to treat just one highly dependent, unapproachable, terrified, often aggressive cat while the owner sobs hysterically makes any effort necessary to prevent such a problem seem worthwhile.

Munchausen Syndrome by Proxy

The final owner-animal relationship is by far the rarest, but bears mention because of its highly negative effects on practitioners and staff alike. Although not recognized in veterinary medicine per se, conversations with practitioners indicate it does occur and that the veterinary syndrome shares much in common with its human counterpart. Munchausen syndrome by Proxy (MBP) was first described in 1977 and since that time an increasing number of articles about it have appeared in professional journals worldwide. Named after eighteenth-century German soldier Baron von Münchhausen, whose exploits were grossly exaggerated, human MBP refers to those parents who feign or create illness in their children to maintain the attention of the physician(s) and medical staff (Meadow 1977, 2:343–45).

Most parents with MBP fit into one of three categories:

- doctor addicts
- help seekers
- active inducers

The doctor addicts believe the child is ill but don't go beyond reporting false symptoms; they may be very health-conscious and go to extremes to avoid the threat of disease. The help seekers may falsify or generate real symptoms and are very grateful and relieved when assistance is offered. The active inducers are the classic MBP parents who cause life-threatening symptoms and undermine the clinician's attempts to alleviate them (Sheridan 1989, 56).

Among those symptoms reported in the literature are fabricated and real apnea, seizures, hematuria, diarrhea, vomiting, skin infections, and bleeding from the respiratory tract, vagina, and rectum. The incidence of proven deliberate poisonings related to MBP leads most to believe these serve as the major cause of any real physical symptoms (Sheridan 1989, 53).

Why would a parent do such a thing to a child? Motivations include a desire to be the center of attention, to master illness, and to gratify ambivalent dependency needs. Unfortunately, the medical profession with all its exciting technology called into play in a crisis situation coupled with a compassionate clinician and/or staff often serves as a perfect source of gratification for these people (Sheridan 1989, 54–55).

In addition to the abuse perpetrated on the child, what makes such cases so traumatic for physicians and nurses is that these people commonly fit the stereotype of the ideal parent. Primarily women with some medical background, they appear exceptionally caring, attentive, and supportive, and many become favorites of the staff because of their willingness to assume more than the usual responsibility for the patient's care as well as to help out wherever needed (Blix and Brack 1988, 10:402–9). Within the veterinary setting some keep journals recording the animal's various ailments, look up the animal's medication in the *Physician's Desk Reference,* ask intelligent questions, and speak knowledgeably about both the drugs and the animal's condition.

Anyone who has agonized over the "people problems" in practice and has read the preceding chapters of this book feeling somewhat abused by the repeated admonition to speak to clients in their own language surely can appreciate the seduction of these owners. They speak to us in our own language; they think everything we do is wonderful and exciting. No matter how discouraged we get, they never lose faith in us. Even when we want to give up and refer them to a specialist, they plead with us to try again. Although they appear very attached to their animals, they display what has been described as a "belle indifference" (Sheridan 1988, 54), which physicians perceive as denial or heroic coping, but veterinarians may attribute to that ephemeral quality we think of as "realism": We want our clients to be attached, but not so much so they will put the animal through unnecessary suffering if its condition becomes hopeless.

These clients are so nice, we give them our home phone numbers and tell them to call us whenever problems arise. If we don't, one of our technicians does. We lie awake at night trying to figure out what's causing the diarrhea *this* time. Why does such a nice animal belonging to such a wonderful owner gets into such problems? What are we missing? What are we doing wrong?

In human medicine, MBP is suspected when children are repeatedly admitted with nonspecific signs by parents displaying the previously described characteristics. The clinician exhausts both the diagnostic and treatment repertoire, the patient may appear clinically normal for a while, but never remains healthy. Eventually, the previously impossible idea that these parents might be fabricating the symptoms or giving the child something to create them gains credibility. Once this occurs, the diagnosis of MBP is usually based on the recovery of the child when separated from the parent(s), although hidden cameras have been used in the hospital setting. These parents often vehemently deny any wrongdoing and become adversarial when the clinician suggests that they might be the cause of the problem (Zitelli et al. 1987, 1102). Because the diagnosis is usually presumptive and most of these parents refuse or resist any kind of psychiatric treatment, very little is known about the psychodynamics of this problem (McGuire and Feldman 1989, 83:292).

What we do know is MBP's effect on the clinician and staff. Because pediatricians and veterinarians both rely on parents/owners for all information regarding the patient, the idea that they would lie makes us feel exceedingly vulnerable. Add the fact that those who we considered ideal would do such a thing and we can see why those involved in such a case inevitably question our judgment and basic instincts about people. Worse, because what little in medical education that focuses on the client-clinician relationship often focuses on the need for clients to trust the practitioner to insure compliance, the idea that we can't trust some of them, that they would deliberately feed us false information that we take and plug into our science and technology like a trained dog, can be a major ego-buster, to say nothing of undermining our faith in all owners (Zitelli et al. 1987, 1102).

Unfortunately, as time-consuming and emotionally draining as MBP can be, veterinarians have even fewer opportunities to definitively diagnose it than physicians with a support staff of nurses, psychologists, and social workers. Of the two "cures" reported by veterinarians, in one situation the client's husband was transferred to another state and the client moved; in the other, the veterinarian sold the practice and moved to get away from the client. Although the idea of anyone so abusing an animal would seem to demand immediate intervention, these clients are extremely difficult to identify conclusively, and that plus their total denial leaves those making such accusations wide open to legal action as well as all the negative publicity that attends attacking a person whom the community at large may very well consider an ideal animal owner.

The relative rarity of MBP demands that practitioners do not use this as a diagnostic dumping ground for all those animals who just never seem to get better, particularly when immunosuppression plays an ever more important role in animal health. Furthermore, we can't overlook that dealing with chronically ill animals can place a tremendous amount of strain on owners not unlike that experienced by parents of chronically ill children that may manifest in ways similar to MBP (Krener and Adelman 1988, 142:946). Consequently, it behooves us to pay particular attention to the owners' needs as well as the animals' in these cases.

The key word in all client-patient-clinician interactions is *balance.* Clinicians who find themselves and/or members of their staffs becoming overly attached to certain clients and patients with chronic and/or recurring problems might want to reevaluate the soundness of their approach. By no means does this mean not caring, but rather caring in an objective, professional manner that gives these animals and their owners the same quality attention given to all clients.

The temptation for practitioners to go the extra mile can prove overwhelming at times. That coupled with a lack of knowledge regarding the different forms the human-animal bond can take may lead us to set precedents during the first client interaction which establish a tone that could lead to problems in the future. Unfortunately, the best protection a practitioner can have against the emotional effects of all the problems discussed in this chapter comes from that almost mystical quality known as professionalism. This is unfortunate because we graduate believing professionalism merely reflects scientific and technological competency. It is only when in practice that (sometimes bad) experience teaches us the importance of presence, that aura of genuine caring with just enough space between us and the client and animal to maintain our integrity and objectivity under the most emotionally trying and seductive circumstances.

Chapter 7
The Role of Guilt in the Treatment Process

The next two chapters will examine the highly unscientific subjects of guilt and love because these emotions can exert such powerful influence over the treatment process. Of the two, the negative effects of guilt can be the more insidious because its use becomes so incorporated into the medical process that we don't even acknowledge its presence. We enter practice with the idea that our job is to diagnose and treat every animal to the best of our ability, which we define as being as close to the academic ideal as possible; we define compliance in terms of our ability to get clients to see and do things our way. When clients resist, we feel disoriented and irritable and seek some way to relieve that tension. Once that happens, the probability of feeding more emotion into a situation already dominated by emotion increases dramatically and the chance of communicating with the client in a meaningful manner decreases accordingly.

Sin and Guilt

In order for guilt to exist, so must sin. In veterinary medicine, owners and practitioners each maintain a list of sins relative to animal health, and these fall into two main categories. First, there are the human sins of omission—those things someone should do but doesn't. Sins of omission include:

- lack of caring
- forgetting vaccinations and other preventive measures
- not giving medication

- overlooking symptoms of illness
- failing to note critical points when discussing the patient history
- failing to conduct the proper diagnostic tests
- lack of sufficient time and/or wherewithal to do things "right"

Second, we recognize sins of commission, those things done to the animal perceived as negative or wrong for one reason or another:

- feeding the wrong diet
- using improper home-remedies
- not treating the animal as directed
- misreading test results
- prescribing the wrong medication
- accepting negative behavior

These two lists deliberately combine owner and practitioner sins to make the crucial point that the identity of the sinner may be quite relative even if our ideas of the sin appear quite clear. For example, the five-month-old unvaccinated pup who succumbs to distemper seems like a clear case of owner negligence until we discover this first-time pet owner never received a vaccination reminder and is a single mother, working full-time and caring for an invalid parent. Suddenly, the practitioner looks at least as guilty if not more so than the client.

In addition, we and our clients also maintain similar lists relative to animals. Among those sins of omission that animals commit, owners and veterinarians list:

- failing to submit to examination and treatment
- failing to accept treatment
- failing to respond to treatment

Interestingly, a list of animals' sins of commission often turns out to be its sins of omission reworded in more active terms. These sins fall into two main categories:

- resisting handling during examination
- resisting treatment

Notice that the animal sins most commonly mentioned by owners and clinicians refer to the animal's behavior rather than its physical state. We do not blame an animal with internal parasites for having diarrhea, even if it has it all over our examination table or boots; we accept that as a normal consequence of the animal's problem. However, we do blame the animal for resisting our attempts to examine it and rarely, if ever, do we see this response as a normal consequence of the lack of proper human interaction every bit as detrimental to the animal's health as the owner's failure to keep its area free of parasite-infested waste.

In addition to maintaining lists of both highly specific and highly nebulous sins that we, our clients, and patients may commit, most people also recognize specific guilty body language expressions in others. The averted gaze of both human and animal commonly falls in this category as do other signs of fear and/or submission: the crouched animal with flattened ears and tucked tail, the owner shifting nervously as Dr. Bowman describes how much easier the problem would be to treat had she seen the animal sooner.

Because of our training as well as our conditioning, we may view virtually every problem encountered in an animal as a sin of some sort. Sometimes the sick or injured animal represents a human sin: somebody did something wrong or failed to do something right and now the animal must pay the price for that. As soon as we identify both the sin and the sinner to our satisfaction, the solution appears perfectly obvious: The sinner must atone for the sin(s) in order to be forgiven. Dr. Bowman clucks sympathetically over the animal with the horrendous parasite infestation—"Poor fella, you're not feeling very good, are you?"—prescribes the treatment with or without remarks regarding the avoidable nature of the problem (depending on how charitable she feels that day), then enthusiastically comments on the animal's improvement when she sees it later: "You look much better now!" Of course, even though Dr. Bowman talks to the animal, we all know she's really communicating with the owner. With not too much practice, most practitioners develop a tone that simultaneously expresses a stated concern for the animal as well as an unstated "This is your fault!" to the client. Similarly, the post-recovery sentiments aimed at the animal also pass judgment on the owner. When these are positive as in the example given, they essentially grant forgiveness to the owner who had sinned by allowing the animal to become ill but then atoned by treating it as directed.

Other times, we perceive the animal's condition itself as a sin perpetrated against the animal by some negative force beyond its control: a virus or bacteria, a faulty immune response. In these situations, we see ourselves engaged in combat with an enemy, seeking to identify it as accurately as possible so we may know its weakness and attack it most effectively and cure the animal. Unlike the previous approach this one does not assign owners an active role in the process, but rather positions them as spectators as we fight a private battle with disease and injury. When we hand them medication to administer, be it at the end of an examination or following weeks of hospitalization or almost daily trips to the farm, we feel we have won the battle or at least have the enemy under control. The idea that the client can't or won't treat the animal as directed strikes us as so incomprehensible, we don't even think to ask.

Positive and Negative Guilt

Whether making a client feel guilty will work depends on whether the guilt serves a legitimate purpose. For example, suppose Dr. Bowman makes that remark about the poor animal with diarrhea feeling so miserable in an effort to relieve her frustration and anger over what she considers an avoidable parasite problem. On the one hand, we can say this serves a legitimate purpose because it relieves Dr. Bowman's negative feelings in a socially acceptable way. She did not, after all, call the client a heartless imbecile and threaten to turn him in to the humane society, which is what she really wanted to do.

On the other hand, is it the purpose of the examination to provide the practitioner with the opportunity to vent his or her emotions regarding the animal's condition, or to exchange meaningful information with the client? If it's the latter, then we can see that Dr. Bowman's comment does nothing to accomplish this purpose. Consequently guilt used in this manner serves no legitimate purpose relative to the treatment process.

Furthermore, such a comment from the practitioner may undermine the treatment process. Suppose the client picks up the snide undertone in Dr. Bowman's remark, thinks, "What's *her* problem?" and decides the veterinarian got out on the wrong side of the bed that morning. This interpretation may affect the quality of the communication every bit as much as Dr. Bowman's view of the client as a heartless imbecile because the client may opt not to ask important questions regarding the animal's problem and its treatment lest he antagonize the prickly practitioner even more. In this situation, not only doesn't the owner associate his negligent behavior with the veterinarian's response, the veterinarian's attitude keeps the owner from asking questions that might prevent him from making similar or other mistakes regarding the animal's health in the future.

At most, Dr. Bowman can say *she* feels better following such an interaction. However, no such claims can be made for either the client or the animal. The client may see Dr. Bowman as worthy of his sympathy—"Poor woman is obviously overworked"—or he may decide to find a veterinarian who isn't so moody. Because neither the clinician nor the client communicate openly, the animal may not receive the optimal treatment or the owner the information necessary to prevent a recurrence of the problem. Worse, when the animal doesn't improve or succumbs to the same condition again, this may reinforce Dr. Bowman's views of the owner as a heartless imbecile and the cycle begins again. Just as likely, though, the client may seek help from another veterinarian because "that grouch Bowman didn't tell me anything!"

At this point we see the second kind of negative guilt visited by the clinician on the client: that which the client takes personally. Although we can use this to our advantage, as we shall see later, some clients respond very defensively to this approach no matter how justifiable we—and even they—might believe it to be. Suppose every time Dr. Bowman came out to the farm she explained the value of good husbandry and made specific recommendations to the owner regarding changes that would help prevent parasite problems. Unless the client truly is a heartless imbecile—and he may be, but fewer exist than some practitioners would like to believe—he *knows* he contributed to the animal's problem. Moreover, he *did* call Dr. Bowman for help, and maybe after going through a fair amount of mental anguish and delay fearing what she might say to him. Consequently, in his mind she should not think ill of him, and he would have every right to respond angrily to her if she did for several reasons:

- He knows he made a mistake so it serves no purpose for her to remind him.
- He does care about his animal because he did call.
- He didn't call her to make him feel guilty; he called her to treat the animal.
- She's a veterinarian, not a judge or his spiritual adviser.

Because Dr. Bowman undoubtedly will expect him to pay for her services, we can see why he would scrutinize her every move looking for some sin on her part, too. Furthermore, if Dr. Bowman becomes sufficiently caught up in her righteous indignation over the client's sins she, too, may forget to ask some crucial question or otherwise err in her diagnosis and treatment of the animal. At that point, the idea that the client would relish pointing the finger at *her* doesn't seem so difficult to imagine.

The worst kind of guilt that practitioners can inflict on their clients follows a client or animal sin that the clinician did nothing to avoid. An excellent—and unfortunately common—example of this is the veterinarian who blames owners for their inability to handle their animals. This practice becomes particularly insidious when the clinician complains to a colleague or staff member rather than the client him- or herself: "That guy can't even handle his own animal!"

However, in many cases what these complaining practitioners have forgotten is that they most likely became veterinarians because they enjoyed being around animals and probably had a fair amount of exposure to them their entire lives. Moreover, their veterinary education and practice experience further enhanced their ability to work with animals. In other words, while many of us would like to believe we were born with "a way with animals" as our mothers claimed, in fact that "way," our genuine affection for and interest in animals, led us to develop the necessary skills over the years to properly handle them.

Conversely, owners may get animals because they *didn't* have much exposure to them and want to add this dimension to their lives. First-time pet owners hardly constitute a rarity in any small animal practice, and most areas can claim at least a few farms owned by former urban professionals—engineers, physicians, managers—who decided to live off the land. Rather than earn our disdain, these people need, and deserve, our most conscientious help in order to make their interactions with their animals rewarding for both. To judge them guilty of any sin—be it improper handling, diet, housing, or treatment—and do nothing to rectify the problem surely stands as the greatest sin. To say we lack the time to discuss the filthy stalls, the standing pools of water in the pens, or the unruly behavior ranks on a par with saying we lack the time to discuss the implications of the animal's bilateral mucopurulent ocular and nasal discharge, and more than a few clients say it ranks even higher.

Consequently, to berate clients for such "nonmedical" infractions as if they lacked a most basic human instinct represents the epitome of professional conceit and serves virtually no positive purpose relative to the treatment process. Owners getting dragged into and out of the clinic, scratched, bitten, kicked, and pinned against the wall *know* they can't handle their animals, and more and more of them resent practitioners who insinuate that the animal's misbehavior during the examination takes up valuable time that should be used to treat the animal's real—that is, medical—problems. When these owners discover through conversations with a sympathetic neighbor or county agent that ways exist to treat and prevent these problems, ironically they may judge their veterinarian lacking in the most basic knowledge, too. It goes without saying that these clients are not pleased when they discover the veterinarian has been criticizing or making fun of them behind their backs.

Using Guilt to Enhance the Treatment Process

More than any other factor, the amount and quality of the information the clinician shares with the client regarding the animal's condition determines whether guilt will serve a useful purpose in the treatment process. In the preceding examples, the practitioner's desire to pass judgment took precedence over the desire to educate the owner. As a result, even if clients were willing to atone for their sins, they possessed no more idea of how to go about this after their contact with the veterinarian than before.

Compare Dr. Bowman's sympathetic murmuring to the animal and alienation of the owner to her providing the owner with concrete suggestions regarding the animal's care. If she truly lacks the time to provide anything beyond that related to the animal's immediate medical problem, she should schedule a specific appointment to address these other issues. If she thinks she'll never have the time or doesn't possess the information herself, she should admit this to the client and refer him to someone who does. In rural areas local extension agents and farriers can serve as valuable sources of client information, yet some veterinarians view these people with suspicion, even going so far as to accuse them of practicing veterinary medicine without a license. Ironically, many times owners turn to these people when the veterinarians fail to meet their clients' needs; these people, in turn, feel obligated to expand their knowledge and skill to fill this void in the veterinary coverage. For example, veterinarians who practice in areas with large beef or dairy cattle populations may know or care little about sheep, goats, chickens, or geese, thereby forcing owners of these animals to seek that information elsewhere.

In addition to providing a sound knowledge base, veterinarians who use guilt effectively in the treatment process recognize its built-in time limitations. Few people like to feel guilty, and the practitioner must decide whether guilt will sustain a particular client through the treatment process. Although some clients may give the impression that they feel so badly about what happened to the animal they would willingly devote the rest of their lives to its treatment, in reality this rarely happens. As noted in previous chapters, financial, time, space, and other life-style and personal factors come into play, and eventually the guilt may give way to resentment toward the veterinarian, the animal, or both. Because of this, guilt works best when used to fuel short-term processes rather than to treat long-term or chronic problems. Dr. Bowman can lean on owners of animals with mild otitis or conjunctivitis with prophecies of more serious problems if they don't medicate the animal as directed for the next week or two. However, the busy owners of seborrheic animals find her dire predictions designed to insure those weekly baths tiresome and even irritating after the first few months.

Although theoretically it would appear that the more serious the problem created by owner negligence, the more determined these owners would be to atone for their sins, such is not always the case. The owner whose animal snaps at Great-Aunt Harriet but doesn't connect may feel much more obligated to treat the problem than the one whose animal draws blood. In the latter situation the combination of guilt and the magnitude of the problem may so overwhelm these owners, the idea of treating the animal seems impossible to them.

In the medical arena, consider the practitioner who insists the owner of the obese animal with congestive heart failure end years of feeding the dog human food—immediately and forever!—or bear the responsibility for killing the beloved pet. Such a potent guilt-laced prescription may so shock owner and animal alike, the bond and behavioral aspects of the problem far surpass its medical implications. The case of the very intelligent, normally stable and genial executive sitting in the examination room beside his obese Labrador two weeks following such a practitioner pronouncement remains firmly fixed in that veterinarian's mind. Tears streaming down his face, the owner pleaded with the veterinarian to understand his anguish: "We've shared a doughnut every morning and a bowl of ice cream every night for thirteen years and it's killing both of us not to do that. I'd rather she died than live the rest of her life like we've spent these last two weeks!"

In this situation, it wasn't that the owner didn't want to make the changes, it was that the practitioner asked him to do too much at one time. As a result, the client not only had to deal with his guilt regarding those practices the veterinarian had confidently assured him were killing his dog, he also had to deal with the guilt that arose when he couldn't carry out the treatment. Once the practitioner worked out a series of small changes implemented over a longer period of time which took into account the behavioral and bond as well as the medical aspects of the problem, compliance ceased to be a problem.

Guilt also can inspire some owners to make lasting changes following sudden, avoidable traumatic injury or serious illness to the animal. The free-roaming animal which ingests a toxic substance or gets hit by a car serves as a familiar case in point. In these situations the animal's suffering, coupled with the owner's mental anguish and the expense and any inconvenience associated with the treatment may serve as a potent incentive for these owners to confine their animals. However, whether this kind of guilt works depends on why the animal was loose in the first place. If the owner forgot to close the gate properly or didn't think there was any traffic in the area, then the memory of the event will fuel that person's desire to make the necessary changes to restrain the animal. However, if the animal ran free because it urinates in the bedroom closet, chews the furniture, or periodically has diarrhea all over the house, the idea of keeping it confined so it doesn't get hurt may not sustain these owners. Similarly, owners of both large and small animals which routinely escape and resist recapture may find it difficult to muster sufficient legitimate guilt to sustain them long enough to make meaningful changes. Once again, whether these owners can change depends on how much concrete information and support the veterinarian gives them regarding the treatment of any underlying problem as well as the trauma or illness that resulted from it.

The Practitioner as Target

Every practice boasts its complement of blamers, and because veterinarians don't like to feel guilty any more than their clients do, taking the time to consider some of the more common ways owners use guilt and how we respond can enable us to cope more effectively with these situations when they arise.

Consider the following statements:

"I would have brought BeanDip in sooner, but I couldn't get an appointment."
"I knew the mare was sick last week, but you were on vacation."
"I couldn't get the pills [ointment, drops] in him."
"That medicine you gave me didn't work."

In all these situations, we could choose to dismiss the remarks based on the belief that the owners who made them hope to project the responsibility for their sins onto the practitioner. However, whether this is actually true may depend on three factors:

• The specific events that led a particular client to come to this conclusion.
• How often we've heard complaints from this client.
• Whether we've heard similar complaints from other clients.

If Jim Cannon inevitably waits until the last minute to seek routine care for his animal then insists this "emergency" must be seen immediately, Dr. Bowman shouldn't feel particularly guilty about her inability to fit him into her schedule. However, if Mr. Cannon is a very conscientious client and especially if Dr. Bowman has heard the complaint from others, the situation warrants further investigation. Perhaps she needs to allow more openings for last-minute problems rather than filling the appointment book with routine work in advance. Or maybe those scheduling the appointments are putting off clients with seriously ill animals because they lack sufficient training to recognize key words or phrases—bloat, colic, down cows, cats straining to urinate—that may indicate serious problems. In these situations, the client who makes us feel guilty can lead us to make positive changes that will benefit all our clients.

Consequently, each client statement that elicits feelings of guilt deserves to be evaluated as objectively as possible. If Dr. Bowman does nothing to discourage her clients from believing she's the only competent practitioner in the county, she willingly must accept any guilt that results when her clients fail to seek other help for their animals in her absence. On the other hand, if she does nothing to foster this client belief and provides what she considers quality back-up in her absence, she has no need to feel guilty.

Then we come to all those client excuses regarding their failure to treat the animal as directed, many of which we've already discussed in previous chapters. When complaints about this subject surface, asking owners to describe or demonstrate the exact nature of the problems they encountered can provide a wealth of information. When Dr. Bowman solicited complaints about commonly prescribed ear drops, she learned the following facts she never even considered before:

• If owners placed the tip of the container as far in the animal's ear as directed, they couldn't see whether the medication was coming out or not.
• A clear plastic seal on one product could be overlooked by owners with poor eyesight or those who removed their glasses to medicate the animal (a common practice).

- Another product required so much force to propel the drops out of the container that some owners were "treating" the animal with puffs of air rather than medication.
- Some containers proved difficult to handle for those suffering from arthritis or those unaccustomed to manipulating small objects.
- The more difficulty the owner experienced medicating the animal, the more the animal would resist, and the more reluctant the owner would be to medicate it.

When we face client accusations related to their inability to carry out our instructions, we must deal with guilt from two directions. In addition to the guilt that arises from the animal's failure to get better, we also must cope with that which results if we then prescribe what we consider a lesser treatment that better meets the client's needs. New graduates often are surprised, and even appalled, when they encounter practitioners who use long-acting injectables to treat conditions for which more efficacious oral medications exist. Although some of these oldsters may not have kept up on the latest treatments, it's also possible they know from experience that there's no way a particular owner can properly medicate a particular animal orally under those particular circumstances. Consequently, it's not a question of giving an inferior treatment when a superior one is available: It's a question of treating the animal versus doing nothing at all.

Passive Aggression

A human behavioral condition known as passive aggression also may play a role in guilt-based client-practitioner interactions. Not only do passive-aggressive people not do what is requested, they provide all kinds of legitimate sounding reasons why they can't *and* attempt to make the person making the request feel guilty for asking them to do anything. The name "passive aggressive" is somewhat misleading because these people are not particularly hostile. In fact, some are so pleasant many times we can't help feeling sorry for their troubled lives or for making demands that further add to their burden. The "aggression" in passive aggression refers to these people's persistent attempts to resist authority indirectly and covertly and get others to assume responsibility for their actions (American Psychiatric Association 1987, 356–58).

Whether a person falls into this category depends on the frequency of the behavior. For example, consider the following conversation between a practitioner and client:

> **Client:** "I'm sorry I'm late again, but my neighbor's house burned down and then I helped an old woman change a flat tire on her car.
>
> **Practitioner:** "How's Fluffy doing?"
>
> **Client:** "Not too good. The dog ate the pills you gave me for her and then he threw up all over the house. And then the kids came down with the flu and my mother's a diabetic and I lost my job because my supervisor was jealous of my ability. That's why I didn't pay my bill the last time I was here."

Granted this is an exaggerated example, but the point is that even though all these reasons for the client's failure to function on various fronts sound so legitimate that we may feel tempted to praise this person's indomitable human spirit, all project responsibility away from that person and onto others. The neighbor and old woman with the flat tire caused the late arrival; the dog, children, and mother somehow conspired against Fluffy's medication in a manner totally beyond the owner's control; the jealous supervisor thwarted attempts to pay the bill.

Because the excuses offered by these people can be very elaborate, one helpful way to get to the heart of the matter is to mentally ask the question, "What is the result of all this?" In the preceding client-practitioner interaction we see that:

- The client is late for the appointment.
- The animal was not medicated as directed.
- The client did not pay.

What makes a person passively aggressive is that he or she is *inevitably* late, doesn't treat the animal as directed, and doesn't pay for services when rendered. Once practitioners realize this, they can free themselves from the feelings of frustration and manipulation these often kind and gentle folk can precipitate. As far as the animal's treatment is concerned, it's best not to rely on these people to do anything, and instead to consider one of those approaches used on large animals living under less than optimal conditions. Whether practitioners wish to extend credit to clients who inevitably find themselves in the midst of financial as well as other disasters seemingly totally beyond their control is a matter of choice. Some practitioners believe that if the money comes in eventually—every cloud must have a silver lining—there's no need to worry about it. Others use the lack of payment as a reason to refuse to provide service to someone they consider a less than rewarding client.

Also note that passive-aggressive veterinarians exist, too. The office manager asks Dr. Dunlevy whether he remembered to make the deposit on his way to a farm call and he treats her to a ten-minute description of the demented horse which kicked him yesterday, the size of the bruise on his thigh today, the agony of walking, his wife's menopausal symptoms, his father's gall bladder attack, and the threat of the demon OSHA inspector who could cast them all out in the streets in an instant if he saw *her* coffee cup on the window sill. Translation: He forgot to make the deposit. Similarly, clients who point out that the unruly animal didn't get the medication because Dr. Dunlevy didn't explain how to give it may need to endure a rambling lecture about the high cost of liability insurance, the excess of conniving lawyers, and how society and the government conspire against the small businessman just trying to do a good job and make ends meet.

Guilt, Law, and Ethics

What about those times when practitioners definitely make a *big* mistake? We become so involved in the surgery that we forget to monitor the anesthesia; we're so convinced the hematuria comes from a bladder infection, the idea that the animal could have been hit by a car never crosses our minds until it collapses and the owner brings it back several hours later. We need only to read the AVMA's *Principles of Veterinary Ethics*, and the writings of Harold Hannah (1992a, 1993), Jerrold Tannenbaum (1989, 1991), James Wilson (1988), and others increasingly concerned about law and ethics in the veterinary profession to realize that there are no simple answers. As Wilson notes in *Law and Ethics of the Veterinary Profession* (1988, 5): "The ethical requirement is to be honest with the client, although honesty could provoke a lawsuit. Morally, there is undoubtedly a heavy burden of guilt as well as a duty to tell the client what happened."

At present, practitioners faced with this problem often feel pulled in opposite directions by legal and moral considerations. The legal view at times seems skewed toward the "above all, admit no wrong" approach which maintains that an admission of guilt not only leaves the practitioner defenseless if the client pursues the issue legally, but practically invites the client to take this line of action. On the other hand, others maintain exactly the opposite view. One lawyer won't defend a practitioner accused of malpractice unless that person made a sincere attempt to apologize to the client. His reasoning? "I don't want to represent anyone who doesn't have the integrity and courage to admit he or she made a mistake." He and others like him believe more people sue because the clinician withheld information or lied to cover the truth rather than because that person didn't perform his or her technical duties properly.

For most of us, however, it boils down to whether we can live with ourselves if we don't acknowledge the error and apologize to the client rather than any legal opinion. Some of us can; some of us can't. Some must confess all to the client and ask for forgiveness. Others find that extending regrets and sympathy to the client for the failure of the treatment or loss of the animal and reserving the confession of all the gut-wrenching details for a sympathetic colleague, spouse, or friend enables them to let the matter go.

Whether we can let the matter go—that is, whether we can forgive *ourselves*—determines the success of any approach. One way practitioners achieve this, whether they admit the error to the client or not, is to do everything possible to insure that they will not make the same mistake again. They read everything they can find pertinent to the misdiagnosed condition; they find the money to replace the unreliable vaporizer; they move those drugs they might confuse to unusual locations to remind themselves to think twice before they use them, no matter how tired they may be. In short, the mistake serves as an impetus for them to expand their knowledge and make changes that will benefit all of their clients. This won't bring the dead animal back to life or lessen the owner's sorrow, but it serves a more constructive purpose than wallowing in guilt and feeling sick every time they encounter that client or a similar case.

What about those animals for whom we want to do more but client constraints make this impossible? In order to better understand these often highly emotional situations, we need to take a closer look at love, the subject of the next chapter.

Chapter 8
The Role of Love in the Treatment Process

In *Dairy Cattle: Principles, Practices, Problems, Profits,* Drs. Bath, Dickinson, Tucker, and Appleman cite an Iowa State study that lists record-keeping as the area of competency most critical to the success of a dairy herdsman. However, the authors also list sincere *love* for the dairy cow as the most important quality for those desiring to develop a herd of superior breeding animals. They go on to note that it is this love that leads people to pay attention to feeding, managing, and "the small details necessary for success" (Bath et al. 1985, 17). The opinion of these four men representing institutions in California, Maryland, Michigan, and Minnesota opens this chapter to dispel any notion that love represents a romantic, companion animal concept generated by doting anthropomorphically oriented owners to complicate the treatment process. In reality, whether we call it love or caring, love serves as the primary force that bonds owner and animal together.

Consider each of the following events that routinely occur in veterinary practice and assign a client attitude toward the animal that would most enhance this process:

1. The client calls for an appointment.
2. The client provides a history of the animal's problem.
3. The clinician proposes a diagnostic sequence.
4. The clinician prescribes treatment.
5. The client carries out the treatment.

Surely every practitioner wants clients motivated by love because these owners pay more attention to their animals and thus are more likely to seek help when things go wrong as well as to do what we ask. To appreciate how much we rely on owner love even though we might not call it that, imagine participating in that same sequence with an owner motivated by guilt, fear, anger, or one who feels nothing for the animal at all. What occurred easily with the owner motivated by love becomes an effort under the latter conditions.

Now add a sixth step to the sequence:

6. The animal dies.

At this point, many who appreciated the positive difference owner love can make in the preceding steps might very well wish the owner didn't care quite so much. However, even though Dr. Gagnon may cringe and think, "God help us all if anything ever happens to that animal!" every time he sees Ms. Emery cuddling her Pomeranian or Suzy Wright with her 4-H ewe, the love between the owner and the animal does affect virtually every aspect of the treatment process from beginning to end whether we acknowledge it or not.

Although some might argue that it's impossible to love too much, if the emotion expressed or felt seems excessive, it probably presents something other than love in the truest sense. As I Corinthians 13:1 so eloquently put it, love is not "a noisy gong or a clanging cymbal." Nor is love a clanging *symbol* although this represents its most common form in those owners whose interactions with animals seem excessive for one reason or another. Recall the discussion in Chapter 6 of the anxiety experienced by animals who become dependent on their owners. In this situation, the animal's sense of self becomes so inextricably entwined with the owner's that it can't function away from that person. However, the owners themselves and many others would define these owners as the ideal and wonder how such a horrible fate could befall an animal so well loved. At the opposite end of this negative spectrum, we see those owners suffering from Munchausen syndrome by proxy who give all the outward appearances of caring very much when in fact they lie and sabotage the treatment process in an effort to maintain the attention of the clinician and staff. In both these situations the owner's love may result in life-threatening circumstances for the animal.

Fortunately, these extreme cases rarely occur in practice. However, clinicians routinely encounter other situations in which the animal becomes tied up in a detrimental process that the owner defines as an expression of love. Once an owner makes this connection, eliminating the practice becomes the same as withdrawing love from the animal or denying the animal free expression of it. Clinicians who define the results of these interactions strictly in medical or behavioral terms and ignore the underlying motivation may find themselves frustrated in their attempts to correct the problem.

Food Equals Love

In the medical arena, perhaps the most widespread and frustrating example of negative love symbolism occurs in those owners who relate food and feeding rituals to love. Such connections prove most resistant to change because these beliefs pervade our society. Guests enter Dr. Gagnon's home and he immediately offers them something to eat or drink. He associates holidays at least as much if not more with their particular culinary delights as with their religious or historical significance. A thick slab of chocolate cake sits on the counter next to an apple: Which one gets the covetous looks? Which one would Dr. Gagnon most likely offer the child who just completed a difficult homework assignment or helped him clean out the barn?

Complicating this process, the medical profession reinforces a very strong connection between appetite and health. If the owner assures Dr. Gagnon that the animal is eating "well," he automatically assumes it is eating "right," and rarely challenges that assumption until what the animal is eating creates problems. Moreover, he views not eating or not eating much as reliable indicators that something is wrong with the animal. When we put the medical belief that a healthy appetite equals a healthy animal with the owners' food-equals-love beliefs, we can see how the owner who loves the animal and wants to keep it healthy will do whatever necessary to keep it eating. Because the food functions as a symbol of both love and good health, the more the animal eats, the healthier and the more loved it must be.

Once people make these connections, we can appreciate how feeding less or something the owners consider less palatable can generate a tremendous amount of anguish because, even though their minds tell them it's the right thing to do, their hearts tell them it's not. Moreover, although practitioners and animal control officers bemoan the sad effects of "Empty Haymow Disease" in underfed large animals, we also see overfed horses, sheep, and other farm animals whose owners we invariably define as caring. Although owners who feed snacks or table food rarely occur in large animal practice, those who toss an extra scoop of grain into the trough aren't that uncommon.

Recall the case in the previous chapter in which the practitioner attempted to force the owner of the obese Labrador with heart problems to change the dog's diet by making the owner feel guilty; the plan failed because the owner saw feeding the animal certain foods as an expression of love. Whether we believe animals capable of experiencing emotion or not, no doubt existed in that owner's mind that his dog shared his view and he responded to it accordingly. Relative to human beliefs about food, love and guilt go hand in hand. Like many working owners, that client got into the habit of sharing food with his pet because he felt guilty about leaving the animal home alone all day. The animal's feeding times, which coincided with the owner's own breakfast and dinner, guaranteed owner and pet two periods of intimate interaction even on the busiest days. Consequently, to assuage his guilt it seemed perfectly natural for this client to give his dog something from his own plate. Soon the ritual expanded to include the shared ice cream at bedtime. However, the owner didn't see these feedings as arising from his guilt; he saw them as arising from his love as well as indicative of the animal's robust good health and love for him. When the naive clinician insisted he must stop the practice immediately or accept responsibility for killing the dog, the owner felt trapped in a no-win situation. Because the food-based ritual provided him with a way to relieve his guilt about leaving the dog alone as well as to express his love, if he eliminated the ritual he had no way to express these emotions. Consequently what the veterinarian perceived as an unemotional, medically sound statement, the owner perceived as a devastating assault.

Ask any owners of an animal on a restricted diet who make the connection between food and love what they read in the animal's expression as it stares at them while they eat. Nine times out of ten, they read condemnation and abandonment into those looks. Is it any wonder these owners agonize over what we consider a straightforward, medically sound diet any loving owner would immediately implement and adhere to religiously?

Moreover, even though obesity looms as the greatest nutritional problem, clinicians also may see love-related beliefs come into play when therapeutic diets are recommended for treating various medical problems. The animal develops heart, kidney, gastrointestinal, liver, or pancreatic problems—perhaps secondary to lifelong injudicious eating habits—and Dr. Gagnon firmly states that the animal must eat *only* a certain food. If the animal finds this fare less palatable than its previous diet, once again the owners get assaulted by beliefs on two fronts:

- They fear the sick animal will think they don't love it any more.
- As long as the animal doesn't eat, by definition it remains unhealthy.

Given these beliefs, can we fault these people for cheating on the animal's diet? Can we blame them for not wanting to admit this to us when they do? Consequently, we can appreciate how owners faced with sick animals may perceive the need to express love as their primary concern, and the success or failure of any dietary changes will depend on the client's ability to replace any detrimental food-based love beliefs with more constructive ones.

Once we recognize the potent influence human beliefs about love may exert, a critical part of the treatment process becomes helping owners either to abolish problematic beliefs or to find ways to maintain them that meet the animal's physical needs in a positive way. Admittedly this can be a most challenging undertaking because the food-equals-love equation assaults us everywhere and may constitute a primary focus in the owner's life. Nonetheless, a surprising number of clients never considered how their own ideas about love affect what they feed their animals, and simply discussing this can help a great deal. Although abolishing any food-equals-love belief that leads the owner to offer large servings, treats, and human food instead of the proper amount of the food that best meets the animal's needs provides the best long-term results, such beliefs may be so firmly entrenched it's often much easier as well as necessary to provide new love symbols rather than try to eliminate the symbolism completely. Because the owner made the original connection, this works best if the owner comes up with the new symbol.

For example, based on the medical principle that the fastest way to lose weight involves decreasing caloric intake while increasing caloric expenditure, theoretically it makes sense to tell owners to show their love for the animal by exercising it rather than sharing a snack with it. This approach may work for those owners who enjoy exercise and see such an activity as quality, that is, loving, time spent with the animal. However, if they perceive exercise as work or an activity that takes up too much time in a life already filled to overflowing, then this becomes yet another burden that adds more negative emotion to the weight-reduction process. Some people find it more enjoyable to play games (inside the house or out) with their pets to exercise them; others so deplore exercise, the weight loss must be handled entirely via dietary changes. In the latter case that may mean offering what owners consider equally palatable alternatives, be these prepared low-calorie diets or thin slivers of gourmet roasted skinless chicken breast instead of cookies.

The key to changing these and all problematic love connections is that the owner must play an active role in either eliminating the symbolism or replacing it with something more constructive. Although this might seem like a time-consuming process, any time spent with these clients discussing their beliefs and helping them work out acceptable alternatives can pay huge dividends in the long run.

Tolerance Equals Love

Another connection people make that can undermine the treatment process relates tolerance to love. We previously mentioned those owners who tolerate dominant animals which leap on people believing this constitutes a legitimate way for an animal to express love. Similarly, we see animals that are so unmanageable and the owners so resistant (albeit many times nicely so) to our suggestions regarding proper training, we must wonder if the misbehavior serves some positive purpose in the relationship. Within the medical arena, we see animals with avoidable or treatable problems that the owners treat haphazardly at best, or allow to reach crisis proportions before treating at all. Animals with ear and skin problems not uncommonly fall prey to this owner idiosyncrasy.

Why would a caring owner *want* an animal to be misbehaved or ill? Listening to people discuss their animals with others in the waiting room or at social gatherings can provide some insight into this seemingly contradictory phenomenon. Many people believe that it takes a more loving person to live with a misbehaved or medically problematic animal than a well-behaved healthy one. Either out of politeness or genuine conviction, those hearing ongoing sagas of medical or behavioral woes often commend these owners for their great love of and devotion to the animal under such trying circumstances. Although Dr. Gagnon would never praise owners who annually ignore flea problems until severe allergic reactions occur, he does offer backhanded compliments to owners of unruly animals: "Ms. Dennis, you must surely love that dog [cat, horse] to put up with that behavior," he jokes good-naturedly. "Frankly, if that animal belonged to me, I'd shoot it."

In addition to gaining points as a superior human being for living with a misbehaved or sick animal, some owners also may tolerate treatable conditions as a means of atoning for various sins. Owners whose animals display negative behavior in their absence are notorious for making this connection. They convince themselves the animal chewed up the rug or vomited on the bed because it loves them so much, and thus quite naturally suffers great anguish and/or a desire to get even with them when they abandon it; they then award themselves points for returning that love even as they clean up the mess yet again. The drawbacks of this approach are twofold. First, it does nothing to solve the problem: The owner's love and tolerance of the behavior does nothing to relieve the daily frustration of the animal who chews the rug. Second, because these owners define their absence and the animal's great love as the cause of problem, they may overlook signs of serious illness as well as behavioral stress in the animal: Rather than trying to get even with its owners for abandoning it as they chose to believe, the animal who vomited repeatedly did so because it had ingested a plastic meat wrapper. The fact that the owners chose to tolerate the vomiting as evidence of their love rather than seek veterinary care delayed the diagnosis and treatment of a legitimate medical problem.

To understand how potent this belief can be, consider the case of Bill Putnam and his off-the-wall yellow Lab, Sunny. In addition to general unruliness, Sunny routinely chewed the furniture and clawed the door when left alone. Mr. Putnam accepted the behavior for three years because he felt guilty for leaving Sunny alone all day, and he believed Sunny was justified in systematically destroying the room where he was confined in his owner's absence. As often happens, when a Significant Other entered the owner's life and questioned his definition of love for his dog, Bill Putnam sought help. Six months later when he called with a progress report on the now well-behaved animal, he still found it difficult to believe he'd needlessly tolerated the negative behavior for all those years.

Like many owners who make unnecessary love-tolerance connections, in order to make lasting changes Sunny's owner first had to accept and trust the love between him and his dog independent of any actions on either of their parts. Then he had to acknowledge and accept that he both wanted and deserved a well-behaved animal in spite of the fact that he worked long hours. Once he made these belief changes, the commitment to the training process readily followed as did the beneficial results. However, without those changes in his beliefs about love, even the most sophisticated training techniques probably would have failed.

Another variation of the tolerance-equals-love theme occurs in cases involving animals suffering from incurable but controllable conditions such as diabetes, or those requiring long-term treatment (severe ear or skin infections, long-standing behavioral problems) where gaining owner compliance may prove to be a struggle. Many times a cycle of periodic crises develops as a result of these owners' failure to handle the multiple aspects of treatment that often attend such cases. Following the crisis they feel guilty and religiously treat and monitor the animal for a while, but then daily life intervenes and they start cutting corners again until eventually they precipitate another crisis. To be sure, in cases such as this the need to evaluate any proposed treatment in terms of the owner's bond with the animal, life-style, and any other owner lim-itations *before* commencing it cannot be overstated. However, conversa-tions with these owners reveal one seemingly paradoxical factor that appears to affect compliance: Those who see the animal as *normal* fare better than those who see it as *sick*.

How can this possibly be? Isn't a constant awareness of the animal's condition necessary to insure vigilance? Evidently not, for several rea-sons. People who perceive the animal as constantly sick often also see it as inevitably on the verge of some crisis. Because of this, they never develop a good sense of the animal's baseline parameters which, in turn, makes it easier for them to overlook changes. Recall those owners of normally healthy animals who seek veterinary assistance based on lit-tle more than their feelings that something is wrong with the animal. Many times the signs they notice are both vague and of short duration, enough so that one practitioner recognized both the subtlety and valid-ity of these symptoms by assigning them a special computer code: ADR—ain't doin' right. However because these owners maintain such a clear image of their normal animal, they immediately notice when something changes.

Owners of animals with chronic conditions who see the problem as normal for that particular animal develop the same kind of awareness that also enables them to respond to changes sooner and avoid crises. Furthermore, such owners do not perceive themselves as saints or mar-tyrs for treating the animal; the animal's daily care becomes part of their normal routine like taking a shower or brushing their teeth. And just as with taking a shower or brushing their teeth, they don't resent or skip doing it on days when they're rushed or too tired; they simply do it without assigning it any emotional charge and in so doing free them-selves of many of the negative feelings that assault other owners of ani-mals with chronic problems over time.

Asking owners to recognize and accept that both the condition and everything inherent in its treatment will comprise that animal's "nor-mal" for weeks or months or even the rest of its life provides them with an opportunity to evaluate their definitions of love and change them if necessary. Those who give themselves points for tolerating various inconveniences caused by the animal's condition prior to diagnosis and/or during the work-up may find the idea of tolerating these for the next five years overwhelming. In this situation, the tolerance first defined as love may yield to guilt and resentment, neither of which bodes well for consistent monitoring and treatment of the condition. Others may maintain such a strictly defined concept of normal that they cannot expand it to include an animal suffering from a particular condition. Owners and breeders of show animals or those who perceive animals as a reflection of themselves more commonly succumb to this orientation. The animal's problem serves as a constant reminder of its imperfection which then negatively reflects on them; they become flawed human beings treating flawed animals, and this less than ideal state also leads to guilt, resentment, and noncompliance.

What makes tolerance as a symbol of love and caring a problem lies in the fact that those who make this connection never really accept the animal and/or any problems it may develop. They believe themselves superior owners for loving the animal *in spite of* the problem rather than *because of* the animal's positive qualities. Consequently, whenever anything goes wrong, this becomes just one more cross to bear and the question becomes whether these owners' and society's (and the veterinarian's) view of them as loving martyrs can sustain them through the treatment process. When it can't or when the animal dies, these owners take it very personally because so much of their definition of themselves as loving people depends on the presence of the animal and this self-sacrificing process.

Tolerance and acceptance form a continuum that leads to success just like forgiveness and forgetting. Some people get stuck at tolerance and never move on to accept the animal and its condition. And like the person who forgives but never forgets an animal's infractions, these owners see their animals as forever flawed and inferior. Although this may make these people feel superior and even saintly at times, for all of their often very intense pronouncements of love, in reality they view their animals as chattel which they use to perpetuate their own self-image.

Fear Equals Love

The idea of linking love and fear intuitively strikes most as incongruous to the point of impossible and yet it does occur in practice. Owners can and do dismiss problems they find frightening by defining them in terms of love. A classic example is the creation of an aggressive animal which the owner defines as "protective." Consider this common canine sequence. The first time the doorbell rings, the new pup, Rex, barks an alarm in response to the novel stimulus, which in the pack amounts to a call for assistance from some older, more experienced member as well as expressing the pup's fear. His owner, Alice Cummings, decides the barking represents the pup's attempts to protect her, and she praises the behavior. Unreasonable as it sounds, Ms.Cummings chooses to believe the ten-week-old, ten-pound pup's *love* for her inspires him to willingly take on any evil on the other side of the door. In addition to reinforcing the pup's fears in this manner, she also assigns Rex a leadership position by allowing him to enter and leave the house before her, jump up on her, and display other dominant behaviors that she also defines as loving.

Inevitably the day of reckoning comes when the owner discovers that she and Rex are playing by dog rather than human rules. As typically happens, this doesn't occur when Rex lunges at a vicious killer, but rather when he lunges at an innocent passer-by. For some owners the sudden realization that their world contains a lot more neutral or positive human presences than vicious killers leads them to establish a more workable relationship with the dog. Unfortunately, however, owners like Ms. Cummings who are fearful enough to foster aggressive behavior also are often much too frightened to accept the fact that they created a potentially dangerous, unpredictable animal. Instead, they make excuses. In retrospect, Ms. Cummings decides the innocent passerby looked shifty-eyed and was obviously on drugs; Rex undoubtedly sensed the deviant meant to harm her even though she didn't. Or maybe Rex snapped because he never saw someone with a beard [on a bicycle, wearing sneakers] before.

Although a common stereotype portrays these fearful owners as shy, frail women or wimpish men, many owners of so-called "one-man dogs" who appear to radiate bravado also may fall into this category. What unites these seemingly incongruous owners is the fear that leads them to reinforce antisocial animal behaviors in an effort to protect themselves from a world they perceive as filled with threats of one sort or another; they then deny their own fear and rationalize the animal's behavior by saying it proves the animal's love for and devotion to them.

The fear-love connection may play a different but equally detrimental role in the treatment of medical problems. Recall those owners who say they love the animal so much they can't bear the thought of putting it through anything as terrifying as neutering, hospitalization, or anesthesia. Although situations certainly exist where various routine procedures or treatments may be contraindicated in a particular individual for legitimate medical or behavioral reasons, these owners project their own fears on the animal in the name of love. As with the "protective" dog which may terrorize the owner as well as everyone else, these cases, too, can assume bizarre forms. The owner of five intact Siamese cats who considered it more loving to confine each to a separate room to pace restlessly, yowl, barely eat and drink, and succumb to various stress-related ailments every breeding season rather than subject them to the horror of anesthesia and neutering comes to mind here.

In *The Prince*, Niccolò Machiavelli notes that love and fear cannot coexist and because we must choose, we will choose fear because that is the *safer* emotion of the two. Most of us find it difficult to admit we're afraid, and to admit to the fear *and* that we defined it as love proves a major assault on the ego. Because of this, it usually takes a crisis situation to stimulate these clients to reevaluate their beliefs. When Alice Cummings sees her grandson following five hours of reconstructive facial surgery, the idea that the child must have done something to antagonize the dog or that Rex attacked the little boy out of his great love for her doesn't carry nearly so much weight. When the beloved ten-year-old Siamese succumbs to a life-threatening pyometra, the once terrifying idea of spaying a healthy young animal suddenly seems like the most loving thing to do.

Abuse Equals Love

Is it possible for love to equal hate? If we view love linearly, the idea that it could evolve into hatred and abuse seems ridiculous. However, just as the velvet-mouthed bird dog can launch a vicious hardmouthed attack against another dog, so love always possesses the potential to manifest abusively.

In the previous sections we discussed how owners can create multiple, often avoidable medical and behavioral problems in their animals all in the name of love. At what point do these orientations communicate hatred or abuse of the animal rather than love? Some argue that this occurs the instant owner practices result in an abnormal blood level or obvious negative behaviors in the animal. Others say that as long as the owners believe themselves motivated by genuine love, nothing they do to the animal can be construed as abusive—misguided perhaps, but not abusive.

A third orientation once again positions the veterinarian in the role of educator and communicator. It maintains that until a knowledgeable person explains otherwise, even the most negative practices may be attributed to owner love if that person believes this true. However, if the owner continues the practice(s) once information proving otherwise is shared *and* workable alternatives are proposed, then the owner's orientation may rightfully be viewed as abusive. In other words, regardless of how detrimental the owner's beliefs are to the animal, no veterinarian has the right to criticize unless he or she has made specific attempts to educate the person about the nature of the problem and its solution.

Although this makes perfectly good sense, we already noted several instances in which veterinarians may forget that everyone doesn't possess their knowledge of animals. Second, abuse is a totally relative concept, just like love itself. Strictly small animal clinicians practicing in large, upscale metropolitan facilities may brand much that occurs in shoestring farm animal practice as abusive, whereas the large animal practitioner might say the same thing about putting an animal through months of hospitalization, chemo- and radiation therapy for a terminal cancer.

Similarly, practitioners may knowingly or unknowingly give their clients a mixed message. Recall those owners who define love in terms of food or tolerance of negative, treatable conditions. Now consider this common scenario: Dr. Gagnon examines an animal that must be stringently restrained so it doesn't fly off the table or snap. At the end of the examination, he says, "Good dog!" and gives the animal a friendly pat and a flavored vitamin tablet or other treat. Via this seemingly innocuous display, the veterinarian communicates his own tolerance-equals-love and food-equals-love beliefs to the client in addition to rewarding the animal for misbehaving. Similarly, giving the animal a treat for behaving *well* also supports the food-equals-love belief in addition to communicating that good behavior during an examination constitutes a rewardable exception rather than the expected rule.

From this we can see that what constitutes love for an animal is arbitrary at best and, like clients, veterinarians often get themselves into problems regarding this emotion because they haven't taken the time to analyze their own beliefs. Because of this, when faced with the obese animal or the owner who picks up the beagle by the ears claiming, "He likes it!" we either respond emotionally or not at all rather than provide the client with solid information. However, the increasing concern about animal rights and welfare demands that practitioners evaluate their own beliefs about this emotion with a view toward answering the question, "At what point does love become abusive?" because not only will the public be turning to us for this answer more and more, our role as the primary educator of our clients mandates we be able to distinguish loving from abusive practices. Moreover, the move toward making animal abuse a reportable offense like child abuse further demands this skill.

So, where do we draw the line? Because more than a few people became veterinarians because they maintain very strong views about animals which usually include what people can and cannot do to them, it may be helpful to look at those practices we label "loving," "unloving," or "abusive" as *different* rather than right or wrong in order to analyze them more objectively. In Chapter 1 we noted that no matter how bizarre or detrimental a relationship might appear, it exists because the owner believes it works, albeit in a way that may totally escape us. Consequently, for Dr. Gagnon to imply or out and out accuse an owner of not loving an animal serves no purpose except for generating whatever sense of power he feels when he makes such a judgment. At most such accusations might result in owner guilt, which we noted may sustain the owner long enough to make short-term changes but often yields to resentment over time. Moreover, the best Dr. Gagnon can hope for in the latter situation is that the client will grow to resent *him* rather than the animal. Were the owner to become resentful of the animal as a result of Dr. Gagnon's accusations, then his judgment would undermine not only the client-clinician relationship but also that between the owner and the animal. When Dr. Gagnon criticizes Ms. Cummings for condoning Rex's aggressive behavior in the name of love, this so embarrasses and frustrates her she kicks the dog as he enters his pen that evening and doesn't feed him for two days. Thus in the process of supposedly making the situation better for the animal by labeling the owner as unloving or uncaring, the veterinarian actually makes it worse.

Interestingly, even though they may possess very concrete ideas about what does and doesn't constitute loving and caring behavior, veterinarians who work out their own beliefs about love tend to respond to those clients who don't meet their ideals with more understanding than veterinarians who don't. This occurs because when we take the time to actually consider the issue objectively, we discover it's not as black and white as we once believed. Furthermore, the more experience we gain, the more variations on the theme of love we encounter. A practice that strikes us as loving in one owner under one set of circumstances strikes us as abusive in another. The daily exercise regime becomes abusive when the owner refuses to accept that the animal's injury makes this no longer possible. But who could condemn the owner of the dying animal for taking it on one last walk through its favorite haunts no matter how medically unsound? The more we consider issues like this, the more options and alternatives we come up with that might benefit our clients.

Reviewing our own beliefs about love also will help prepare us for a future filled with increasingly complex human-animal relationships. For example, a trainer asked one veterinarian for a professional opinion regarding the following case: From observing the dog and owner—a highly regarded professional in the community—during private lessons, the trainer was convinced he was abusing the animal at home. However, she also recognized the role animals can play as emotional safety valves in some stressful situations and her client's two young children appeared healthy and happy. If she notified the local overworked, underpaid animal control officer, she knew he would immediately impound the animal and publicly denounce the owner which could leave the children vulnerable. What should she do?

Aside from opening a major Pandora's box of beliefs and emotions for both this trainer and practitioner to work through, this case once again points out that no clear line exists between "animal problems" and "human problems" anymore—if it ever did. And although working through our own beliefs about love won't give us all the answers, at least it will help guarantee that when we encounter love-related problems in practice, we will provide these clients with objective information and solid recommendations rather than value judgments.

Chapter 9
The Practitioner as God

Now that we've examined the effects of the human orientation toward the animal and the treatment process, we need to turn our attention toward the practitioner. In the next three chapters, we will consider the three most common orientations clinicians take toward their patients and clients:

- God
- Best friend
- Facilitator

Two reasons exist for practitioners to consider the distinguishing characteristics of these orientations as well as their advantages and disadvantages. First, although we may not realize we assume these roles, most of us subconsciously if not consciously select one of them depending on the circumstances. Recognizing which one we use when not only enables us to respond more quickly, it also enables us to fine-tune an approach if necessary to meet specific client needs. Second, most of us find one orientation more comfortable than the others and automatically assume it at times of stress as well as when we believe it will serve us and our clients best. As long as this orientation does best meet the needs of the stressful situation, no problems arise; however, if it doesn't, it may undermine our ability to communicate with the client. Because both the necessity for quality communication and the difficulty of achieving it increase proportionately with the stress of the situation, we can appreciate why choosing the orientation that would best meet the client's needs rather than mechanically assuming a fallback position would be particularly beneficial at such times.

The God Clinician Prototype

Of the three orientations, the god clinician is both the most familiar and the most inflexible. The familiarity comes from the fact that it serves as the standard built into medical education. The traditional medical process progresses linearly from diagnosis through treatment with seldom any mention of the client at all, let alone of the one who says, "Excuse me, but I don't want to do that." At most, veterinary students might encounter such an owner during clinical experience, but many times people who bring animals to teaching hospitals do so with the idea they will do whatever the resident experts recommend. In satellite practices, students may see clients only for routine procedures and thus get only secondhand information, if that, regarding "difficult" owners. In this context, they may perceive the problem as the failure of a particular client to recognize the practitioner's authority rather than that the practitioner may have used the wrong approach with that person.

The inflexibility of the god role arises from its adherents' claim to a certain omniscience, omnipotence, and omnipresence relative to their patients and clients. The omniscience comes from our education, the omnipotence from our technology, and the omnipresence from our twenty-four-hour-a-day coverage of one sort or another. Although the use of such terms might imply imperiousness or arrogance, most who assume the god role see themselves more as benevolent monarchs. As long as patients and clients do what Dr. Hardy wants, everyone gets along just fine. If they don't, he expects certain gestures—a direct look, a few firm words—to bring the miscreants into line. If the patient or client ignores these and continues challenging his authority, Dr. Hardy feels justified in becoming angry.

Considering the similarities between this orientation and that of the dominant alpha pack figure, we can see why more men than women adopt this as their primary orientation. Although women may claim this role, most in private practice find that, although it has its place, many clients find it at least disorienting if not threatening. Consequently these practitioners adopt one of the other client orientations because it yields consistently better results. While some may view this as a sexist issue, any approach should facilitate communication with the client and enhance the treatment process, not make a personal or political statement. When the latter occurs, miscommunication and a breakdown of the treatment process often follow, regardless what orientation the practitioner assumes.

God-Playing and the Patient

Relative to our patients, most of us feel superior by virtue of our veterinary education and experience. Although this may sound facetious, in reality most of us lay claim to a certain Dr. Doolittlism by virtue of these attributes that we believe place us in a higher position relative to the animal kingdom than the average client. How does this belief affect our interactions with our patients? It can go either way because a certain aura of dominance serves as a major distinguishing quality of this orientation. Because all of our domestic animals except the cat are social or pack animals, they will attempt to position people—including the veterinarian—as dominant or subordinate to them in any given interaction. Two factors will determine if the animal recognizes the god clinician as dominant at that time:

- The animal's own orientation.
- The animal's perception of the clinician's position as definitive.

If the animal perceives itself as subordinate to the clinician but not particularly threatened, then it will submit to handling. This approach works particularly well with stable but slightly rambunctious animals. The untrained male Airedale initially acts up to test the pack structure, but an icy stare and firm, deep, but not loud "No" from Dr. Hardy settles the animal immediately. However, if Dr. Hardy claims the god role but cannot muster the presence and tone of voice to communicate dominance to the animal, the Airedale will continue challenging him throughout the examination.

If the animal perceives itself as very submissive, the god orientation may magnify any fear response. The shy Doberman which merely freezes with dilated pupils, pounding heart, and racing respiration when faced with a less dominant presence, may dribble urine, defecate and/or express its anal glands when confronted by Dr. Hardy. If these animals perceive themselves in an environment where escape is possible, they may try to run. If thwarted in that regard, they may become aggressive. Unlike the previous situation, the more god-like Dr. Hardy acts, the more frightened and unmanageable these animals may become. The direct gaze and firm command that worked so well with the unruly but stable Airedale reduces the Doberman to a ball of frazzled nerves and negatively affects all baseline physiological parameters.

Very dominant animals pose the greatest challenge to the clinician who routinely assumes the god role because the clinician must present him- or herself in a manner that the animal perceives as more dominant, and what works with one animal might not work with another. In general, we may say that most dominant animals respond to people based on their prior experience. Although this may evoke the image of an animal abusively strong-armed by an owner or herdsman which now seeks to unleash its rage on the veterinarian, most interactions between owners and dominant animals tend to be much more benign. Many times owners of both farm and companion animals find it much easier to work around dominant animals rather than confront them. Because of this, the god veterinarian may be the first, and even the only, person these animals encounter who wants to assert dominance over them.

In these situations several factors come into play. First, does the veterinarian possess a sufficiently dominant presence to carry it off? Although some of the tiniest women can project a tremendous amount of authority, conversations with numerous female practitioners indicate that, in general, dominant untrained male animals do not acknowledge women as dominant. The question then becomes whether the animal will ignore the woman and let her proceed with the examination or feel obligated to make some sort of dominant display in response to hers. In this situation the more authoritatively the woman acts, the more likely she will precipitate a negative display.

Male practitioners encounter such negative responses from dominant untrained animals more often than women because most animals instinctively perceive adult males as dominant. Consequently, these animals are more likely to test a man as well as be less tolerant of his handling. Once again, how much resistance an animal offers depends on the perceived difference between its own position and that of the veterinarian. If Dr. Hardy clearly communicates that he's in charge, then even the most dominant animal will settle down. However, if the animal perceives the gap as narrow and most certainly if it perceives itself as equal, then it will challenge him.

Another, more troubling variation on the theme of dominance is becoming more and more common. In a significant number of households, more submissive dogs hold what amounts to pseudo-dominant positions that they assume because humans tolerate this behavior, usually in the name of love (as discussed in Chapter 8). As we would expect, a more submissive animal thrown into a dominant role by circumstance may not respond the same way to a challenge as one more comfortable with this position. Although some readily will cede dominance to a practitioner they perceive as dominant, a lack of confidence in their own roles may lead others to overreact, often adopting a get-them-before-they-get-me attitude. If we add the presence of an apprehensive owner the animal can see but from whom it is physically separated, we can appreciate how such animals may feel driven to mount a defensive display.

One final note about assuming this role with feline patients: Because cats are solitary animals by nature, dominant human displays that may quiet and comfort social animals may exert no effect on or upset an apprehensive cat even more. Those who use this approach routinely discover that those feline patients who find it threatening do not hesitate to respond aggressively. Because cat owners often mention the animal's behavior as a major reason why they don't seek routine veterinary care for it as they do for the dog, it makes sense to do everything possible to make these visits as atraumatic for owner and animal as possible. Practitioners who routinely use the god approach may need to develop techniques that enable them or their technicians to quickly and completely immobilize the animal. Once so restrained, most cats will give up; however, if they sense any hesitation in the handling, they will become even more unmanageable. For certain, whereas social animals may be intimidated by yelling or hitting, such activities may serve only to drive cats more deeply into the attack mode.

From this discussion we can see that those clinicians who adopt this approach as their primary orientation toward patients would be wise to ground themselves firmly in the basics of animal behavior and handling because this orientation can lead to problems with certain kinds of animals. Furthermore, because the failure of the animal to submit passively serves as a major source of stress in stressful patient-client-clinician interactions, routinely adopting this orientation without the corresponding knowledge of behavior at such times may make a bad situation worse.

The Advantages of Playing God for the Practitioner

Just as animals may respond differently to the clinician who assumes an all-powerful role, so do clients. Some prefer clinicians who take charge of everything associated with the animal's care, whereas others accept this at some times but not others. Surely every practitioner can lay claim to at least one client who believes the veterinarian can do no wrong and will do whatever told: Dr. Hardy tells the owner to medicate the dog's infected eye a minimum of four to six times a day and she sneaks the animal into work so she can do this. Other clients may never question anything the veterinarian says or does during routine examinations, but challenge everything that occurs when the animal succumbs to illness or injury. Still others do just the opposite: Ms. Anderson constantly challenges Dr. Hardy's authority regarding routine preventive procedures, but submits completely when her animal's health appears to be in jeopardy.

A major advantage offered by clients willing to perceive the practitioner as a god is that the clinician needn't explain things such as the rationale behind a certain procedure and/or treatment. This can be of particular benefit to practitioners lacking a clear idea of the animal's problem. It also benefits those who lack basic communication skills which, according to studies supported by the Pew National Veterinary Education Program, does not occur infrequently. Obviously, the less one communicates, the fewer communications skills one needs. In "Attitudes of Veterinarians toward Emerging Competencies for Health Care Professions," the authors noted that less than 50 percent of the veterinarians graduating between 1980 and 1990 rated their training in communication skills excellent or good (Stone et al. 1992, 201:1851). Furthermore, not communicating with clients can save the practitioner a tremendous amount of time. Recall all the different aspects of owner-animal relationships as well as various owner characteristics and lifestyles that may undermine the treatment process. It takes time to address each one of these, and those clients willing to accept whatever the clinician offers free the practitioner of this burden.

A second advantage of this orientation some practitioners find particularly appealing is that owners who accept it are less likely to raise the issue of cost, if for no other reason than they tend not to raise issues at all. Needless to say, those practitioners who find it difficult to talk about money consider this a definite plus.

This approach also can work very well with those clients the practitioner doesn't like for one reason or another. Most commonly these are the owners who take what the clinician considers a chattel view: Dr. Hardy finds Ms. Anderson's views of her animals as four-legged showing and breeding robots offensive and his god orientation permits him to focus the majority of his attention on the animal rather than her. Not only does this limit his interaction with the client, it gives him an opportunity to focus entirely on an animal which may experience few other opportunities for intimate human contact. Similarly practitioners may find the god approach an effective way to deal with the occasional lewd client: A direct stare in the owner's direction followed by total involvement in the examination of the animal and precise remarks strictly related to the animal's condition and any treatment make a very clear statement regarding where the practitioner intends to focus his or her attention.

This orientation also enables practitioners to rule out the owner as a variable in the treatment process. Dr. Hardy believes that the client's lack of time, space, or the physical, mental or emotional wherewithal to accomplish his wishes are the owner's problems, not his. Those not comfortable with this approach may find this a rather insensitive view, but the majority of clients do find some way to accomplish the treatment more or less and one way or another because they do want their animals to get well.

Running concurrently with that advantage is the one most commonly mentioned by those who favor the god approach: It permits the practice of medicine closest to the academic standard which these practitioners perceive as the highest quality possible. Because the Pew Commission studies indicate that more than 80 percent of us consider our training in diagnosing and treating disease excellent, we can see the appeal of an approach that emphasizes this over client communication (Stone et al. 1992, 202:1851). Clinicians who routinely assume the role of god always do the optimal work-up and always prescribe the optimal treatment: Because Dr. Hardy doesn't allow subjective owner considerations to compromise his standard of medical excellence, regardless of how the case turns out, he always possesses the consolation of knowing he did everything medically possible.

The Advantages for the Client

Even as some practitioners like to keep the client out of the picture, so some clients want to be out of the picture, too. Those with complex lifestyles may prefer to turn the animal's care over to the practitioner completely to the point some may say, "Just give me a call when the dog [or horse or cow] is ready to go home." Although this would seem a more common response among those sharing the weakest bond with the animal, just the opposite may hold true. The traveling sales rep drops his vomiting dog off at Dr. Hardy's clinic Monday morning on his way out of town with instructions for the clinician to "do whatever you think best" because he fears the high school student who cares for the animal in his absence might not carry out any treatment as conscientiously as he would. Similarly, the owner of a prized ram which falls ill during the peak of lambing season may turn its care over to Dr. Hardy even though he would involve himself totally in the treatment process at other times.

Other owners prefer to be out of the treatment loop because they find the whole idea of medicine almost mystical and prefer to keep it that way. Many times these people hold this view of human medicine and simply transfer it to veterinary care. As one of Dr. Hardy's clients so aptly put it, "When I'm sick, I like to think I'm being cared for by someone on a first name basis with God, and I want the same thing for my animals, too." Clinicians who totally engross themselves in the examination of the animal and then present a list of commandments and a bill to the owner at its conclusion fit these people's ideas of how a medical professional should act.

Clients lacking communication skills find this practitioner orientation as beneficial as those practitioners who adopt it for the same reason. Within this group we find naturally shy clients as well as those who find various aspects of the veterinary experience intimidating. Both kinds of owners believe the practitioner will tell them everything they need to know, and anything else isn't important. In general, these owners want to get the examination over with as quickly as possible and welcome the take-charge approach of the god clinician who asks few questions except those pertaining strictly to the animal and its condition.

Owners who don't pay much attention to their animals and prefer to keep it that way also like clinicians who exclude them from the treatment process as much as possible because such practitioners often free them from the embarrassment of displaying their own ignorance. When Dr. Hardy has his technician immediately take Bob Chapman's pup and place it on the examination table, he spares the owner from demonstrating he knows nothing about handling it. When Dr. Hardy dispenses pills for the dog without ascertaining whether or not Mr. Chapman can medicate his animal, he spares the owner from having to admit he has no idea how to do it. When Dr. Hardy automatically assumes the owner will neuter his pet, the client can avoid the issue rather than confronting it directly. Mr. Chapman finds such an interaction relatively stress-free because Dr. Hardy's remote approach to him mirrors that which he takes toward his animal.

Finally, those clients who don't like to make choices also favor this clinician approach. Kathy Goodall's calendar bulges with all the activities associated with her career, motherhood, and an active interest in sports and community affairs which she perceives as orchestrated or mandated by others. She doesn't want to be asked whether she would prefer a full work-up or to take a wait-and-see approach to her animal with vague symptoms; she finds the idea of choosing between a medical or surgical approach to the animal's problem overwhelming. "You do whatever you think is best" and "Just tell me what you want done and I'll do it" are her most common responses to Dr. Hardy.

Clients also may prefer clinicians who assume the god role when they wish to avoid making certain decisions, such as when the animal succumbs to serious illness or injury. Many different factors can come into play in these situations, and we'll discuss these in more detail in Chapter

15. Suffice it to say that the confusion and negative emotions owners may feel at such times will compel some to try to distance themselves from the treatment process as much as possible. This may reflect the aforementioned owner desire to believe the animal in the care of a very superior being at this critical time because the magnitude of the situation exceeds their ability to comprehend it. For others the idea of making choices regarding the animal's future is so frightening, they prefer to let the veterinarian take care of everything.

The Disadvantages of the God Orientation for the Client

Of all the practitioner orientations, the god practitioner shares the least amount of information with the client. Consequently, those clients who want any kind of intimate involvement with the treatment process will feel slighted by this approach. Consider the following list of characteristics which clients rated on a scale of zero to ten in terms of importance when selecting a veterinarian:

- High quality of medical services   9.7
- Doctor gives clear explanations   9.5
- Doctor shows love   9.5
- Polite veterinarian   9.3
- Doctor listens to owner's opinions   8.9

Although medical competency ranks the highest individually, four of five owner concerns relate to the clinician's ability to interact with the animal and owner (Charles, Charles Associates 1983, 13). Consequently, clients who seek these other qualities do not respond well to practitioners using even the most pleasant god approach. As one client put it, "I wish he'd stop poking at the animal and listen to me and explain things for a change!"

Several categories of clients may experience more difficulty with this practitioner orientation than others. Among these, we see breeders who may have an economic as well as personal interest in their animals that goes far beyond that of the casual owner. Not only may they be quite knowledgeable about their particular breed and animal, they also may be very eager to learn all they can about the animal's problem and its treatment. They find veterinarians who believe all cows, sheep, horses, or dogs are the same at least frustrating if not irritating. Nor do they appreciate having their observations and comments regarding their own breed or animal dismissed as inconsequential.

Clients who want to make their own decisions also find practitioners who take the god approach less than satisfactory. They see the animal and its care as an integral part of their lives rather than an isolated entity, and they may need to consider multiple factors not directly related to the animal when choosing a treatment. Consequently, they need a practitioner willing and able to discuss all available options rather than presenting them with a *fait accompli*. This isn't to say these clients don't place much weight on the veterinarian's recommendation when it comes to choosing the option. However, they want and need to take a much broader view of the treatment process than the god approach allows.

The third group of clients who do not respond well to this practitioner role is that growing segment of the population interested in wellness. Many practitioners find preventive medicine boring because they see it as mostly talk and little action. However, no matter how we look at it, no antibiotic or surgery will clean up the standing water in the sheep pen, correct the poor ventilation in the barn, or keep fleas from becoming a problem again next summer. Those clients who desire this kind of veterinary service at most will get a list of commandments from the god practitioner. Although that's better than nothing, these clients consider themselves information-oriented consumers and they want the answer to the question "Why?" as well as "How?" Because practitioners who assume the god orientation see "Because I said so" as the standard reply to "Why?" we can appreciate why these owners prefer those with other orientations.

The Disadvantages of Playing God for the Practitioner

Although playing god can do wonders for the ego, unfortunately people are much less tolerant of what they consider less than 100 percent results from human gods. Even as we routinely accept hurricanes, floods, earthquakes, and other disasters as acts of God which serve only to strengthen rather than undermine the faith of the faithful, disasters that befall patients of god clinicians may not receive such a charitable review. Moreover, what the client considers a disaster may be quite different from what the clinician does, to the point that the practitioner doesn't consider it a disaster at all.

For example, a common practice scenario involves new graduates who launch state-of-the-art work-ups with the idea that these represent the practice of quality veterinary medicine. When owners go white and sag against the wall when they see the bill and then become belligerent about paying it, Dr. Hardy feels genuinely surprised and hurt by the reaction. It never dawned on him that the client didn't know the cost of the procedures or would hesitate to pay it. When this occurs, several factors may come into play that only make a bad situation worse. Dr. Hardy may respond to his clients' indignation indignantly because, after all, *he* cared only about making the animal well and did the very best he could to insure this. Lack of experience may even lead him to note that obviously any owner who doesn't share this view doesn't care about the animal, a value judgment guaranteed only to alienate these clients more.

If Dr. Hardy refuses to discuss the issue, believing he did the very best job possible and deserves payment for it, then the clients have two choices: They either will pay or they won't. If they do pay, not only will they be unlikely to seek Dr. Hardy's services again, they most likely will not hesitate to tell anyone who will listen about his "outrageous" fees. If the clients refuse to pay, they will repeat their tale to everyone encountered at every step during any collection process. Regardless of the monetary outcome, Dr. Hardy will lose because of the damage done to his professional reputation. Ironically, even as he insists he cares so very much, these clients will insist just the opposite. For a practitioner who envisions himself as the ultimate caring authority, being portrayed as a money-grubbing charlatan is a most disheartening experience.

Clients who accept god practitioners also often expect miracles, and their definitions of a miracle may differ greatly from that of the practitioner. Some can't comprehend that they should have to do something for the animal themselves after they gave the veterinarian carte blanche to do anything he or she wanted. Kathy Goodall looks at Dr. Hardy incredulously following his extensive work-up of her animal with chronic problems: "You mean I still have to give him pills? I thought once you did everything, I wouldn't need to do that any more!" Considering that Dr. Hardy believed it quite miraculous that he managed to isolate the obscure cause of the problem, his client's lack of enthusiasm leaves him feeling confused and depressed. Even more disconcerting are those clients who cede all responsibility to the clinician and expect their animals to recover totally from even the most serious conditions: "How come he's still limping after all those plates and wires you put in his leg?" Once again even though the practitioner may have performed exceptionally well from a medical or surgical point of view, the client sees both the results and the clinician as flawed.

God-Playing and the Lack of Communication

In all these cases, the problems that arise may be traced to lack of communication. However, unlike other situations in which this occurs, this lack of communication occurs by choice. The practitioner chooses not to communicate with the client and, whether or not the client initially shared this view, when results don't meet client expectations, the client sees the practitioner's lack of communication as the cause of the problem: "He didn't tell me how much it was going to cost." "She didn't tell me how to get the pills into him." "He didn't say the animal would limp."

How much of a problem is this? Going back to the Pew Commission report, even as less than 50 percent of the practitioners surveyed felt they received good or excellent training in communication, almost 100 percent rated such training as important or very important (Stone et al. 1992, 201:1851). Another almost perennial indicator appeared that same year in an article with the highly suggestive title "Communicate to Avoid Malpractice Claims." Its authors reviewed malpractice claims processed by the AVMA Professional Liability Insurance Trust and compiled this list of client complaints:

- not aware of or unable to understand the prognosis
- lacked comprehension of examination findings
- received inadequate explanation of procedures needed for definitive diagnosis
- shocked and surprised over charges
- felt anger from unrealized expectations or unexpected results

Note that all of these relate directly to the practitioner's failure to communicate effectively with the client (Dinsmore and McConnell 1992, 201: 383).

Practitioners who encounter problems when using this orientation must confront a major paradox: The only way to resolve the problem involves open communication, and we assumed the god role because we weren't trained or don't like to communicate in general, or with that client in particular.

Consider the case of the competent but naturally shy Dr. Hardy, who finds it difficult to explain the implications of a routine case to a neutral or even positively responsive owner. When things go wrong as a result of his lack of communication, he must face the ultimate communications challenge: dealing with an irate client. Does it come as any surprise that Dr. Hardy may opt for a fear response?

- He may freeze and refuse to react to the client, telling himself he's above such behavior.
- He may flee, saying he has no time for people who don't understand veterinary medicine.
- He may fight, feeling the client has no right to challenge his authority.

Ironically, even though all three approaches are evasive, fear-based tactics, Dr. Hardy perceives all of them as worthy of his superior status. In reality, however, none of them compels him to communicate in a meaningful way with the client and he finds that very acceptable because he knows he doesn't do that well. Consequently, even though it might appear that the results are less than satisfactory because the client feels Dr. Hardy didn't measure up to expectations in one way or another, these responses do permit him to maintain the image of himself as a god, which, in turn, frees him from the responsibility of making any changes in the way he practices.

Similarly practitioners who assume this role to avoid more intimate interaction with a particular client find themselves in equally distasteful situations when something goes wrong with the case. The practitioner who thought it would take too much time to show the bubbleheaded owner how to restrain her cat to medicate its eye finds himself trying to explain this to her over the phone as his office manager points to the clock and the waiting room full of patients. The Don Juan who felt rebuffed takes great pleasure in stopping in with questions that could have been answered during the course of the examination. The farmer who claims he never would have put that much money into his cow had he known the prognosis tells his tale of woe to everyone who belongs to the Grange as well as to his son's 4-H pals to the point the practitioner feels he must publicly justify his actions. In all of these situations, the clinicians' attempts to distance themselves from the client generate more—and more negative—interaction than would have occurred had the practitioners assumed a more responsive orientation.

Consequently, because lack of communication inevitably looms as the number one complaint when things go wrong, wise practitioners never assume the god orientation because they don't want to communicate unless they feel totally comfortable with their ability to completely control the situation. For some, this means only assuming it for the most routine cases: vaccinations, hot spots, milk fevers. Others will expand its use depending on their knowledge and experience. However, even the shiest, most highly skilled practitioners dealing with the most obnoxious clients agree that the more complex the case, the greater the need for consistent quality client communication throughout the process, no matter how difficult this may be for the clinician.

The God Dilemma

Of all the aspects of the god role that can confound practitioners, none creates the mental anguish that arises when the clinician discovers he or she cares more than the client. Although this can occur any time, it happens more often to those who assume the god role because the orientation involves the least amount of contact with the owner. The veterinarian provides the highest quality service only to discover that the clients care little about the aftercare of the animal. Or maybe the clients do care, but they can't carry out the clinician's instructions given their life-style or other limitations. Dr. Hardy does a first-class job of working up a dermatology problem only to discover the owner lacks the facilities to bathe the Newfoundland weekly and the financial wherewithal to hire someone else to do it. Suddenly he finds himself backtracking, proposing what he considers a lesser treatment when the medically optimal one fails. Not only does this require more time and client interaction, the god practitioner who thought he practiced the highest quality medicine winds up looking like he doesn't know what he's doing. Moreover, he also may feel manipulated by the client, which further undermines the client-clinician relationship.

However, sometimes practitioners feel so very strongly that only one right way exists to treat a case that they believe doing anything less amounts to providing inferior care to the animal. Those who feel this way do neither themselves nor their clients any favors by practicing what they consider substandard medicine. If Dr. Hardy believes his clients routinely thwart his attempts to practice quality medicine, both they and he would fare much better if he found other work in a more compatible setting. For those who feel obligated to maintain the highest medical standards for their patients regardless of the client's ability to fulfill any obligations these might entail, it makes sense to remember that that choice consists of a two-step process: the choice itself, and the consequences of that choice. Practitioners who passively or actively make choices for their clients willingly should assume full responsibility for the consequences of those choices if the client cannot or will not. If Dr. Hardy insists his client *must* treat an animal a particular way because it deserves the very best and then turns his back on that animal when the client can't carry out the treatment, few would classify him as a decent human being let alone a god.

Chapter 10
The Practitioner as Best Friend

For many practitioners, the idea of functioning as the patient's and client's best friend serves as the ideal role to assume. Although some periodically bemoan what they perceive as the veterinary profession's lack of self-esteem, many times this refers to our inability or unwillingness to see ourselves as equal or at least comparable to physicians. However, many veterinarians don't want to lump themselves with physicians because they see the latter as arrogant and insensitive as well as inflexible. If any doubt exists in their minds regarding the value of this difference, they need only listen to those clients who wistfully note that their animals get better treatment than their owners do when they require medical care. In these clients' minds, the fact that their physician can summon millions of dollars worth of technology in their behalf compared to that which the veterinarian can muster means little; the lack of intimate concern looms a far more relevant issue than the presence of the technology.

Interestingly, as the veterinary profession aligns itself more closely with a human medical standard which claims prestige as a function of science and technology, the once solid reputation as genuinely caring individuals we once could claim among the general public has begun to waver. Although very few question our medical competency, like the physician's patients, more and more veterinary clients complain that the veterinarian doesn't care about either them or their animals: "He treats sheep like chunks of meat!" "She doesn't like cats. I can tell by the way she handles them." Along with that we hear the now familiar litany of complaints regarding the practitioner's lack of communication.

At the same time, however, we also need to maintain that ineffable quality known as professionalism. Professionalism used to mean wearing a shirt and tie (or dress and hose when women entered the profession) and assuming the god role common to physicians. However, both large and small animal clients tend to be more sophisticated as well as more educated today. Moreover, unlike the physician of old who lived in the big house on the hill, we not uncommonly encounter clients as equals at PTA meetings, the supermarket, block parties, softball games, town meetings, church, or when we take our children to the dentist's or pediatrician's office. Because of our integration into the overall fabric of our clients' lives, the rather superficial view of professionalism has had to give way to the development of other, often intangible qualities as both the nature of practice and the desires and expectations of the client base change. Now we must find some way to strike a balance between genuine caring and the distance necessary to maintain objectivity. Where the god approach attempts to maximize the distance, the best friend orientation seeks to maximize the caring, often with equally troublesome results.

The Best Friend Prototype

Best friend clinicians come in two forms: prepackaged and real. The prepackaged best friend results when the practitioner lacks sufficient self-confidence and he or she adopts someone else's ideas of friendliness, usually those gleaned from client relations seminars or books on the subject. At its worst, we walk into a practice owned by Dr. Sam Sears and feel like we've entered a movie set. Cheerful smiles adorn all in the front office and each animal gets fifteen to thirty seconds of oohing and aahing. Everyone on the staff goes by first names and their solicitous attention toward the client borders on irritating. The veterinarian, known as "Dr. Sam," greets each client with a bright smile and a firm handshake and treats the patient to another quantum of attention. The examination proceeds as if from a script with Dr. Sam telling the client—whom everyone automatically refers to by first name—what is going to happen with stops at specific points in the process to solicit client input. At the end of the examination, a cheerful farewell speeds the clients on their way.

Although strictly large animal practitioners might find such an orientation beyond comprehension, mixed animal practitioners who discover their large animal base eroding may take this approach because they perceive both small animal owners and practitioners as more emotionally involved. In an effort to compete successfully with strictly small animal practices, they follow a formula that they hope will convey their sensitivity to the small animal client. Similarly, those who discover their basic god orientation losing out to the more cheerful competition down the road may make a concerted effort to generate a more client-friendly image.

For those who experience little difficulty talking to clients, the idea of pursuing such a course might seem bizarre, but it makes good sense for those uncomfortable dealing with the public. Communication is a skill like any other, and just as new graduates may refer to notes and textbooks which they rigidly follow until a certain medical or surgical procedure becomes fixed in the mind, so those inexperienced in client communication may need to follow a set protocol until they develop this skill, too.

What differentiates the real best friend orientation from the prepackaged one is the naturalness and intimacy of the former approach. Those who routinely assume this role take a genuine interest in both animals and people and don't hesitate to become involved with either. Whereas the god practitioner tends to focus on the animal to the exclusion of the client, the best friend clinician not only focuses on both, that interest may exceed the limits of the normal treatment process. Not only do these practitioners discuss topics that relate directly to the animal and the treatment process, they also discuss mutual friends, local politics, children, football, church picnics, and any other subject of interest to them or their clients.

Patient Responses to the Best Friend Practitioner

Because most practitioners admit they became veterinarians because they like animals and enjoy working with them, it would seem that taking a best friend approach toward patients would be the most natural as well as the most advantageous. And, indeed, the majority of animals do respond positively to what they consider a friendly human presence. However, the key here is to conduct ourselves in a manner the *animals* consider nonthreatening. For example, some apprehensive animals may respond very positively to the clinician's cheerful chatter because it distracts them from more worrisome aspects of the treatment process: Within minutes of entering the exam room, Dr. Ward's cheery comments convert the Goldman's trembling golden retriever into a tail-wagging, devoted pal for life. However, other animals may find such an approach distracting to the point of threatening: The more Dr. Ward chatters, the more shy and retiring Ms. Blake's shy and retiring cat cringes and tries to pull away.

As we would expect, animals at the opposite ends of the dominant-submissive spectrum create the most problems. Some dominant animals may perceive both variations of the best friend orientation as either submissive or barely dominant, whereas some submissive animals may perceive that same practitioner role as dominating to the point of being frightening. Under such circumstances these animals may challenge the practitioner who does anything the animal considers threatening—which may be nothing more than establishing direct eye contact, placing hands on the animal's neck or shoulders, or picking up a paw. When the animal reacts defensively, the veterinarian must confront two problems simultaneously. First, he or she must deal with any threat posed by the animal itself. Second, the clinician must decide whether to maintain the best friend orientation or assume another role.

Consider pseudo-best friend Dr. Sears, who decided to enter private practice after completing a residency in physiology. Because he considers himself a naturally reserved person and experienced little client contact during his education, he adopts this orientation because he realizes many clients prefer this to the god role that comes more easily to him. When the Crocketts' Rottweiler, Satan, curls his lip and lets out a low growl when Dr. Sears gives him the prepackaged jolly routine, Dr. Sears must decide whether to continue the interaction in this less-than-natural role or assume the god role he finds more comfortable. Even though he may make his choice in a matter of seconds, some animals perceive even a slight hesitation as further proof of submission, which only complicates the situation. Moreover, although dominant animals may yield to practitioners who initially assume the god role, switching to it from another orientation may dilute any positive effects it may offer.

Or consider Dr. Ward, who wants to believe all her patients consider her one of their best friends. When Satan growls at her, she may choose to deny the behavior: "Silly old Satan, are you talking to yourself?" Or maybe she opts to excuse it, even positioning herself as the villain: "I bet I held your paw too tightly, didn't I? I'm sorry." In this situation, the veterinarian creates a no-win situation for herself. Because she doesn't recognize the critical stabilizing role dominance and submission play in interactions with social animals but rather sees dominance as wrong and unnecessary among good friends, she wouldn't consider responding dominantly to gain control over the animal.

If Dr. Ward feels frightened as well as betrayed, she may freeze, unable to comprehend that the animal would treat her that way. She may evade the situation, perhaps suggesting tranquilizers for Satan in the future. Or she (rarely) may fight, perhaps yelling at the dog in a manner she hopes conveys dominance. Although any of these approaches may yield positive results, the fact remains that all do arise from fear and none of them does anything to generate the lasting changes necessary to positively affect the animal's behavior.

Similarly, Dr. Ward's best friend approach may create problems with submissive animals who find this orientation more threatening than comforting. Rather than converting the Caswells' Akita into another tail-wagging fan, Dr. Ward's cheerful chatter causes the animal to growl and retreat. Needless to say, Dr. Ward feels crushed by this response. Worse, because she perceives her orientation as totally benevolent and nonthreatening, when it fails she can't imagine any way she could treat the animal that would threaten it less.

From this we can see that, once again, the patient response to the clinician depends as much on the animal's personality as the clinician's. In general, the orchestrated best friend approach doesn't work well because those who adopt it commonly do so because they lack self-confidence in dealing with people rather than animals. Although Dr. Sears responds to each animal according to its personality in the own-er's absence, the orchestrated best friend role he assumes with clients requires sufficient concentration that he treats animal and owner alike when he interacts with both in the examination room or stall. Even if the approach doesn't threaten the animal, its unnaturalness may com-municate a certain apprehension that many practitioners believe ani-mals can sense.

As with the god practitioner, whether the best friend orientation works depends on the practitioner's ability to read the animal's behav-ior and change his or her own behavior accordingly. The more rigid the definition of what constitutes a right, normal, or good manner in which to approach an animal, the less likely the practitioner will meet the specific needs of a particular animal.

The Advantages of a Best Friend Veterinarian for the Client

The major advantage of the best friend orientation compared to the god role lies in its ability to foster more open communication. When clients feel the veterinarian's interest in them and their animal goes beyond what many consider the aloof state called professionalism, they more likely will share their concerns about aspects of the animal's prob-lem that reflect their own needs as much as or even more than their ani-mal's. Shy and retiring Ms. Blake would never consider challenging a god practitioner's instructions to give pills three times a day to her cat,

Tiger. However, because she considers Dr. Ward a friend, she doesn't hesitate to raise the issue of both her work schedule and her reluctance to open the animal's mouth.

Similarly, clients who see the practitioner as a friend may feel more comfortable asking questions about the animal's condition. Just as Ms. Blake finds it much easier to discuss her own needs with Dr. Ward, so she finds it easier to ask specific questions about her cat's infection: Is it contagious to her other cats? When can she expect Tiger's appetite to improve? Can she do anything to prevent the problem in the future? As we have noted time and time again, knowledge is power. The more knowledge clients possess regarding all aspects of their animal's condition, the more confidently they approach its treatment.

Clients' greater willingness to communicate with a veterinarian they consider a friend also may lead to greater commitment to the treatment process. Whereas clients of god practitioners might accomplish the treatment out of fear or awe, those of best friend practitioners may feel a genuine desire to please the veterinarian. Although it would seem that fear would serve as the most potent motivator, as we saw when we discussed the role of guilt in the treatment process, the more negative the motivating emotion, the more difficult it is to maintain the motivation. Suppose that every time Ms. Blake needs to medicate Tiger, she must drag him out from under the farthest corner of the bed and be wary of claws throughout the entire process. As she dons her heavy gloves and prepares to capture the terrified animal yet again, which practitioner relationship would best sustain her: her fear of Dr. Ward's anger if she doesn't medicate the animal exactly as directed, or her belief that the treatment reflects her good friend Dr. Ward's very best attempts to meet her own and her cat's needs?

The Advantages for the Practitioner

The practitioner who assumes the role of best friend often finds it much easier to gain meaningful information from the client regarding the animal's condition. Consider shy Ms. Blake, who only will speak to a god practitioner when spoken to. Under those circumstances what history the practitioner gains from the client will depend solely on the questions asked. Although the science of taking a history constitutes a part of every veterinarian's training and theoretically results in a protocol that covers all the medical bases, anyone who has been in practice even a few weeks realizes that it involves a great deal more than ticking off items on a preprinted form. Surely every practitioner has followed such a protocol to perfection only to stare at the nonspecific results in confusion.

When that happens, we face two choices: We can launch a series of diagnostic tests in hopes these will provide the answer; or we can question the owner more thoroughly in hopes of gaining more definitive information about the animal and its environment. Although the scientifically conditioned response leans toward the diagnostic work-up, more than one practitioner has felt foolish when the client later volunteers that the problem began shortly after he began getting hay from a new supplier, got another cat, stripped the white paint off the woodwork in the old house, or drained the antifreeze in the car. Not only may the animal's condition persist or deteriorate during the interval between the initial examination and this revelation, the practitioner may find him- or herself in the less than elegant position of starting the work-up process all over again based on this new information.

Unlike clients who perceive their clinicians as gods, those who see them as good friends routinely share information that adds to the knowledge base from which the practitioner can draw when treating the animal. Because Ms. Blake feels comfortable talking to Dr. Ward, she asks what a cat's normal temperature is as she watches the clinician insert the thermometer. When Dr. Ward responds, she asks whether she could do that at home herself. Dr. Ward then notes that Ms. Blake could, but Tiger seems pretty feisty to her, which causes Ms. Blake to share her concerns about medicating a cat with such a temperament since she lives alone. Thus in her role as best friend, Dr. Ward learns about Ms. Blake's interest in monitoring her cat's health at home, its behavior, her fears regarding medicating it, and her single status. Moreover, Dr. Ward learns all this in the brief time it takes to take the animal's temperature. Compare this to the client standing silently as the god veterinarian performs this task: The more comfortable the client feels with the practitioner, the more naturally and quickly the information flows.

Ironically, even as those who assume the god role like to believe that their word is law, in reality the best friend clinician can claim this distinction just as often if not more. This results from yet another of those paradoxes common to practice: When clients feel they can openly challenge any aspect of the treatment process without incurring any negative results, they do so less and less. This results because each challenge teaches the practitioner more about the client as well as the patient, and this information automatically becomes incorporated into the treatment process. Consequently, when Dr. Ward prescribes pills three times a day for Tiger, Ms. Blake accomplishes this arduous task religiously because she knows Dr. Ward wouldn't ask her to do this if there were any other alternative.

Even in those relatively rare cases in which practitioners encounter clients who like to challenge them simply for the sake of the challenge, best friend practitioners often fare much better than god-players. In this situation, the ability to meet the challenge cheerfully not only may add some useful information to the client and patient knowledge base, it doesn't provide the owner with the irritated response necessary to perpetuate the adversarial stance.

Practitioners who see their clients and patients as best friends also often notice changes more quickly themselves or are more likely to be apprised of them by the client. When Ms. Blake brings Tiger in for routine vaccination, the cat's coat appears much duller and dryer than usual, and Ms. Blake herself appears thin and pale. The god practitioner who sees Ms. Blake as a conduit of strictly feline-related information and a treatment mechanism sees the cat's coat as a symptom and Ms. Blake's own appearance as none of his business. He may request a stool sample, dispense a medicated shampoo and conditioner, or suggest a work-up to determine the cause of the problem. However, because Dr. Ward considers both Ms. Blake and the cat her friends, she inquires about Ms. Blake's health as well as the animal's and learns the owner now cares for her invalid father as well as works full-time, which allows no time for her to groom the long-haired cat daily as in the past. Via one simple, nonmedical, good friend question, Dr. Ward learns of a major change in her client's life that will definitely affect both the animal and the treatment process.

Finally, some practitioners may adopt either the genuine or the prepackaged best friend role when faced with clients whom they find distasteful for some reason. Although few clinicians consider it an optimal response, they find it more acceptable than the less communicative god role. When confronted with clients who treat their animals like objects, Dr. Ward puts on a happy face and chatters gaily to cover her own discomfort.

The Disadvantages for the Client

Although some reserved clients open up more to a best friend clinician, others find this same orientation unprofessional. Some people consider referring to others as Mr., Ms., and Dr. a sign of respect and good manners and they feel as uncomfortable when Dr. Sam refers to them as by their first names as they do calling him "Dr. Sam." Consider very proper

Ms. Blake and her best friend clinician, Dr. Ward: Every time Dr. Ward refers to Ms. Blake as "Helen," Ms. Blake misses half of what the clinician says as she deals with her irritation. When this practice results from a general policy rather than   genuine friendship, clients may find it even more troublesome. Although shy Lester Charles Tobias considers Dr. Sam Sears a competent enough veterinarian, he cringes every time he takes his dog to Dr. Sam's clinic because everyone there refers to him as "Lester" or "Les." His real friends know he hates the name Lester and goes by Charlie. On the one hand, Charlie considers this such a minor point, he can never get up the nerve to correct Dr. Sam; on the other hand, he can't deny that he finds Dr. Sam's behavior more indicative of ignorance than friendliness.

Other people find the best friend approach too intimate for various reasons. Some who maintain a chattel orientation toward their animals often want to get any examination and treatment over with as quickly as possible and they consider any but the most minimal interaction with the practitioner unnecessary. When Ms. Blake's ailurophobic brother brings Tiger in for examination, Dr. Ward's cheerful fussing over the animal and questions regarding Ms. Blake's health and welfare strike him as totally superfluous. Breeders, handlers, and hunters who assume the chattel orientation may see the best friend clinician's interaction with the animal as an attempt to distract it or ruin its training; these people may attempt to control the animal either by voice command or physically whenever it tries to respond positively to the clinician. Still others see the practitioner's apparent concern for both the animal and the owner as intimidating. To them, such friendliness constitutes an invasion of privacy: What business is it of Dr. Ward's what medical problems befall Ms. Blake or her invalid father?

Perhaps the most common client complaint regarding this practitioner orientation involves the amount of time it takes. As people's lives become more complex, they have less time for idle chitchat. Unfortunately, clients who feel this way may never share their views with the clinician for a very selfish reason. Most people don't mind spending a few extra minutes chatting with their veterinarians about the previous weekend's football game or the result of the school board election; what bothers them is waiting while the veterinarian talks to *someone else* about these same or other incidental subjects. Ms. Blake sits in the waiting room with Tiger and notes that Dr. Ward is running almost an hour behind. She tells herself the poor dog now seeing Dr. Ward probably has serious problems, even though it looked perfectly healthy to her. When the client finally emerges laughing and tells Dr. Ward he'll get in touch with the other members of the volleyball team and finalize the schedule they worked out, Ms. Blake finds her patience wearing thin.

A less common but more troublesome complaint clients mention about good friend clinicians is the temptation to overcommit themselves to these veterinarians out of friendship. Note that these clients complain of *over*-commitment not commitment: They feel the clinician asked them to do something in excess of that which meets their definitions of best for them and the animal, but they feel obligated to agree because of their friendship with the veterinarian. Ms. Blake agrees to bathe Tiger weekly even though she lacks the time, skill, and desire to accomplish this task rather than disappoint her good friend Dr. Ward.

Some—and perhaps even many—practitioners might feel that the end justifies the means and as long as the cat gets the necessary bath, it doesn't matter who or what motivates the owner to accomplish this. However, when clients feel they do anything for any reason other than that they believe it best for the animal and/or themselves, compliance decreases and the probability of negative feelings aimed at the practitioner increases. As Ms. Blake misses a chance to go out with her friends because she must bathe the cat, she experiences a faint irritation at Dr. Ward for placing her in this position. When Tiger leaps from the tub, scratches Ms. Blake on both arms and streaks through the house spraying suds in all directions, the owner's irritation toward her good friend Dr. Ward escalates to resentment and then anger.

Granted, the majority of these clients realize they should have been more honest with the practitioner. However, they also note that the very familiarity of the relationship led them to believe that the practitioner was fully aware of their limitations. Because they consider the veterinarian the expert regarding all matters pertaining to the animal and its treatment, a surprising number do believe that the clinician knows more about their ability to accomplish these animal-related tasks than they do. As we noted, sometimes the extra boost of confidence supplied by a best friend clinician can lead clients to successfully complete treatments they might have considered beyond their capacity. Nonetheless, sometimes clients know their limitations better than the practitioner and those who take on more than they can handle out of friendship often wind up disenchanted with the veterinarian.

The Disadvantages of Playing Best Friend for the Practitioner

Compared to the god approach which focuses primarily on the animal, the best friend approach necessitates that the practitioner focus on the animal, the owner, and those other subjects the clinician considers conversational icebreakers or of interest to the client. Note the use of the word "conversational": Although best friend practitioners may communicate more with their clients than those who assume the god role, some may wind up conversing more but communicating less relative to the animal and the treatment process. Consider what happens when Dr. Ward becomes involved in her discussion of the trials and tribulations of dealing with an elderly parent with Ms. Blake as she examines Tiger.

Instead of focusing on getting a good history, Dr. Ward sprinkles questions regarding the cat throughout the conversation regarding Ms. Blake's father. When the cat-related questions occur within the context of a discussion of another subject, Ms. Blake doesn't give them much thought before answering because her mind is on her father and what she wants to tell her sympathetic friend Dr. Ward about him. Second, as the veterinarian focuses on her client's personal life, she pays less attention to the owner's responses regarding the cat. When Ms. Blake notes that Tiger "ate less than usual yesterday," Dr. Ward ignores the comment in her haste to tell Ms. Blake about an uncle who suffered from the same condition as Ms. Blake's father.

The physical examination of the patient may suffer as much as the history taking when the practitioner assumes the best friend mode. To be sure, some people can do two things well at once, most often when one of these is a repetitive or habitual act. Although some practitioners do consider the physical examination of an animal a habitual act, particularly when the animal is being seen for some routine reason, in reality a significant number of important findings in practice fall under the heading of "incidental." Dr. Ward feels the small lump in Tiger's pinna and intends to mention it to Ms. Blake, but then tears come to Ms. Blake's eyes as she speaks of her father's failing health and Dr. Ward forgets all about it. Or maybe Dr. Ward becomes so involved in her conversation with Ms. Blake, she doesn't notice the lump at all.

The final disadvantage of the best friend orientation relates to how seriously the practitioner takes the role. We already noted how, if clients perceive the veterinarian's interest as superfluous and time-wasting chatter, it will alienate rather than appeal to them. However at the opposite end of the best friend spectrum, we see those clients who truly appreciate the veterinarian who cares very deeply about them and their lives, and all that caring can take a tremendous emotional toll on the practitioner even as it does nothing to enhance the animal's health. As Dr. Ward looks over her schedule of daily appointments, she not only thinks of Ms. Blake's father, she thinks of the Greens building their new house, the Grays' son with AIDS, the Browns' bankruptcy, and the Whites' recent divorce. Although all of these situations certainly may affect both an animal's health and the treatment process, practitioners who adopt this approach may see their interest as a critical part of good client relations whether this is relevant to the animal's health or not.

"Shouldn't I care about my clients?" asks Dr. Ward.

It's a matter of both definition and degree. To some extent the best friend role can assume its own godlike qualities. The combination of medical and nurturing/nursing skills can make a veterinarian a very appealing authority figure to many people. Consider Dr. Ward, who as a new graduate wanted all her clients to like her. Her genuinely caring attitude attracted many who came to her because of her interest in them as well as their animals. Now Dr. Ward's clients number in the thousands and she worries about a significant number of them. Even if this doesn't distract her from the veterinary process, it takes times and energy.

Just how easily and deeply a practitioner can become involved was pointed out to one veterinarian by a concerned staff member. While the practitioner was at lunch, the employee taped this very telling sign on the examination room door: "Counseling 5¢."

By virtue of education and personality veterinarians who assume this role run the risk of becoming quasi-counselors. However, lacking the proper training, we don't know how to distance ourselves and/or maintain our objectivity in such situations. Dr. Ward feels flattered that Ms. Blake trusts her enough to share her deepest fears about her father's illness and what lies ahead for him. She expresses genuine concern during Tiger's examination, and throughout the day her thoughts return to poor Ms. Blake and what will happen to her when her father dies. As she drives home, she thinks about Ms. Blake again, and again later as she lies in bed unable to sleep. Dr. Ward also worries about the Greens selling their old house before their new one is completed and racks her brain trying to think of anyone she knows who might be interested in buying it. Her thoughts about the Grays and their son with AIDS are legion, as are those about her patients with malignant lymphoma, FIV, nonspecific lameness, and unresponsive hepatitis.

Is it any wonder Dr. Ward might consider a drink and a valium before going to bed every night?

As owners' lives and their relationships with their animals become more and more complex, the desire to become more intimately involved with clients as good friends will appeal to more nurturing individuals even as it will drive the more reserved deeper into the god mode. Both orientations carry their risks and although some might feel the greater legal risk posed by the uncommunicative god role looms as the greater evil, the emotional toll extracted by the best friend approach may prove equally if not more problematic.

Chapter 11
The Practitioner as Facilitator

As technology becomes more and more expensive and more and more alternatives fill the medical and surgical repertoire, many practitioners find they need to add the role of facilitator to their practice art. And, just as we noted in our discussion of veterinarians as gods and best friends, whether or not this role works depends on the needs of the patient and the client as well as those of the veterinarian.

The Facilitator Prototype

Choice serves as the basis of the facilitator role. Whereas god practitioners mentally work through various probabilities related to the treatment process, pick the one they believe best for the patient, and then present it to the owner with or without the corresponding rationale, facilitators share this process with the client. Rather than saying, "This is what we're going to do," Dr. Henley says, "Here are some things we could do." Although the best friend approach may involve the client more in the treatment process, unlike best friend clinicians those who use the facilitator approach do not become involved in their clients' personal lives, save as these directly affect the animal's health and welfare. The facilitator approach also differs in that practitioners may combine it with one of the other approaches, especially that of the best friend, whereas the god and best friend orientations are mutually exclusive.

Like the god and best friend orientations, that of facilitator requires its own special brand of knowledge as well as perception of the patient and client. If we view the god role as expressing the maximum interest in the science and technology of medicine and the best friend as expressing maximum personal interest in the patient and client, the facilitator falls between the two. Relative to the knowledge base, the practitioner who routinely assumes the facilitator role may represent either a compromised or enhanced state compared to the other clinician orientations. For example, sometimes veterinarians will offer clients options because they don't believe one approach will work better than another. This may occur for three reasons:

- They don't possess a clear idea of the medical problem.
- They lack a clear idea of the animal's needs.
- They lack a clear idea of the client's needs.

Although this makes the facilitator role appear like an escape hatch for the clinically inept, in fact even the most qualified veterinarian will see cases posing such a dilemma. A common example mentioned by practitioners are those situations in which the owners know their animals so well that they can detect changes before any signs manifest clinically. Cats on the verge of feline infectious peritonitis not uncommonly fall in this category. In these cases everything about the animal appears essentially normal save for the owner's feeling that something is wrong, a feeling the practitioner may or may not share. Under these circumstances the probable treatment options span the range from doing nothing to working up virtually every system in the animal's body; however, any tests done at this time rarely reveal any abnormalities. Because no clear idea of the problem exists, the animal's needs similarly lack definition. Finally, how can we assess the owner's needs in terms of the animal and the treatment process when we lack a clear idea of the animal's problem?

In these situations, the facilitator shares his or her thought processes with clients regarding probable causes and treatment options with the idea that the owners then will pick the one that best meets their needs. Practitioners used to assuming the god role may find such an approach incomprehensible, but to some extent we may say that these cases dwell entirely in the realm of the incomprehensible. More than one veterinarian who summarily dismissed such clients as overreactors or hypochondriacs has been humbled when these animals succumb to serious illness a week later—particularly if that practitioner learns of the animal's condition from his or her colleague to whom the client took it because "that vet down the road doesn't know anything!"

At the opposite end of the spectrum, facilitators may represent the maximum amount of knowledge involving the problem, patient, and client. In this situation so many options may come to the practitioner's mind, no single one stands out clearly as the ideal. The combination of a behaviorally stable animal with chronic skin or ear problems owned by the intelligent, caring, financially secure client falls into this category. Dr. Henley's knowledge of the patient and client assure him both could handle virtually any treatment and his knowledge of the animal's problem assures him no one "right" treatment exists. Each one poses advantages or disadvantages of one sort of another.

Finally, facilitators may act as clearinghouses for an ever growing array of other animal health-care professionals and specialists. These now may play such an important role in veterinary practice that we will discuss them in detail in Chapter 12. For now, suffice it to say that facilitators see these people as comprising another set of options they can offer their patients and clients.

The Facilitator and the Patient

Not surprisingly, whether the facilitator approach works with a patient depends on the practitioner's knowledge in two areas:

• Animal behavior
• The animal's needs relative to its problem

If the veterinarian chooses this role out of ignorance, once again the approach can create more problems than it solves.

The facilitator who responds to the animal from a solid knowledge base reads the animal's body language and observes it with the owner or handler and then chooses that approach which creates minimal stress on the animal while permitting the practitioner to work safely and efficiently. Although many fine texts and articles exist on various aspects of animal behavior, experience also serves as an excellent teacher. Moreover, practitioners may greatly enhance their interactions with a particular animal by following one simple rule: *When entering the examination room, stall, or pen, stop and observe the animal momentarily.* This simple act, which may be accomplished while sharing opening comments with the owner, enables the practitioner to pick up early signs of apprehension or aggression in the animal from a distance. The veterinarian can then assume the approach best suited to that animal *before* intimately interacting with it. Compare that to the clinician who comes into the room or stall and immediately begins examining the animal. When the animal responds negatively, these practitioners wind up reacting— and often out of fear—rather than setting the tone of the encounter.

Lacking such knowledge of behavior, facilitators may come across as indecisive to animals who feel threatened in any way by the treatment process. If the animal perceives the practitioner's behavior as submissive, this can precipitate the advantages and disadvantages noted previously: Some animals may see this as a reason to mount a challenge while others may see it as a reason to let the clinician do whatever he or she likes. However, the inconsistency of the facilitator approach may disorient a patient even more than if the practitioner assumed a threatening position and maintained it because many animals derive a certain stability from knowing their place even if they may not particularly like that position. Compare the clinician who definitively handles an animal to Dr. Henley who attempts to match his response to the animal's actions. In his attempts to find an approach the animal accepts, he winds up chasing the patient around the stall or tabletop.

Experienced practitioners immediately will note that sometimes moving with the patient isn't such a bad idea, and rightly so. However, these clinicians refer to that often precisely choreographed examination and treatment of the animal which responds best to minimal restraint. Some cats who become very defensive when restrained will tolerate all sorts of manipulation if allowed to move freely. In addition to adopting this technique with large animals possessing similar personalities, practitioners also will use it when the on-site handler is unskilled or unreliable. Although perhaps an unorthodox approach, the ability to match one's own tempo to that of an unrestrained animal and efficiently and effectively examine and treat it pleases the aesthetic sense as few other patient interactions in veterinary practice can.

Whether or not the facilitator approach works also depends on the practitioner's knowledge of the animal's needs relative to its problem. For example, every drug dispensed consists of three critical components:

- Its pharmacological properties
- Its administration schedule
- Its form

When treating a particular condition, a comparison of the pharmacological properties of several drugs may indicate one drug's obvious superiority. However when Dr. Henley takes the owner's schedule and lack of handling skills into consideration, a drug that requires less frequent administration becomes a more likely candidate. When he then factors in the animal's temperament which negates all but the use of liquids, the identity of the "ideal" drug may change yet again. Consequently, in order to be viable, any options presented by the facilitator must take into account the relationship between the owner and the animal and the animal's behavior as well the medical parameters inherent in the treatment of the problem.

The Advantages of the Facilitator Orientation for Clients

Because facilitators focus more on options than absolutes, they become favorites of clients whose lives are not only complex but also constantly changing. The owner who stayed at home with her children last year may sell real estate this year, and her success may affect how much money and time she can spend treating her animals. She appreciates knowing all the options because then she can choose the one that best meets her needs at that particular time.

Similarly, as clients become more educated and sophisticated, many take a more intellectual approach to the treatment process. They prefer the facilitator orientation because it gives them a broader view of the problem and its treatment. The owners of the dachshund with a disk problem more fully appreciate the variables inherent in the condition when Dr. Henley describes a range of medical and surgical treatments than when he describes only one approach. Although these owners may accept his recommendations for treatment every time, to them discussing the options plays a crucial role in the treatment process, and they consider this information as much a part of the veterinary experience as the examination and any medication prescribed. Consequently, even though ultimately the facilitator may treat the *animal* in exactly the same way as the god practitioner, these clients believe—and will tell their friends—that the facilitator is a much better veterinarian.

Another advantage offered to clients by the facilitator role is that it can nonjudgmentally present options spanning the entire anthropomorphic to chattel-oriented spectrum. We noted that, just as practitioners may feel more comfortable with one orientation toward animals than another, so may clients. However, like us, clients will assume a different orientation if it better meets their needs at a particular time. Usually anthropomorphically oriented Mr. McLaughlin may take a chattel approach to a problem that occurs the week after he loses his job, whereas normally chattel-oriented Ms. Edwards may choose a highly anthropomorphic option when her animal becomes ill the day after her mother's funeral. In these situations the god orientation may result in a treatment that doesn't meet the clients' needs, while the best friend orientation may put clients in the awkward position of having to provide information they consider embarrassing or irrelevant to the treatment process. By providing options, the facilitator allows the owner to depart from an established relationship norm with the animal and insures that those unwilling to bring up the underlying reason(s) directly will get the treatment that best meets their needs.

The very nature of the facilitator orientation also makes it easier for some clients to communicate more freely about the animal's problem and their own needs. When Dr. Henley discusses options, Ms. Edwards feels more comfortable mentioning an alternative therapy she read about in a natural health magazine than she would have had he presented her with only one treatment possibility. She also finds it easier to apprise him of her own particular needs and limitations when she realizes he recognizes more than one treatment approach as valid: Whom would you rather tell that you can only afford to spend so much money or time treating your animal every day—a facilitator or a god?

Finally, facilitators who discuss options with their clients tend to offer more services. Obviously the practitioner who only treats a particular condition one way—his or her perceived right way—wouldn't bother maintaining much in the way of drugs or equipment to treat the problem in a manner he or she considers lesser. For a significant number of clients in our service-oriented society, the more options offered by a particular practitioner or practice, the greater the convenience. Given the choice between receiving several options that may be fulfilled by one practitioner and seeking these from several different sources, they much prefer the one-stop shopping approach.

The Advantages for the Practitioner

Veterinarians who desire to offer clients options of necessity must take a broader view of many medical conditions. In order to do this, they must gain not only a greater appreciation of the scientific and technological aspects of a particular problem, but also its more subjective bond and behavioral components. This, in turn, may entail the use of nontraditional as well as traditional sources of information. Those practitioners who take this approach believe it helps them stay more current relative to both their patients' and their clients' needs, as well as provides them with a more stimulating and eclectic knowledge base. Not only does Dr. Henley attend scientific presentations and read scientific journals, he calls on a wide variety of resource people for additional information when the need arises. When a combination of animal needs and owner limitations appears to make treating a particular problem impossible, a call to a former classmate-turned-faculty-member produces yet another option to add to his repertoire. In addition to better serving his clients and patients, Dr. Henley finds such exchanges personally rewarding.

As noted previously, practitioners who give their clients options tend to offer more services; the more services offered, the more opportunities to develop new skills. For those who become bored doing the same things the same way day after day, finding new and different ways to treat problems makes the work challenging and enjoyable. Where god practitioners will expand their drug or equipment inventories because they believe it will enable them to treat a problem better, facilitators will do so because they believe it will enable them to treat the problem *differently*. Consequently, the facilitator's pharmacy may contain ten different kinds of flea-control products that address client needs relative to cost, ease of administration, and environmental and other public health issues as well control fleas.

Because of their expanded view of the treatment process, practitioners who assume the facilitator role also tend to be more tolerant and flexible. Consequently, situations that irritate practitioners who maintain a more rigid view may not bother these individuals at all, and some even see them as a welcomed challenge. We noted in our discussion of the god role how the absolute approach can lead to frustration and resentment when the client says, "No, I can't do that." However because facilitators routinely incorporate such variables into their practice philosophies, such an owner response serves as a stimulus to expand their knowledge even more: "Hmmmm," says Dr. Henley thoughtfully, "let's see what we can come up with that will still do the job, but won't cost quite so much."

Finally, the facilitator role gives practitioners an opportunity to learn about their clients' and patients' needs in a more professional context than the best friend approach. When Dr. Henley discusses options with his clients, their questions may reflect intimate personal concerns but only as these relate to the treatment process. Compare this to the god orientation in which such information may never be shared, or the best friend approach in which far more of it may be shared than necessary.

The Disadvantages for the Client

Whether the facilitator approach works for clients depends on two factors:

- The client's willingness to make choices.
- The client's perception of the practitioner as knowledgeable.

Some people simply do not like to make choices, and they find facilitator practitioners at least irritating if not downright threatening. When Dr. Henley launches into a description of the options available to treat their animal's intermittent diarrhea that run the gamut from benign neglect to exploratory laparotomy and everything between, the Johnsons shake their heads in bewilderment. They feel so overwhelmed by all this information that they send Dr. Henley on his way, telling him they'll call him when they make up their minds. Once he's gone, they agonize over the various options fearing they'll pick the wrong one. Finally Mr. Johnson throws up his hands in exasperation: "I paid that guy to tell me what to do, not ask me. Let's get someone out here who knows what he's doing!"

Similarly, those who take a less intellectual approach to their animal's care may consider the facilitator's options an attempt to make them feel inferior. Although few practitioners would intentionally do this to a client, sometimes we forget that many among the general public do not understand our technobabble as readily as our colleagues and staff. Out of the seven options Dr. Henley offers Ms. Edwards and her animal with chronic otitis, six of them make no sense to her. She picks the one that does make sense even though it doesn't meet her and her animal's needs because she's too embarrassed to admit to Dr. Henley that she has no idea what he's talking about. Needless to say, if that particular treatment turns out to be problematic in any way, she will not feel kindly toward Dr. Henley for two reasons: first, because he made her feel dumb and, second, because the treatment failed to meet her expectations.

Other clients may interpret all those options to mean that no good treatment exists for their animal's condition or that their veterinarian doesn't know it if it does. After all, why would anyone bother offering all those choices if there was one approach that would do the job? The Johnsons call in a practitioner known to his colleagues as "Bicillin Bill" because he treats practically everything with that drug. The Johnsons think he's wonderful: "So confident," gushes Ms. Johnson. "He knew just what to do to treat our mare. From the way that Dr. Henley was talking, we were afraid she'd never get better."

Interestingly, for as many clients who perceive the facilitator approach as too intellectual, an equal number see it as indicative of the veterinarian's lack of knowledge. This holds especially true for those who prefer to deify medicine and its practitioners. Rather than seeing Dr. Henley's options as representing the most extensive knowledge base, they see them as indicative of his indecision. As we noted in the previous example with the Johnsons, this practitioner evaluation often comes from clients who don't want to make choices themselves. Rather than admit this, they much prefer to blame the practitioner whose options put them in the awkward position of having to recognize this.

Another variation of this theme occurs when clients face terminal illness or injury and/or the possibility of euthanasia. Many different factors can come into play at such times, and these subjects will be dealt with in depth later. For now, simply note that even the most intelligent, alternative-loving clients may take a very dim view of the veterinarian who throws options out like so many cards on a table and then stands back and waits for them to make the life-or-death decision.

The Disadvantages for the Practitioner

When we take the increased complexity of owner life-styles and human-animal relationships and couple it with the increased complexity of our science and technology, we can appreciate how those practitioners who try to cover all the bases for their clients face an increasingly difficult task. This holds particularly true for those who adopted this orientation as a practice builder rather than as a result of any conscious plan. Consider what happened to Dr. Henley. As a new graduate, he decided that the best way to attract clients was to give them what they wanted. Although that seems like a very caring approach, his lack of experience in dealing with clients and in business matters led him to set three precedents that later plagued him:

- He became accustomed to reacting to his clients.
- He maintained a large inventory of drugs and equipment.
- He did things he found disagreeable for one reason or another.

Nobody questions the value of tailoring one's practice to meet patient and client needs. However as the number, complexity, and cost of options continue to escalate, practitioners who allow clients to dictate their responses can soon find themselves feeling out of control. In an effort to meet the needs of a clientele that includes faculty members from the local college, human health-care professionals from the hospital, organic-vegetarian New Agers from the mountaintop meditation center, and poverty-level pet owners and farmers among others, Dr. Henley subscribes to fifteen different journals and belongs to an equal number of local and national organizations that address various patient and client needs. When a physician's dog succumbs to malignant lymphoma, he feels obligated to read up on human as well as veterinary approaches to the problem. On his way to the meditation center, he scans a holistic health journal as he drives.

Because there are only so many hours in the day, Dr. Henley eventually reaches a point at which he can't keep up with the burgeoning information within the profession, let alone that addressing all those other areas of concern to his clients. Eventually he discovers that he knows less and less about more and more, an awareness that hardly complements his desired image of himself as someone able to meet all his patients' and clients' needs.

In addition, Dr. Henley maintains an inventory that bulges with drugs and equipment he may use once a year, if that. The drugs often become outdated, but he replaces them "just in case" someone might request them. His collection of flea-control products, anthelmintics, and medicated shampoos takes up so much space that his practice looks like a retail outlet. His staff refers to his "toys," that collection of in-house laboratory equipment and other diagnostic aids that gather dust in various corners awaiting the day when they and their operating manuals will be pressed into service once again. Like more than a few practitioners, he owns several pieces of equipment (including his computer) whose potential he barely taps because he lacks the time to learn the techniques necessary to use them properly. Eventually and just as all his journals and memberships make him feel like he knows less and less about more and more, these increasingly exotic drugs and technologically complex marvels with their inch-thick manuals leave him feeling he can do less and less with that more and more.

We can easily appreciate how Dr. Henley's lack of a coherent plan regarding what options he would offer his clients led to the establishment of unsound and costly business practices and caught him in a vicious cycle. As the practice grew, he felt obligated to offer more options, which led to the purchase of more drugs and equipment, which increased his costs, which meant he had to see more clients, which meant more options, drugs, and equipment. Eventually he reached a point at which he was working long hours to finance his options rather than having those options generate income for him. Worse, the long hours meant he no longer had time to network with all those resource people and to read all the journals which made those options viable alternatives for him and his clients as well as served as a source of enjoyment for him. And surely it goes without saying that veterinarians who recommend treatments or procedures about which they possess only the most rudimentary knowledge pursue a most questionable legal and moral course.

Another disadvantage of the facilitator option is that those who use it must possess good communication skills. Obviously if clients don't understand the options, they won't be able make any meaningful choices. We already discussed what happens when clients remain silent because they feel intimidated by medical jargon. However, others may ask the practitioner for clarification, and a lack of communication skills in this situation can result in a time-consuming process as the veterinarian flounders around for the real-world words to translate the technobabble. Consequently, it behooves those who use this approach to work out a protocol that clearly addresses the advantages and disadvantages of any option in a manner the client can readily understand.

Facilitator clinicians who decide to be all things to all people almost invariably must also face the troublesome dilemma of what to do when clients ask them to do something they don't want to do. Although Dr. Henley personally doesn't condone ear cropping and tail docking, when he first started his practice and was trying to make ends meet, he rationalized doing it, saying he couldn't afford to alienate the breeder who owned a very large kennel. Later, as his practice grew, he kept doing it, saying that, even though he didn't agree with it, he did do it very carefully and better he should do it than someone without his skill and concern for the animals. Then one day he heard himself described as "the best ear cropper and tail docker in the state," a remark that caused him to lose more sleep than some of his toughest medical cases.

Practitioners who successfully use the facilitator option focus on those options that work best *for them* as well as for their clients and patients and let the others go. This doesn't mean abandoning those clients who wish other alternatives, but rather referring them to others more comfortable with those options rather than trying to be everything to everyone. Above all, they never offer an option that they cannot fully support emotionally as well as intellectually and physically because they know it won't work for them. Even if they accomplish the treatment flawlessly—and sometimes especially if they do so—the idea that they compromised their values will come back to haunt them again and again.

Striking a Balance

Most likely during the discussions of the three common practitioner orientations, some elements of each seemed quite familiar whereas others seemed quite alien. We noted previously that maintaining a different orientation toward the animal and the owner can be quite difficult if one or both of these do not come naturally. In reality, however, most of us ultimately create a professional identity that vacillates among these orientations as well as contains elements of more than one at the same time.

For example, let's observe Dr. Rawson on a typical day. She treats her first patient—a wriggly, blissfully happy German shepherd pup—as a best friend, but adopts the god role with the pup's owner—a taciturn old farmer—because she knows he expects her to take full control of the situation and tell him only what he needs to know. Later, she admits a dominant male Doberman for surgery who belongs to a shy young woman with her arm in a cast. In this case, Dr. Rawson assumes the god orientation with the dog to establish her authority but then addresses the owner as a best friend, inquiring about the young woman's arm and discussing mutual acquaintances as well as allaying the client's fears about the dog's surgery. Still later she goes over the available options with the owner of a terminally ill animal. In this situation, she initially combines elements of the best friend and facilitator approaches, then switches to the more authoritative god role when the client goes over the same issues again and again without coming to any meaningful conclusions.

What about Dr. Rawson's needs? "What works for my patients and clients works for me," she says, but only because she has worked out a clear definition of what both quality practice and a quality life mean to her as well as to her patients and clients. Consequently, when owners demand something she cannot do for whatever reason, she can refuse without feeling guilty or fearful of the client's response. Not only that, she can refuse in her role as god, best friend, facilitator, or some amalgam of the three.

For students with little experience in patient and client relations, this might seem like so much magic, and to some extent when practitioners strike the perfect balance between authority, friendship, and flexibility and their own, the patient's, and the client's needs, the result does seem that way. However, it falls within the province of professional responsibility to assume that role or those roles that will do this as a means of insuring adequate quality communication. As we have noted time and time again and will most certainly note yet again, failure to communicate with clients in what they consider a meaningful way creates more problems for more veterinarians than any other factor encountered in practice. Consequently, whether we deliberately create a public persona that conveys what we consider a professional image or evolve one on a trial-and-error basis over time, in order to succeed it must fulfill three criteria:

- We must feel sufficiently comfortable in any role we assume that we can relate to the animal confidently and effectively.
- The role must enable us to communicate in a meaningful way with the client.
- The role must not lead us to do anything we find professionally or personally unethical.

A fundamental truth of medicine that goes back to Hippocrates if not further maintains that the success of any treatment relies on the patients' faith in their own ability to get well first, and in the clinician's ability to perform his or her duties second. Although faith in the practitioner as a healer serves its purpose, it must not exceed the patients' faith in their ability to heal themselves.

As veterinarians we face a far greater challenge than our colleagues in human medicine: Because of the nature of the human-animal bond, we must not only reinforce our patients' faith in their own healing abilities, we must also reinforce our clients' faith in their animals' ability to achieve and maintain a state of health consistent with a quality life. And we must accomplish this even as we reinforce our client's faith in their ability to assist the animal in this process. To do this we must find some way to communicate with both of them in a nonthreatening manner. Once we find the approach that enables us to accomplish all this with that particular client and that particular patient, then, and only then, will we earn their faith in us and our ability to perform our duties, too.

Chapter 12
The Art of Referring

Although traditionally most veterinarians view specialists as those whose knowledge in a particular area exceeds their own, as both the science and technology of medicine and human-animal relationships become more complex, veterinarians also must view these individuals as extensions of themselves and their practice philosophy. In addition to enabling the practitioner to provide a full range of services for clients and patients, to the client these people represent the referring clinician every bit as much as they represent their specialties. Over the course of a decade, Dr. Wallace refers Sue Martin to five different specialists. However, throughout that time Ms. Martin sees Dr. Wallace far more than any one of these and she relies on him to act as an intermediary between her and any specialist if necessary. Because Dr. Wallace recommends these people, any experience the owner and her animal have with them reflects on Dr. Wallace for good or ill. Consequently it behooves Dr. Wallace and all practitioners to recognize when, to whom, and how they refer a patient and client.

As the profession continues to evolve, practitioners must decide what services they can reasonably and effectively provide their patients and clients themselves and which ones they should refer. In our discussion of the facilitator role, we noted how trying to be all things to all people is not only not cost-effective, but also emotionally draining and may result in substandard care for patients and clients alike. By focusing on those areas that meet the majority of client needs while providing sufficient professional stimulation and enjoyment and referring the rest to competent individuals, the practitioner can remain a "full service" veterinarian in the clients' eyes.

The term *specialist* will be used in this discussion to mean anyone practitioners believe can provide necessary or desired services beyond their expertise rather than in the more limited context used within the profession itself. Thus a groomer or farrier functions as a specialist as does a veterinary ophthalmologist or orthopedic surgeon. Rather than reflecting any disrespect, the use of the term reflects the prevailing perception of the majority of clients that anyone their veterinarian refers them to is a specialist.

When to Refer Clients

Because faith serves as the core of the healing process, clinicians should consider referring patients and clients any time anything undermines that faith. Circumstances involving a loss of faith include:

- The clinician's loss of faith in his or her ability to treat the animal successfully due to a lack of knowledge or skill.
- The clinician's loss of faith in the client's willingness to carry out the treatment.
- The client's loss of faith in the practitioner to treat the animal successfully.

In addition, clients' relationships with the animals and their beliefs regarding specialists can also serve as legitimate reasons to consider referring.

Ideally, the best time for practitioners to recognize that they lack sufficient knowledge and/or skill to carry a case through to its conclusion occurs before the treatment begins. Dr. Wallace takes the history, performs the physical and possibly a few preliminary diagnostic tests, realizes the animal's or client's needs exceed his ability, and refers the case. Although this seems obvious, more than one veterinarian has launched a major diagnostic and treatment campaign only to discover the case featured complex aspects that were previously overlooked. This occurs particularly often among those who put more faith in technology to give them the answers than in a solid history and thorough physical examination. When the work-up doesn't provide the answer, these people find themselves in the awkward position of either starting over or referring.

Similarly, practitioners who see referring as a sign of their inadequacy rather than as a valuable service they can offer their clients may waste precious time and even worsen the animal's condition before they admit they lack the necessary knowledge and/or skill to treat it. At this point, the specialist may need to repeat much of the work-up as well as factor in all the effects of any attempted treatments, which leads to additional expense for the client as well as prolongs the treatment process for the animal. Surely more than a few practitioners can claim a permanently limping patient they wish they had referred to a more skilled orthopedic surgeon.

Regardless where in the process practitioners realize they lack the necessary knowledge or skill, these observations should be shared openly and honestly with the client. This does not mean waiting until no doubt exists in the practitioner's mind; it means sharing the thoughts about referring with the client as soon they occur. This not only avoids shocking clients who believed the veterinarian could successfully treat the animal, it avoids all the negative effects that result in the client-clinician relationship when the owner raises the issue of the practitioner's ability to treat the problem. Compare the relationship with Ms. Martin that results when Dr. Wallace shares his concerns about the nature of her animal's problem and the possibility of referral during the first or second visit to that which results when he raises the issue after weeks of unsuccessful treatment: Which approach more likely communicates caring to the client?

Practitioners also should consider referring clients whom they feel will not carry out the treatment for them. This in no way means using specialists as dumping grounds for the worst clients, but rather recognizing that some people will do more for a specialist than they will for a regular practitioner even if both ask the same thing. When Dr. Wallace tells Ms. Martin to medicate her animal's eye four to six times a day, she looks at him incredulously and reminds him that she works, has three kids, and coaches a softball team. When she hears the same thing from a specialist fifty miles away who charges her twice as much, she finds the time to medicate the animal as directed. Admittedly, referring such cases doesn't do much for the ego of the referring veterinarian, but if the animal gets better one can hardly question the soundness of the practice. Moreover, if the animal gets better the client will credit not only the specialist, but also the veterinarian who recommended that person.

It should go without saying that clients who have lost faith in the practitioner's ability should be referred graciously and to the very best person possible. Unfortunately, this may not happen if the clinician responds fearfully to the situation. When Sue Martin brings up her concern about her animal's lack of response, Dr. Wallace feels threatened for several reasons. First, the fact that she brought it up before he did makes it appear that she knows more than he does. Second, he fears she will challenge his handling of the case. Third, he wonders what she will tell whomever next sees the animal—that he did his best or that he's incompetent? Dr. Wallace sees all of his client's remarks hovering over his head in a black cloud labeled "possible litigation." Unfortunately, the common responses under these circumstances include freezing (denying the problem exists), fighting (blaming the client for her lack of faith or not doing her part), or running (telling the owner she can do whatever she wants with the animal). However, any fear-based response can only make the situation worse because it further inhibits communication at a time when it's needed the most. Rather than argue or deny the reality of the situation, Dr. Wallace should accept his client's view gracefully and make every attempt to insure she and her animal see someone who better fits their needs.

Clients who lack faith in the practitioner also benefit from referral whether or not the clinician believes that lack of faith is justified. This most commonly occurs with clients who routinely use specialists for their own problems or who move from large metropolitan areas to those they consider less sophisticated or, a common New England hazard, quaint. Under these circumstances, practitioners who try to prove their competency may find themselves fighting an uphill battle. People who routinely use specialists also may do so because they believe this makes their—or their animal's—problem more special. Consequently, when practitioners insist they can treat the condition, these people may feel more threatened than grateful for that information, and some may even go so far as to say that the clinician's belief that he or she can treat the animal proves his or her lack of knowledge.

Owners who believe the practitioner or practice too unsophisticated for whatever reason make very poor clients. Their lack of faith leads to a lack of compliance, which leads to lack of positive results, which reinforces their lack of faith. In effect, they prove their point—that the clinician can't handle the problem—even though the veterinarian might very well have treated the animal successfully had it belonged to someone else. Granted, the temptation to prove one's ability as well as prove these clients wrong can be very powerful; however, practitioners should only yield to this if they feel confident that they can override any negative client influence. If they succeed, they may or may not win a client. If they fail, for sure they'll lose one. However, if they refer they will gain the client's respect and, over time, perhaps even their trust to do more and more for their animals.

Relationships and Referring

Other bond and relationship factors may come into play when determining whether or not to refer a client. In Chapter 6 we noted how some animals strongly attached to their owners tolerated hospitalization very poorly. To send these animals for treatment at a teaching hospital a hundred miles away serves no purpose unless that treatment can be accomplished in a very short time or provisions can be made for the owner to stay with the animal. Under these circumstances, it often works better for the practitioner to maintain phone contact with the specialist and implement his or her suggestions as best possible in surroundings more familiar to the animal. If the practitioner has discussed the problems inherent in the relationship with the client from the beginning, such a hybrid approach to treatment will come as no surprise. If the practitioner has not, the consequences of the relationship as well as the animal's medical problems will have to be dealt with simultaneously.

Even though some clients wouldn't consider taking a terminally ill animal to a specialist, that's the only time when others would. Several different motivations underlie this behavior. Some clients may challenge the practitioner's pronouncement of the animal's condition as terminal. This may result because they lack faith in the practitioner or because they are not ready to face the possibility of losing the animal at that time. Either way, referring these clients provides a valuable and necessary service for patient, practitioner, and client alike. If the second veterinarian confirms the diagnosis, the client who lacked faith will see the referring clinician in a more positive light. What if the second veterinarian doesn't share the referring clinician's hopeless prognosis? In this situation, the act of referring itself communicates caring. Dr. Wallace tells Sue Martin he believes her animal's condition hopeless, but he'd be happy to refer her to someone who might see something he overlooked. When she reports that the other veterinarian did discover such an oversight, he shares in her joy that the animal might recover.

Owners of terminally ill animals also may appreciate referral to specialists for several nonmedical reasons. At such times people may be overwhelmed by feelings of helplessness and want to play a more active role. For some, making a five-hour drive or spending so much money to hear a specialist tell them the same thing as the referring veterinarian makes them feel they went the extra mile for the animal. This may serve a particularly important function for those clients who believe they contributed to the animal's illness in any way: They see any inconvenience and expense as a form of atonement which comforts them during this difficult time. Just as some owners would never consider allowing anyone to treat their terminally ill animal other than the veterinarian who cared for it all along, so an occasional client will request referral so that the regular clinician doesn't attend the animal's demise. All of these clients openly admit this has nothing to do with the competency of the regular practitioner, and everything to do with superstition and emotion: They don't want to associate the regular clinician and/or his or her facility with the death of the animal. Were the animal to die there or in that person's care, they believe they would be reminded of this every time they saw that veterinarian or entered that clinic.

Selecting Specialists Within the Profession

Because anyone to whom the clinician refers a client indirectly represents the referring practitioner, it makes sense to choose these people wisely. Regardless how competent and credentialed a specialist might be, his or her value to the referring veterinarian and clients depends on the specialist's ability to interact effectively on three levels:

- With the referring veterinarian
- With the patient
- With the client

Few things in practice can prove more frustrating for client and practitioner alike than dealing with a specialist who either doesn't communicate or communicates poorly. This holds particularly true if the specialist expects the client and/or referring practitioner to treat the animal or perform any follow-up procedures. Unfortunately, and particularly when dealing with specialists within the profession, some practitioners feel they and their clients must take whatever the specialist offers and be grateful for it. However, as the number of people with advanced training increases, so do the number of choices available, and practitioners should make a conscious effort to choose those specialists with whom they can communicate well and who will best meet their clients' needs.

Ideally the practitioner should have some contact with the specialist before referring any clients, even if only an introductory phone call. During that conversation, the clinician should ascertain the following:

- The range of the specialist's services
- The specialist's personality
- The specialist's ability to communicate
- The fee schedule
- Any pertinent details regarding scheduling or other aspects of the referring process

During this conversation the practitioner should evaluate the specialist both as a potential professional colleague as well as from the view of any potential client. For example, during a state veterinary meeting Dr. Wallace makes a special effort to seek out Dr. Hanrahan, an orthopedic surgeon in a teaching hospital. During his conversation with her, Dr. Wallace determines that she is extremely proficient medically and technologically but definitely assumes the god role. She uses jargon that leaves him feeling more than a little inadequate and makes it quite clear that her services not only cost a great deal, they are also in great demand.

Dr. Wallace then speaks to another orthopedic surgeon, Dr. Nielsen, who does referral work for several practices around the state. Dr. Nielsen can't summon all the technology that Dr. Hanrahan can, but he is cheerful and outgoing and appears eager to work with Dr. Wallace should the need arise; he supplies Dr. Wallace with a fee schedule and the names of other practitioners who use his services.

From these brief meetings, Dr. Wallace collects some valuable information for himself and his clients. In the file he keeps of specialists, he notes Dr. Hanrahan's excellent medical skills as well as her aloof personality and lack of communication skills, the probable expense, and the difficulty in securing an appointment with her. Similarly, he notes all the information Dr. Nielsen shared as well as his own observations regarding the surgeon's personality and ability to communicate.

Later, when presented with a patient with an orthopedic problem that exceeds his ability, Dr. Wallace refers to his file. At that time, he may select the specialist he believes best fits the patient's and client's needs or he may discuss the possibilities with the owner. When Sue Martin presents her top breeding animal with multiple pelvic and femoral fractures, the case falls at what Dr. Wallace considers the outer limits of Dr. Nielsen's ability, but he must weigh that against Dr. Hanrahan's limited ability to communicate, which could be a serious drawback given the nature of the problem. He discusses the pros and cons of both surgeons with the owner and she ultimately decides to use Dr. Hanrahan with the understanding that Dr. Wallace will act as a go-between if necessary.

Getting input from clients following an appointment with a particular specialist also provides valuable information. Sue Martin later tells Dr. Wallace that she got lost three times trying to find the hospital and then had to wait more than an hour for Dr. Hanrahan, but the surgeon treated her animal very well even though she did more or less ignore the owner (which fortunately Dr. Wallace had warned her might happen). And although Dr. Hanrahan does find it difficult to communicate in person, she did supply the client with some excellent printed material and sent Dr. Wallace a full written report of the animal's condition, treatment, and prognosis within a week of the initial visit. By adding these observations to his records, Dr. Wallace gains a more complete view of Dr. Hanrahan which enables him to better determine when and who to refer to her. It also reminds him to provide clear instructions regarding how to locate any specialist so his clients don't get lost.

Finally, Dr. Wallace adds his own input to Dr. Hanrahan's file following his interactions with her. Although initially intimidated by both her reticence and use of jargon, he persists in his efforts to gain useful information for his clients and eventually develops what he considers a workable relationship with her. However, because Dr. Nielsen's personality and practice philosophy more closely reflect his own, Dr. Wallace refers all but the most complex orthopedic cases to him. Interestingly, this improves his relationship with Dr. Hanrahan because what she considers "routine cases" bore her and she learns she can always count on Dr. Wallace to send her something challenging. By keeping such specialist files, practitioners in even the most remote areas can build up an impressive collection of outside resources over time.

A significant number of veterinarians in practice also develop particular interests to meet their own and their clients' needs. Although they may not possess the academic credentials of a professional specialist, their knowledge and expertise can be extensive and they can serve as valuable resources in areas lacking board-certified specialists or for those clients who cannot afford these services. By tapping into the grapevine at state and local meetings, the names of practitioners with personal interests in birds, ferrets, cats, dermatology, or surgery may be added to those in the referral file using the same process of interview and client feedback.

Some practitioners object to the use of such veterinarians for reasons of political correctness; they maintain very strong beliefs regarding who and what constitutes a specialist and will not refer clients to anyone who does not meet this criterion. Returning to the recurrent theme of faith as the core of medicine, no one should refer to anyone in whom one lacks faith (regardless of his or her credentials), if for no other reason than that clients see that person as an agent of the referring practitioner. If clients can't afford the services of a specialist who meets the referring clinicians' definitions, then these practitioners face three choices:

- Treat the animal themselves.
- Send the animal to an acceptable specialist and absorb the cost.

• Let the clients fend for themselves.

Some practitioners resist referring clients to colleagues who possess self-developed specialties for fear they will lose the client to the other veterinarian. Although that may happen, it still seems preferable to be known as "that nice Dr. Wallace who referred me to Dr. Wood who loves and knows so much about horses" rather than "that grouch Dr. Wallace who couldn't care less about my horse."

The final form of referral within the profession, the second opinion, many times does not occur as a formal referral at all. In fact, sometimes the second clinician may not even be aware that the client is seeking another opinion until halfway through the examination, if then. To some extent, not knowing may enable practitioners to view these cases more objectively than they would if they knew their good friend or worst enemy had seen the case previously. On the other hand, animals are dynamic physiological and behavioral organisms and the more we know about what went on before, the more informed our analysis of the current situation and its prognosis. Consequently if the owner doesn't volunteer the information and the clinician suspects the animal may have been seen by another veterinarian, he or she should come right out and ask about this.

A helpful technique employed by some practitioners when dealing with those seeking a second opinion is to inform these clients that the previous veterinarian will be contacted. When they hear this, clients who criticized the first practitioner may suddenly remember they didn't medicate the animal quite as directed or never paid for the work done. Although just saying such a call will be made can yield valuable information, the call actually should be made. Some practitioners hesitate to do this, fearing their colleague's wrath. However the animal's health, professional courtesy, and basic good manners demand that it be done. Admittedly practitioners do exist who respond defensively and refuse to supply information, but the majority realize that on any given day they could see one of their colleague's clients for a second opinion, too. To them the second opinion amounts exactly to that: another person's opinion, not a condemnation of the first person's diagnosis and treatment of the problem.

Referring to Specialists Outside the Profession

In addition to specialists within the profession, practitioners may need to call on those representing a wide range of other areas. These include trainers, groomers, handlers, breeders, county agents, farriers, animal control officers, wildlife rehabilitators, and herdsmen, as well as some of those representing the alternative therapies that we will discuss in more detail in the next chapter. How many of these people a practitioner uses depends on the practitioner's feelings regarding such services as well as the needs of the clients.

Obviously clinicians who don't believe in a service offered by a particular specialist will experience difficulty recommending it or that person to their clients. More than a few veterinarians chafe at others doing work they consider within their domain, such as county agents or breeders who offer what the practitioner considers medical advice. However, before condemning these people, it might be wise to investigate the circumstances that lead others to seek them out. Although the idea of getting cheap or even free advice or service may serve as one motivator, conversations with animal owners indicate this doesn't serve as the primary one. More often than not, these people say they seek out these individuals because the veterinarian cannot or will not provide them with the information or service they desire. Comments such as "I would call Dr. Wallace if I felt he knew or cared more about goats than the county agent," or "I like Dr. Wallace, but he's so busy it takes ages to get an appointment and then he never has time to answer my questions" occur frequently when these owners describe why they use these other specialists.

Rather than berating both the specialists and the clients who use them, practitioners would serve themselves, their patients, and their clients better if they focused on why the clients use them. In the aforementioned case, Dr. Wallace might decide he needs to develop his small ruminant skills or he might decide he lacks both the interest and client base necessary to support this endeavor. In the latter case, it makes sense for him to develop a good working relationship with the county agent who does possess these skills and enjoys this work so he can assist that person professionally whenever necessary. Compare that to the antagonistic approach in which both the clients and the county agent dread asking Dr. Wallace for help because they know he will subject them to at least his "practicing medicine without a license" lecture if not his wrath.

Veterinarians whose clients repeatedly turn to nonprofessionals for what the practitioners consider professional services also should consider whether it's time to hire an associate to better meet these clients' needs. When Dr. Wallace discovers he provides the least information and service to his large animal clients, he ponders the economics of hiring an associate with interests in that area versus selling that part of his practice or phasing it out. If he opts for the latter he should discuss his plan with colleagues who do large animal work, then send out a mailing to his large animal clients informing them in advance of this change as well as providing them with the names and phone numbers of clinicians able and willing to meet their needs.

Dealing with specialists whose services don't conflict with ours can be a most rewarding experience because these people can provide us with an expanded view of our patients and clients as well as the treatment process. Here again, personal interviews and client feedback can serve as invaluable assets when compiling information about these specialists. Because Dr. Wallace does no grooming in his practice, he develops relationships with two groomers who not only provide this service but also will give medicated baths according to his instructions to animals whose owners can't bathe them at home. He realizes he lacks a knowledge of behavioral problems and maintains a list of resource people that includes trainers and handlers as well as veterinarians. When he encounters a problem he feels might be associated with a particular product, he doesn't hesitate to call the manufacturer's professional service representative. In all of these situations Dr. Wallace knows he could develop the necessary knowledge base and skills to provide all these services for his clients directly, but he lacks the time and/or interest, and he trusts others to do it for him. Like many practitioners, he looks at those specialists outside the veterinary profession as condiments to the basics: The practice could probably survive without them, but there's no doubt they enhance the quality of the service he offers.

How to Refer

Just as knowing when and to whom to refer clients consists of more art than science, so does knowing how to refer. The first issue referring practitioners need to address is who contacts the specialist—the practitioner or the client? Because of the complexity of many owners' lives, the correct answer is often both. The practitioner provides the specialist with any salient information about the animal and client as well as makes arrangements to send any necessary records to the specialist if these won't accompany the client. The clients set up the actual appointment that best fits their schedules.

Some referring practitioners prefer to handle all the preliminaries to make it as easy as possible for their clients to secure the additional assistance for the animal. When Dr. Wallace refers patients to Dr. Nielsen, he calls Dr. Nielsen and discusses both the nature of the animal's problem and any special needs of the clients. At that time Dr. Nielsen provides a broad overview of his probable approach to the case and sets up an appointment to see the animal. Dr. Wallace then shares this information with the owners and arranges for them to pick up a copy of the animal's records and directions to Dr. Nielsen's facility on the day of the appointment.

Compare this to what happens when Sue Martin tells Dr. Wallace she'll arrange everything herself and he lets her because he's very busy. Her poor sense of direction lets her down again and she arrives late for her appointment and in a state of agitation. Dr. Nielsen looks on his schedule beside the owner's name and reads only "HBC, fx leg." This approach does a disservice on two fronts. First, Dr. Nielsen must spend time ascertaining the nature of any other, possibly relevant injuries the animal sustained when hit by the car as well as the nature of the fracture. Not only does this take time—which the client will pay for—the majority of this information will come second-hand. If Dr. Nielsen considers this insufficient, he may opt to work up the animal from scratch or call Dr. Wallace to gain the necessary base-line information. More time and more money trickle away and Dr. Nielsen has yet to address the reason for the visit.

From this we can see that referring a client to a specialist without adequate preparation is neither a cost-effective nor caring thing to do. Clients shouldn't have to pay for the same preliminary work-up twice any more than the animal should need to go through the procedure twice. Similarly, why not take full advantage of a specialist's skills by giving that person as much information as possible? It not only makes the specialist look better, it makes the referring veterinarian look better, too.

Sometimes practitioners do not contact specialists until after clients verify that they've made the appointment. This most often occurs when the clinician questions the client's commitment to the process. Sue Martin has been complaining about one of her animal's recurrent skin problems for more than a year and Dr. Wallace questions whether she really wants to do something about the problem or just feels obligated to mention the possibility of treating it. He provides her with the specialist's name and phone number and tells her to let him know when she sets up an appointment so he can then contact that person and discuss the animal's history. He considers this a more valid approach than taking time to call a specialist to discuss a patient and client who may never show up. Unfortunately, if the owner makes the appointment and forgets to notify Dr. Wallace because he distanced himself from the entire procedure, she and her animal will once again arrive sans history.

One final variation on this theme deserves comment: Sometimes practitioners do not share a history with a specialist because they believe they have no history to share. "I don't know anything about behavior problems," explains Dr. Wallace. That may well be, but Dr. Wallace presumably does know his patient, his client, and the relationship between the two, and this information can benefit any specialist. Consider the following practitioner comments regarding clients and patients:

- "She's a nice lady, but you have to tell her things at least twice."
- "Whatever you do, don't turn your back on that horse."
- "The owner's an M.D. with a Ph.D. in reproductive physiology and this is a top show animal."
- "Money's no object, but they travel a lot and a hired man cares for their animals most of the time."

Although none of these statements provides information regarding any specific medical or behavioral problem, each one gives valuable insights that could effect how a specialist might choose to relate with these people and animals. Consequently, practitioners never should underestimate their ability to share meaningful information with a specialist any more than they should underestimate the specialist's ability to share meaningful information with them. Perhaps the most rewarding relationship a veterinarian can experience with a specialist occurs when the latter willingly educates the former in the process of treating the patient. Not only does this improve the quality of the service the referring veterinarian can offer his or her clients, it insures that the specialist will get the highest quality information and the most challenging referrals from that practitioner.

Chapter 13
The Art of Alternative Therapies

The subjects of the next two chapters, alternative therapies and animal rights, tend to arouse such emotional responses it seems unlikely any consensus opinion regarding either will emerge from the profession for a long time. However, as anyone in practice knows, clients tend to care less about what the profession thinks than about what their particular practitioner thinks. Because all indicators point toward increased public awareness of and interest in both these areas, it behooves clinicians to work out their own feelings and formulate their own opinions so they may articulate these clearly to others if necessary.

Ironically many practitioners avoid confronting these subjects both personally and with clients believing that offering no opinion poses the safest course. However, just the opposite holds true: Those who take this route often feel the most threatened when a client brings up the subject. At that time, the practitioner may revert to the familiar freeze, fight, or flee fear mode and alienate the client. On the other hand, clinicians who possess a personal and practice philosophy regarding these issues stand a much better chance of stating this clearly and objectively. Moreover, when practitioners share their views in this manner, they also stand a much better chance of proposing a differing view without alienating the client.

Practitioners who maintain strong positive or negative opinions about these subjects also should try to view these issues objectively regardless of their specific orientations. Undoubtedly those who harbor such intense feelings will dismiss this as unnecessary, citing all the scientific evidence that supports their particular view. However, surely in our calmer moments we share the observations of scientists Albert Einstein, Werner Heisenberg, and Erwin Schrödinger, among others, who noted we are as apt to create our science to prove our beliefs as create our beliefs based on the proof of our science.

In the following discussion, the general terms *alternative* and *alternative treatments* will be used rather than dealing with specific approaches within that category for a very simple reason: What makes an alternative an alternative is the lack of formal professional acceptance. Consequently and as we already are seeing with acupuncture, today's alternative approaches may become part of tomorrow's traditional treatment regime even as today's mainstream treatments may find themselves on the fringes of the accepted treatment repertoire tomorrow.

The Alternative Issue

The real dilemma facing most practitioners is not the scientific validity of any one alternative, but what to do when faced with the possibility of using or accepting the use of such an approach on a patient. When this happens, veterinarians may find themselves confronting one of two equally distasteful probabilities:

- They know little or nothing about the alternative in question.
- They possess no faith in the alternative.

Although those who support the alternative would argue that the second naturally follows the first—that is, that ignorance leads to lack of faith—those who do not support it would argue the opposite saying their knowledge of alternatives leads them to lack faith in these approaches. However, while the argument rages, what do we say to the client who asks about using an alternative and what do we do with the patient for whom traditional medicine appears to have no answer? Tell them to come back next year when we might have an answer?

Granted this may constitute the proper scientific approach, but according to some estimates as much as 37 percent of the American public seeks alternative treatments, and as a group these people tend to be more educated and affluent than average ("Alternative Medicine" 1993, 11: 6). Although some practitioners might consider it neither personally nor financially discomfiting to turn away or even scoff at these people as a matter of principle, as their numbers continue to grow they will become harder and harder to ignore. Moreover, for many people alternatives comprise exactly that—*alternatives*, not total replacements for traditional medicine. The Shays still have faith in Dr. Kent as their veterinarian, but they have lost faith in his treatment(s) of their animal's condition. This subtle but critical distinction bears repeating:

Many clients who seek alternatives do so because they have lost faith in the *treatment*, not the veterinarian. Practitioners should keep this in mind when owners ask them about homeopathy, chiropractic, or the Bach flower remedies.

Another dilemma posed by alternative treatments centers around the troublesome question: If we must choose, to whom do we owe our allegiance—the animal or the owner? If we maintain strong beliefs about what constitutes an acceptable treatment and the owner desires to try something else in which they possess more faith, should we go along with this to please the client? Students or those practitioners in large, fully equipped facilities with access to a seemingly infinite supply of sanctioned treatments certainly could argue that no need exists to turn to an alternative. However, what about all those practitioners like Dr. Kent who lack such facilities and whose clients can't or won't drive miles for the latest science and technology, or who can't afford such care? When they ask Dr. Kent about using alternative therapies, should he turn his back on them saying, "I care too much about your animal to treat it that way and since I can't do anything more, I'm not going to do anything at all"? Or how about, "It's stupid and inhumane to subject an animal to that kind of treatment and I'll have no part of it"? Or maybe, "Go see some New Age crackpot if you like, but don't come crying to me if your animal doesn't get any better"? Clients who suggested alternative approaches got exactly such responses from their veterinarians.

Within an academic setting where client interaction may be tangential at best, one can easily maintain the illusion that veterinarians exist to meet the needs of their patients, and the animal and clinician form a dynamic duo for the purpose of establishing and maintaining the animal's health. However, in many other practice environments the duo gives way to a trinity of veterinarian, patient, and client, all of whose needs must be met simultaneously in order to maintain a stable relationship. If we place greater emphasis on the animal's needs than the owner's, we can lose the latter's faith and commitment, on which we must often depend for the success of the treatment process. If we care more about the owner, the animal might suffer; and if we subordinate our own needs, both the client and the patient may suffer even as we do.

When Dr. Kent insists on treating Ms. Shay's animal with yet another antibiotic, the owner's personal feelings about the drug cause her to cringe every time she administers it; not only does the animal recognize and soon anticipate her negative response, the owner periodically skips giving the medication to avoid the negative feelings doing so evokes. However, if Dr. Kent feels obligated to go along cheerfully with his client's request for an herbal remedy and the animal's condition deteriorates, the animal must bear the consequence of his desire to please his client. If Dr. Kent believes the Shays forced him to try the alternative, he may feel manipulated and resentful, both of which will negatively affect how he responds to the owners.

Faith and the Placebo Effect

Several times the role of faith in the treatment process has been raised, but it deserves closer scrutiny for those seeking to formulate a workable philosophy regarding the use of alternatives in practice. Obviously, if veterinarians do not believe that the patient's and client's faith plays any role in the healing process, then the only faith they need worry about is their own: As long as the practitioner believes in the treatment, his or her faith will carry the animal and owner through the process to a successful conclusion. However, if we believe we need our patients' and clients' faith as well as that in our own ability to successfully treat the animal, then the idea of treating an animal in a manner in which the client believes but we do not poses a major problem. At that point elements of ethics and morality as well as science and medicine come into play as we view the animal with the nonresponsive problem before us.

Previously, the concept of faith as the foundation of the healing process was proposed more as a matter of fact. However, does it *really* possess any validity in veterinary medicine? Can we know what faith means to an animal or owner any more than we can know what time means to a pig? To some extent a scientific analysis of the role of faith can be gained by reading the literature on the placebo effect. In their article on the use of placebos in veterinary medicine, Pesut and Kowalczyk traced the evolution of the term from its Latin roots meaning, "I shall please," to that of "a commonplace method or medicine" in *Quincy's Lexicon* in 1787, to that of an epithet attached to any medication given more to please than treat the patient (Pesut and Kowalczyk 1983, 182: 675). This change in definition accompanied the shift in the physician's belief in the patient as the center of the healing process to that of science as the cure. Thanks to the vast numbers of wounded and sick available during the French Revolution, by 1807 surgeons were elevated to the same level as physicians, specialists appeared, and faith in science rather than the patient became firmly entrenched in the practice of medicine (Burke 1985, 195–237).

Since that time, however, the tide has shifted again and studies of placebos have taken them out of the epithet category and elevated them to the level of a scientific curiosity and beyond. Nonetheless, cures that occur without the assistance of medical science still cause more consternation (and sometimes even resentment) within the majority of medical community than joy for the patient. However, practically all practitioners acknowledge that the patient's will to live plays a critical role in the treatment process. Unfortunately, though, many times we don't do this until our science fails: "I'm sorry, Ms. Shay," says Dr. Kent, "I did everything I could, but Elsie just gave up."

As mind-body studies gain credibility our awareness of how placebos work expands. Pavlov's and others' experiments with morphine demonstrated how, just as those famous dogs salivated when they heard that bell, animals previously treated with morphine grew sleepy and vomited as soon as they saw the researcher preparing the injection (Pesut and Kowalczyk 1983, 182: 677). More recent studies of endorphins and the nonaddictive pleasure center of the mid-brain offer other intriguing insights into the phenomenon (Levine et al. 1978, 2:654–57; Thomas 1992, 32–37). And most certainly the studies proving the intimate anatomical connection between the central nervous system and the immune response, as well as those proving how emotions affect the immune response for good or ill, show great promise (Berlfein 1988, 22:16; Cogan et al. 1987, 10:139-44; Pert et al. 1985, 135:820S-26S; Schleifer et al. 1983, 250:374–77). When we recall Gantt's study of the Effect of Person, Cornhill's low-cholesterol petted rabbits, and Robert Ader's ability to produce conditioned immune responses in animals using placebos (Ader and Suchman 1985, 8:379–426), it becomes increasingly difficult to rule out the critical role any patient's mind—regardless of species—plays in the treatment process.

Once we recognize the mind effect, then the idea of using placebos—those treatments some may define as scientifically useless or invalid—becomes a viable alternative. Although many veterinarians would claim never to use placebos, in fact many in practice routinely do. The use of antibiotics to treat viral infections falls into this category. Granted many clinicians would resist that definition saying they prescribe these drugs to the animal with clear nasal and ocular discharges to ward off any secondary bacterial attack, but the fact remains the animal doesn't have a bacterial infection and therefore the antibiotics serve no scientifically valid purpose. However, Dr. Kent dispenses them because the animal looks so miserable he as well as the owners feel he should do *something*.

Another variation on this theme—the use of antibiotics following sterile surgery—also places faith squarely in the center of the treatment process. In this case the practitioner lacks sufficient faith in some aspect of what should be a noninfectious procedure that he or she feels the need to prescribe medication "just in case." Perhaps Dr. Kent fears his new technician didn't prepare the animal or the instruments properly;

maybe he questions his own pre-op or surgical technique; perhaps he questions the animal's ability to keep the area clean, or the owner's ability to monitor its post-op recovery properly. In all these situations, personal feelings and intuition rather than science determine the treatment.

These cases bring up the fascinating—if troubling—possibility that *all* treatments incorporate placebo elements because the placebo effect amounts to no more or less than the physiological effects of faith. One physiology professor kept a bar of soap on top of a Bible among the scientific and medical texts on the shelves in his office. When students would ask the meaning of the unusual display, he said it symbolized the first principle of medicine: Cleanliness is next to godliness. In other words, faith in the body's ability to heal itself plays the most crucial role, cleanliness ranks number two, and medicine and surgery share the third position. Every time we perform a procedure or treat a patient "just in case," we use that procedure or treatment to compensate for a lack of faith in ourselves, the client, or the animal's ability to achieve or maintain a state of health. Unfortunately, some of us also use these to compensate for laziness and a disregard for the basic rules of cleanliness, too.

Does using a treatment to maintain or restore faith constitute practicing quality veterinary medicine? Although science may argue that a certain number of animals must respond a certain way to prove the efficacy of a certain treatment, all most clients care about is whether it works for them and their animals. Moreover, most practitioners take this view at one time or another. Many of us do dispense antibiotics to treat viral conditions or following anything but the most routine sterile surgery because it makes *us* feel better. We don't do this to flout science, but rather because every practitioner knows the power of the self-fulfilling prophecy. Just as Dr. Kent knows that the animal which belongs to the client who worries about its sutures becoming infected will more likely experience this problem, so he knows from experience that once the thought of secondary bacterial infection crosses his mind—and even if no logical evidence supporting such a thought exists—he had better cover the animal with antibiotics.

Similarly, we see timid animals who barely can cope with normal existence or that increasing population of purebreds of all species who lack even the most rudimentary awareness of self-grooming and cleanliness in addition to often precarious immune responses, and we reach for treatments we know we shouldn't need given the medical definition of the problem. No doubt if we didn't treat them, scientifically speaking we could prove that the treatment would have served no purpose and we did the right thing; that is, only a certain small, perhaps even statistically insignificant percentage of them would succumb to illness. However, a reality of practice is that when the scientists' statistically insignificant percentage of the total population turns out to be 100 percent of the Shays' cow or cat, the science doesn't carry a lot of weight with the client or the practitioner, to say nothing of the animal. For those who have encountered even one such case, the belief that "useless" prophylactic treatment could have prevented the problem remains both very real and very strong. Consequently, even though science may argue that we treat these animals in that manner for ourselves and the clients, most of us also believe we do it for the animal.

But are we deluding ourselves when we believe that those treatments that science says don't work *do* work for us and our patients? The answer to this question lies in the answer to another. What is the practitioner's purpose? To make the animal better—or perhaps more correctly, to attend the animal's recovery—or to fulfill scientific process? For those who believe their purpose is to fulfill the scientific process of veterinary medicine, then obviously only those approaches sanctioned by that science possess any validity. The more objective practitioners who maintain this view share the sentiments expressed by one academic during the early days of acupuncture: "I'm not saying it doesn't work. I'm saying it can't." In other words, these people believe that if the treatment doesn't fit the definitions and rules of veterinary medicine, it cannot exist. Because virtually all placebos and alternatives require new definitions and rules, and because the scientific method practically mandates that these evolve from the old, we can see why official approval of many of these may be years away.

When to Use Alternatives

If we see our purpose as helping the animal regain and/or maintain its health rather than fulfilling process, then it seems that any treatment which accomplishes that purpose is valid. Most practitioners who use alternatives do so for two reasons:

- Traditional approaches aren't working in a particular case or type of case.
- The client requests an alternative.

Because the use of an alternative—be it an herb, prophylactic antibiotic, extra-label use of a traditional drug, or self-styled variation in an established surgical procedure—immediately puts us in a precarious position relative to the law as well as science, we need to approach these situations as objectively as possible. For example, before Dr. Kent considers using an alternative when traditional approaches fail to achieve the desired results, he owes it to himself, his patient, and his client to review every step of the process that led him to this conclusion:

- Was a thorough history taken?
- Was the physical examination thorough?
- Were the proper diagnostic procedures accomplished and their results interpreted properly?
- Was the proper treatment properly prescribed?
- Did the animal receive the treatment as prescribed?

Put another way, Dr. Kent can't say the treatment didn't work if he didn't know what he was treating and/or the animal didn't get the treatment. On the other hand, if conditions are such that he and his client believe he took the traditional approach as far as he could and must either abort the treatment process or use an alternative, then it would seem more caring to opt for the alternative.

Most practitioners who use alternatives do not set out to flout the system. More often than not, they find themselves in a situation like that of Dr. Kent, who felt he had done everything possible to diagnose and treat Ms. Shay's cat's intermittent diarrhea within the limits she imposed. The owner tearfully tells him she must get rid of the animal if a cure can't be found because she can't have the cat soiling everywhere with two toddlers in the household: Isn't there anything else he can try?

The scientific approach says that, if Ms. Shay really cared about the cat, she'd drive the 150 miles to the nearest teaching hospital and spend however much necessary to solve the problem "right." However, and like many in private practice, Dr. Kent doesn't recognize this as the only viable solution, nor even the most common one. The majority of his clients depend on him as their sole source of care for their animals. If he doesn't provide it, his clients will turn to others for that service—not because they don't care about their animals, but because they do.

Consequently, Dr. Kent looks at his tearful client and the big cat cheerfully batting his hand and recalls the colleague he met at the last state meeting who almost furtively mentioned she had started to use homeopathic remedies in some cases in which she had taken traditional medicine as far as she could or the client would allow. He tentatively suggests this approach to Ms. Shay, sharing all his skepticism as well as his belief that the treatment will do the animal no harm and might do it some good for reasons he doesn't understand. Ms. Shay says that anything is worth a try and, feeling somewhat like Adam in the Garden of Eden about to reach for that apple, Dr. Kent picks up the phone and calls his colleague. She describes her experiences, suggests articles and books for him to read, and gives him the names of other practitioners to call for additional information.

As with all treatments, the probability of any alternative curing an animal is fifty-fifty: It either works or it doesn't. However, treatments can work in more ways than one. Ideally the animal's symptoms resolve in a time period coincident with or sufficiently close to the treatment period that the clinician and client believe the treatment cured the condition rather than just happened to be present in the animal's body when its immune response handled the problem. Most practitioners prefer this form because it most closely fits our training which identifies us as the *source* of the cure. Granted, whenever the issue of alternatives that work is raised, skeptics inevitably argue that they only seem to work because the animal would have gotten better anyhow, but this same probability also may affect the efficacy of traditional treatments, too. The reality for Dr. Kent and Ms. Shay remains that those traditional treatments either didn't work or didn't happen to be on the scene when the animal healed itself, and because of this the veterinarian and client sought an alternative approach.

However, treatments also work even if they don't work in a physiological sense. Even though Dr. Kent's first homeopathic remedy doesn't improve the cat's condition, the fact that the veterinarian is willing to consider alternatives convinces Ms. Shay to keep the animal. In this situation we could go so far as to say the alternative saved the animal's life even though it failed to cure the diarrhea. While perhaps a blasphemous notion from the scientific view, the idea that the practitioner cares, not only about the animal but also about the owner and any limitations he or she might bring to the treatment process, can carry a tremendous amount of weight. Moreover this often translates into enhanced regard for and faith in the veterinarian and, consequently, any treatment that person might propose.

Clients Who Prefer Alternatives

In addition to more or less accidently falling into the use of alternatives when traditional approaches don't work, practitioners see increasingly more clients who bring up the subject as the result of their own experiences. Ms. Corcoron's physician recommends a mostly vegetarian diet and she wonders if it would benefit her pets as much as it benefited her; Mr. Burrows experiences a negative reaction to steroids and doesn't want any used on his animals. In these situations, the ability to communicate with the client again becomes critical. Ms. Corcoron and Mr. Burrows both need reliable information from someone sympathetic to their concerns. Ms. Corcoron doesn't need diatribes against the evils of vegetarianism; she needs solid facts about if and how she can incorporate her vegetarian beliefs into her pets' diets. Nor will Mr. Burrows appreciate Dr. Kent's statistics that prove his fears groundless because he knows what he experienced and has already decided no animal of his will ever receive steroids. He doesn't want statistics; he wants information about alternatives to these drugs.

When clients raise the issue of alternatives, quality communication may lead the client to accept the traditional approach or the clinician to accept an alternative one. Many problems arise when veterinarians maintain rigid beliefs and consider it their duty to *make* their clients see things that same way. If Dr. Kent sees himself as a source of objective data as opposed to his client's emotional New Age ravings, he'll respond quite emotionally—and negatively—and alienate that person.

As noted previously, practitioners never should do anything that violates their beliefs. However, it makes more sense for those who do not believe in alternatives to recognize their clients' beliefs as different rather than wrong because then they can refer them to others in a professional manner. Doing so acknowledges the clients' reality as valid for them if not necessarily for the practitioner. Second, and more important, it doesn't alienate the client. Rather than putting good manners above good science, this creates one major positive effect: By supporting these clients, we remain available to assist them and their animals if problems arise.

Compare the following scenarios:

- Dr. Kent tells Ms. Shay her ideas about alternatives are stupid and she responds angrily and seeks out the help of a budding herbalist in the next county. When the well-meaning but inexperienced person prescribes the wrong herbs and the animal's condition worsens, Ms. Shay feels she can't turn to Dr. Kent for help. Not only does she feel embarrassed, she sees him as the cause of her problem. After all, if he had cured her animal, she wouldn't have needed to seek help elsewhere.
- Dr. Kent tells Ms. Shay he personally has no faith in herbal remedies, but he gives her the name of another practitioner he

knows with an interest in alternative approaches. Or, if he doesn't know such a person, he calls or refers his client to the American Holistic Veterinary Medical Association for a possible reference in the area.

In the first scenario, Dr. Kent keeps his principles, loses a client, and possibly jeopardizes the animal's health on two fronts. First, by not taking an active role in helping his client find a competent practitioner with knowledge of the alternative's veterinary applications, he contributes to the animal's treatment by a less-than-qualified person. Second, by alienating Ms. Shay, he makes it extremely difficult for her to ask him for help when problems arise. Once again, we might say that his response constitutes good science and even good (traditional) medicine, but is it good veterinary practice? Ms. Shay would undoubtedly say no and we anthropomorphically may assume her now sicker animal would agree. Dr. Kent, like each of us, must answer for himself.

The Ideal versus the Real

Regardless of whether they view the ideal as using only those procedures and techniques sanctioned by those they consider valid authorities or adopt a "whatever works" approach, practitioners once again can save themselves a lot of mental anguish by working out their personal feelings about alternatives in advance. Those who do not support their use should be able to articulate clearly and unemotionally to their clients why they maintain this view. They should also decide if and to whom they want to refer those clients who do not share their views. Above all, they should avoid taking an adversarial stance on the issue. Even though many choose to define such an approach as justifiable indignation, most clients perceive it as overreaction and fear, and those veterinarians who believe they represent the highest standards of the profession wind up looking less than professional.

Those who feel alternatives pose valid adjuncts to the practice of quality medicine must decide which, if any, of these alternatives to pursue themselves and which to refer to others within and outside the profession. Those who decide to develop these skills will find colleagues with similar interests and the aforementioned American Holistic Veterinary Medical Association invaluable sources of information and support. Those who support the concept but prefer to refer these clients to others should follow the same procedures discussed in the preceding chapter. Although always a consideration, the recognition that anyone to whom a practitioner refers a client serves as a reflection of that veterinarian becomes particularly important when dealing with nontraditional approaches.

Chapter 14
The Art of Animal Rights

Listening to a group of veterinarians talk about animal rights immediately brings to mind the tale of the three blind men trying to describe an elephant based on that part of the animal's anatomy they could feel from where they stood. Just as the number of animal rights organizations has almost doubled in the last twenty years, so has the number of professional and lay articles and books addressing the issue ("ALF Claims Research Raid" 1992, 4; "All They Are Sayin'" 1989, 106:15; Arkow 1987, 191:937–42; Boyce 1993, 203:356–57; "Committee on the Use of Animals in Medicine" 1991; Coniff 1990, 92:120–32; Jasper and Nelkin 1992; Kronfeld and Parr 1987, 191:660–64; Morris 1991; Ritvo 1982, 95:54–62; Rollin 1981; Singer 1975; Tannenbaum 1986, 188:1258–63 and 1991, 198:1360–1376).

Unfortunately, more than a few in the veterinary profession feel obligated to take an either/or position in a battle that pits adherents of animal "welfare" against those of "rights" as defined by the American Veterinary Medical Association in *The Veterinarian's Role in Animal Welfare*:

> Animal welfare is a human responsibility that encompasses all aspects of animal well-being, including proper housing, management, nutrition, disease prevention and treatment, responsible care, humane handling and, when necessary, humane euthanasia.
> Animal rights is a philosophical view and personal value characterized by various animal rights groups. (1993, 1)

While this part of the elephant appears relatively straightforward, anyone in practice knows it means little to the general public who see the two terms as inextricably intertwined and often use them interchangeably. Beliefs regarding the rights of animals determine beliefs regarding animal welfare and vice versa; to denigrate or elevate one is to denigrate or elevate the other. As one client put it, "Why would anyone bother providing proper housing, nutrition, and veterinary care to something they believed possessed no rights?"

Perhaps the reason the subject strikes such an emotional chord within the profession is that it, like the bond and the alternative approaches, doesn't adhere to the linear rules of science. Although some feel the only route to validity involves somehow shoehorning animal rights into those rules to come up with the equivalent of normal bovine rectal temperature or canine blood values, most clients don't care whether it fits those rules or not. Each person maintains his or her own set of beliefs regarding what constitutes his or her specific animal's as well as other animals' rights, even as they maintain other beliefs that determine what constitutes animal health, illness, or suffering. For practitioners, problems arise when these beliefs conflict with our own or we haven't taken the time to work through our own beliefs so we can respond to others objectively.

Veterinarians can and do meet clients who consider themselves animal rights advocates and can produce the proper membership cards to prove this. Moreover, more and more veterinarians belong to such organizations, too. However, the majority of both clients and practitioners—regardless of any memberships—maintains often very specific views about animal rights that represent a synthesis of science and philosophy and often form a flexible fusion capable of changing at a moment's notice in response to the increasingly complex real world of human-animal interactions.

Common Views toward Animal Rights

Most people assign animals rights as a function of their own beliefs and experiences with animals rather than as a result of any methodical thought process. This seems logical because we can only guess what a cow or dog, let alone a red eft or garter snake, considers its legal or moral rights. And just as our orientations toward animals may vacillate between anthropomorphic, chattel, and integrated views depending on the species, individual, and circumstance, so our views regarding animal rights may fluctuate wildly. When questioned carefully, it turns out that the neighbor whose car sports the "I brake for animals" bumper sticker really only brakes seriously for mammals and birds, only reluctantly for small rodents, and never for rats. Another who professes no species bias admits that her adherence to this principle depends on visibility and her driving speed; a walk down her road one rainy spring day reveals a whole population of dead frogs, newts, and other small animals whose existence, let alone rights, she never acknowledged as real.

What rights people ascribe to animals fall into three general categories that reflect their beliefs about themselves as well as—and maybe more than—animals:

- Animals possess more rights than I do.
- Animal possess the same rights as I do.
- Those animals to which I attribute rights possess those similar to the ones I attribute to my own animals.

The idea of assigning an animal more rights than claimed for oneself seems incomprehensible until we consider what potent symbols animals have become in our society. Perhaps the most dramatic example of this is the oft-told tale of the gray whales trapped under the ice off Point Barrow, Alaska. In the overall evolutionary scheme of things, animals—like people—who make unwise choices should bear the responsibility for those choices. However, most of us believe or want to believe in the existence of some Almighty Force(s) which will assume responsibility for us when we err, and we project this belief onto the animal kingdom. That three-week, million-dollar effort that drove off predators and eliminated all the other negative consequences of a less-than- prudent whale choice appealed to that part of us that wants to believe in miracles. As one adherent of this orientation noted, "If it happened to those whales, maybe someday it will happen to me, too."

Those who adopt this orientation see animal rights as a combination eternal happy life and health insurance policy, a state of bliss beyond human capacity that many would like to claim for themselves. They believe that all animals have the right to a perfect life in a perfect environment (the definitions of which vary greatly) and state-of-the-art care. If the people these advocates hold responsible for the animals' care don't meet these expectations, they accuse them of violating the animals' rights.

As clients, these individuals' emotional and sometimes messianic approach can prove a major irritant to the practitioner who lacks a clear philosophy of animal rights. However, most of these people do not see themselves that way at all. Dr. Kennedy is the most educated, professional "animal person" activist Cindy Schaeffer knows, and she wants to know what he thinks because she sees his views reflecting those of an otherwise inaccessible scientific, medical, and food-animal-owning community. If he criticizes her for failing to differentiate between animal rights and welfare, she will consider his response pompous and esoteric at best, and irrelevant and intimidating at worst. If he responds angrily or dismisses her concerns, she will only become more antagonistic.

More commonly, people assign their own rights to animals, and their definitions of these may vary greatly. Because polls label the majority of those associated with the animal rights movement as white, affluent, educated women, this often creates the false impression that animal rights advocates want to give animals white, upper-middle-class rights. In reality, the rights attributed to animals by the inner-city teenager differ from those of the Cape Cod yuppie gallery owner and those of the aging hippie writer in Montana; nonetheless all three consider themselves animal rights proponents. Because these people assign human rights to animals, not surprisingly many who fall into this category tend to take a more anthropomorphic view toward their own animals. Consequently, successfully communicating with them requires an appreciation of the owner's needs as well as the animal's and species' under discussion.

Veterinarians who lack knowledge regarding a specific species or use of animals should resist any temptation to bluff their way through any confrontation with people of this orientation because they, too, can be quite proficient when it comes to amassing data that support their position. Far better for Dr. Kennedy to admit he knows little about factory farming and request copies of Ms. Schaeffer's data to review. Sometimes simply expressing a willingness to consider a different view satisfies these people; other times practitioners do the research necessary to formulate their own views, which they then share with their clients. Although some may consider this a waste of time, those who use this approach believe that, in the long run, it saves them time because it gives them a broader view of the problem as well as enables them to maintain a more stable relationship with the client.

The third and most common view of animal rights shares much in common with the integrated view of animals. As long as the animals—both domestic and wild—remain within the physical, mental, and emotional boundaries the person imposes, they live in harmony; if an animal or species exceeds these, the person feels justified in forcing it to play by human rules. Dr. Kennedy grants his family pets, cattle, chickens, and horses rights to what he considers a quality life as long as they behave in a manner that does not threaten the health or safety of his family. He can easily expand this definition to include various wild creatures which appeal to him for one reason or another. However he feels no obligation to spiders, which he dislikes for purely emotional reasons and in spite of the fact that one of his clients considers them the most special inhabitants of the animal kingdom.

Patient Rights

Once we gain an appreciation for the wide range of complex views people hold toward the subject of animal rights, we need to consider what, if any, role these rights play in the treatment process. Of all written on the subject of animal rights, Jacob Antelyes's "Animal Rights in Perspective" most profoundly addresses the world of the private practitioner. According to Antelyes (1986, 189:757–59), all animals, regardless of their commercial value or the wealth and status of their owners, have a right to:

• Respect
• Food and water
• Privacy
• Freedom from avoidable pain
• Purposeful death

Of all the rights of animals and especially patients, respect looms as the most important. Interestingly, a strange paradox has emerged with the move to replace live animals in the veterinary curriculum with inanimate models and computer simulations. No matter how we look at it, neither of these can elicit the awe and respect inherent in exposure to the living animal. Inevitably the plastic models get picked up by bored students and tossed around or poked at in frustration as they try to remember the names of obscure anatomical features. Unlike living animals, models and computer simulations can be put back on the shelf or turned off when we get tired: We don't need to worry about feeding and exercising them, monitoring their recovery from anesthesia, or dealing with the messy emotions that attend the euthanasia of an experimental animal. Neither models nor computer simulations possess distinct personalities and behaviors that make us evaluate our own feelings about animals in general and this one in particular, a tragic loss of learning experience for those who intend to enter private practice. Neither of these alternatives possess owners whose beliefs and emotions can scramble the animal's physiology and behavior to an incredible degree, so we can maintain a view of medicine as static and linearly predictable rather than dynamic and often up for grabs thanks to the owner's—and our own—beliefs and limitations. And finally, neither of these alternatives can begin to duplicate what goes through the mind when all these subjective factors converge as that knife cuts through the linea alba and we view all that miraculous anatomy and physiology, not only in terms of our scientific and medical responsibility to it, but also in terms of our responsibility to the owner and to that animal as a unique being far greater than its component parts.

Granted, the use of such alternatives spares animals mistreatment by uncaring individuals, but this would seem to raise a much more troubling issue: How did such people get into the veterinary curriculum in the first place?

Every animal that comes under the care of a practitioner has a right to that person's respect as well as the respect of everyone associated with it in the treatment process. As Antelyes puts it so eloquently:

> *The patient displays the awesome miracle of being alive. This very life, marred by infirmity, qualifies it for dignified nursing care and medical attention, delivered with decency and sincerity. Limitations notwithstanding, respect for the living animal is paramount.* (Antelyes 1986, 189:758)

The Patient's Right to Food and Water

From the veterinarian's point of view, an animal's right to food and water usually means providing a well-balanced diet that best meets that particular animal's needs, and access to clean, fresh water at all times. However, for all animals and particularly the ill or injured, providing even the best quality food and the purest water constitutes only half of our obligation; we must also insure that the animal eats the food and drinks the water.

Such a consideration seems obvious, yet we need only recall all those small animal problems that can be traced to injudicious owner feeding practices or read Fraser and Broom's *Farm Animal Behavior and Welfare* (1990) to realize how human and animal behavioral responses can stymie this process. Spot's owners buy him the finest dog food and religiously offer him the proper amount as directed by Dr. Kennedy. When the dog gains weight, they offer him the highest quality low-calorie diet, and then the finest therapeutic diet when his obesity results in medical problems, both as directed by their veterinarian. Throughout this nutritionally sound sequence, the owners continue feeding their pet ice cream, pizza and other foods from their own plates to keep his spirits up. Meanwhile some farm animals offered the highest quality foods barely get by because neither the farmer nor Dr. Kennedy notice the social dynamics in the flock or herd that determine who gets to eat what, when.

It falls within the responsibility of practitioners to insure that at least those sick animals under their care receive proper nourishment. Unfortunately, and often for the sake of convenience, the science of practice again displaces its art. If the congested cat doesn't eat, we ignore the fact that its appetite strongly depends on its sense of smell as well as its sense of territorial security and we reach for a drug instead. Protocols involving intravenous feeding and other forms of artificial alimentation immediately fill our minds when clients or technicians utter the words "not eating," rather than a critical analysis of the many subjective as well as medical factors inherent in this phrase.

All these views of food and water consumption overlook the critical need and right of the patient to good nursing care and the practitioner's responsibility to provide for that. A conscientious technician or owner can do more to stimulate the appetite and insure the proper nutrition of an injured or ill animal than any drug. However, if practitioners define the feeding and watering rights of animals to mean offering food and water twice a day and giving IVs or appetite stimulants to those who don't eat or drink within a certain interval, the idea of hand-feeding, doing what we can to make the animals feel more secure, or allowing owners to visit hospitalized patients will seem excessive and a waste of valuable time.

Regardless of whether we take a pharmacological or behavioral approach to eating and drinking or a combination of the two, every patient deserves to be discharged from our care capable of eating and drinking on its own or assisted by someone instructed in the proper techniques to insure the fulfillment of this basic right.

The Right to Privacy

Veterinary medicine takes the same if not a more cavalier attitude toward patient privacy as human medicine. Although we say we hospitalize animals to facilitate their recovery, just as often it's to facilitate our treatment of them; it's much more convenient to have them confined to an area where we can work on them as it fits our schedule. The idea of saying, "Let's hold off taking Snoopy's blood until he wakes up from his nap" sounds as ludicrous to most veterinarians as it does to most physicians: We don't have time to let the needs of the patient interfere with the process of medicine. In fact, every veterinarian to whom the author mentioned the idea of waiting for an animal to wake up couldn't imagine why anyone would want to do such a thing. Rather than being uncaring, however, just the opposite held true: To them "waking up" referred to recovery from anesthesia. It never crossed their minds that an animal might be sleeping because it needed rest.

If we see making the patient better as our purpose, we should grant animals privacy for three reasons. First, although more convenient for us, hospitalization is a stress for most animals above and beyond that created by any illness or injury from which they may suffer. All animals are territorial and taking them out of familiar surroundings and confining them in a strange environment often produces an energy-consuming fear response and all the negative physiological changes that accompany that.

Second, whether social or solitary in nature, few animals readily adapt to the presence of other animals until they have had the opportunity to collect sufficient sensory data not only to identify the others but also to position themselves relative to them. Barring this opportunity, they exist in a state of behavioral suspension. More submissive animals huddle, fearing reprisal from the more dominant occupant of the stall or cage beside or above them; more dominant ones may try to assert their authority from a distance, with some going so far as to attempt to spray the cage doors on either side or urinating on other cages as they pass them. Lacking a clear idea of their position, many animals will not eat or drink; and more dominant ones may pace restlessly—if space allows—while more submissive ones may tremble and try to hide.

Third, in "Animal Behavior and the Fever Response," veterinary behaviorist Benjamin Hart notes that fever, anorexia, and depression play critical physiological as well as behavioral functions in the healing process, permitting the body to focus all its energy on getting well (Hart 1985a, 187:998–1001). For those schooled in a tradition that perceives fever, anorexia, and depression as signs of disease rather than a coordinated beneficial response of a healthy body to disease and behavior of little or no consequence in the healing process, the idea of providing animals with security and privacy to focus on recovery probably seems inconsequential. However, all animals have a right not to be stressed by other animals and untrained or uncaring people just as they have a right to clean, well-ventilated quarters.

Reduction of stress and increased privacy for companion animals may be achieved by putting boxes, large bags, or even small kennels in cages to provide havens for frightened animals. Admission forms that list other animals in the household can provide clues to the patient's likely response to those of the same or different species and these can be taken into account when housing these animals; many cats find hospitalization with dogs less stressful than that with other cats. Draping the fronts of cages housing very dominant or submissive animals also will help relieve environmental stress. Finally, dimming the lights in the wards when not needed addresses the right of animals to privacy and may produce benefits for the staff as well. Veterinarians who use this technique note that both they and their employees find walking through these wards a very peaceful respite from the bright lights and activity of the treatment room and surgery.

The Right to Freedom from Avoidable Pain

It goes without saying that every animal deserves prompt relief from pain by the most effective means possible. A rather sad consequence of the fusion of the animal rights movement with the scientific approach to medicine has resulted in a trend toward the increased use of pharmacological analgesics at a time when awareness of the mind-body connection leads more and more in human medicine to move away from them (Campos 1989, 60:781–92; Grant 1987, 21:21; Kehoe and Blass 1986, 100:624–30; Philips 1987, 25:365–77; Schwartz 1991, 266:3064). Numerous studies link the perception of pain to fear (Arntz et al. 1990, 28:29–41; "Comforting Words" 1991, 6:1; Gutfield et al. 1991, 43:18; Long 1986, 20:28; Miller 1986, 20:83); to remove the pain but do nothing to address the underlying fear treats the symptom but not the cause. Other studies indicate a wide variation in individual response to pain and that most patients given control over their medication take less than the clinician would prescribe. This results because patients who feel more in control experience less fear and hence less pain, and clinicians tend to prescribe higher dosages because they fear the patient's pain response—or rather the implications of it relative to their skill (Berntzen and Gotestam 1987, 55:213–17; Litt 1988, 54:149–60; Parker et al. 1991, 266:1947; Radnitz et al. 1988, 26:253–60).

Similarly, we must question the wisdom of removing self-limiting pain: It may make us and the owner feel better that the animal with the fractured leg appears oblivious to its condition—until it overtaxes the limb and complicates the injury, or underestimates its ability to maneuver and falls and hurts itself again.

Third, all painkilling substances possess their own pharmacology, which must be factored into the treatment process: Does the analgesic serve a beneficial purpose if it removes pain but taxes a compromised liver or kidneys or interferes with the effect of other medication?

The most troubling consequence of an increased dependency on the use of pharmacological analgesics, however, is far more insidious and detrimental to the healing process. Compare these two clinical situations:

- Dr. Kennedy completes his surgery and injects the patient with an analgesic as part of his post-op routine. After the animal recovers sufficiently from anesthesia, his technician puts it back in the cage or pen and both she and Dr. Kennedy feel secure in the knowledge that it will experience no discomfort.
- Dr. Kennedy completes his surgery and after the animal recovers sufficiently from anesthesia, his technician puts it back in its cage or pen. Throughout the day, Dr. Kennedy and other members of the staff check on the animal, petting or stroking it and giving it words of encouragement, rearranging or replacing bedding, and doing other small things to make it more comfortable. Those from the office staff routinely spend their breaks in the wards, offering words of comfort and reassurance. As soon as the animal is ambulatory, the technician helps it learn the limitations of its condition and how to avoid discomfort by not exceeding those limits. Her knowledge of animal behavior enables her to choose exactly the right tone of voice to convey support and encouragement rather than pity, and she or Dr. Kennedy instructs owners how to do likewise.

This in no way means analgesics do not serve a purpose in veterinary medicine. It does mean that each animal has a right to have its response to pain evaluated individually and both the behavioral and physiological aspects of that pain addressed in a caring manner. Granted, it takes much less time to perceive and treat pain as a strictly physiological phenomenon, but those who say they can't spare the time or that they take this approach out of their concern for the animals would be wise to review the growing body of literature that questions this orientation. If we put this in the context of granting animals rights equal to those we would claim for ourselves, which form of pain medication is the most comforting: An injection or pill, or the companionship of a supportive individual? As human patients vote for the presence of their dogs over their physicians, it would be a shame to perceive a strictly pharmacological approach to pain control as a triumph for animal rights.

The Right to a Meaningful Death

Death and euthanasia are almost anathema to the traditional medical educational process yet play such a critical role in veterinary practice that they will be discussed in detail in Chapters 16 and 17. At this point, we will only consider one often overlooked implication of the animal rights movement that deserves attention because of its ramifications for those in practice.

If we perceive animals as possessing rights equal to our own, then euthanizing animals puts us in the position of euthanizing the moral equivalent of another human being. Consequently, we can appreciate why many veterinarians who feel this way refuse to euthanize animals, saying it violates the animal's rights. However, those who take this approach must take it the next logical step: What will happen to this animal if Dr. Kennedy doesn't euthanize it? Will it suffer needlessly from a condition the owner cannot or will not treat? Does his choice not to euthanize the animal include a moral responsibility to treat it at no cost if the owners cannot afford to do so? What if he tells the owners to find a home for an animal with behavioral problems and they say they tried, but couldn't? Isn't it his responsibility to find a home for that animal or take it in himself? What if he, with all his training and experience, tells them that, if they want the animal killed, they should take it to the local shelter where the job could very well be done by an overworked, underpaid person in limited facilities using less than optimum procedures and drugs? Doesn't that violate the animal's rights? Or what if the owners abandon the animal because the landlord will evict them if they don't get rid of it?

The troubling nature of these questions in no way undermines a need to respect the rights of animals. On the contrary, it points out that of all human beliefs we project on animals, none looms so great as the fear of death. Consequently, as concern for animal rights continues to increase and because euthanasia remains a fact of life, practitioners should recognize how their beliefs about animal rights affect their response to this aspect of practice. We cannot refuse to euthanize an animal saying this violates its rights, then condemn it to an environment that violates its right to respect, food and water, privacy, and/or freedom from avoidable pain and fear.

Finally, we must realize that clients expect the veterinarian to show the proper respect for the dead animal and the rights they assign to that animal whether the practitioner's view of animal rights coincides with theirs or not. Without a doubt and whether we speak of companion or food animals or anthropomorphically or chattel-oriented owners, nothing so upsets clients as the feeling that the veterinarian did not show proper respect for the dead or dying animal, even if these people did not overtly show it themselves. They expect such respect from of us and morally it would seem that they and their animals deserve it.

Animal Rights and the Food Animal Client

Of all practitioners, those who work with food animals need the most comprehensive and tolerant view of animal rights because, like laboratory animal practitioners, they will attract more than their share of animal rights activists. In the case of food animals, this may result from these predominantly urban advocates' perception of all domestic animals as companion animals. Whatever their thinking, their focus on food animals will continue to increase, and practitioners and their food animal clients either can passively react or actively respond to these and other individuals concerned with animal rights.

Unfortunately, more than a few active responses to the movement rely on that aforementioned enigmatic differentiation between "welfare" and "rights," which is more likely to perpetuate or enhance the distance between food animal producers and animal rights advocates than resolve any issues. Recall how Cindy Schaeffer considered Dr. Kennedy's discourse on the subject obscure as well as patronizing. Worse, in her mind his definitions of "welfare" and "rights" translated "no rights" and "rights," which to her meant he believes animals can claim no rights at all. However Dr. Kennedy *does* grant animals rights—and probably more than most people—but he gets so caught up in his food animal clients' them-against-us mode and his own politically correct definitions when he encounters the likes of Ms. Schaeffer, he forgets all about this.

To become involved in such us-against-them battles and support similar attitudes in food animal clients would seem an unwise professional approach for several reasons. First, as the movement attracts more and more people, it leads more and more away from meat as a primary protein source for philosophical reasons. Moreover, it seems unlikely that the defeat of any animal rights legislation will alter this trend because the philosophical change has already occurred. In fact, it could be argued that such a defeat actually would gain more anti-meat converts because the media most likely would portray the adversarial stance as animal lovers against insensitive, bottom-line agribusinessmen and those veterinarians who chose to support the latter's view. Because the public traditionally has perceived those in our profession as animal lovers—and our professional organizations have made every effort to capitalize on and promote this image—an antagonistic response of a few could have major consequences for the entire profession.

Further fueling the trend away from meat eating is that growing body of studies linking this to health problems (Raloff 1990, 138:74; Sussman 1990, 109:67; Willet et al. 1990; 323:1664–73). When we add the public concern about contamination of the food supply as well as studies that raise the disturbing possibility that prophylactic or injudicious use of antibiotics may lead to the presence of resistant pathogens in our meat and poultry supply, alternative protein sources gain appeal (Belongia et al. 1993, 269:883; Centers for Disease Control 1992, 267:3263 and 1993, 269:2194; Freese 1993, 202:1733–34; Hunter 1991, 74:8; Kaneene and Miller 1992, 201:68–76; Lance et al. 1992, 201:864–68; Lautner 1993, 202:1727–29; Wilkes 1993, 202:1725–27). Granted, Dr. Kennedy could make a concerted effort to refute this data, but it pervades the general as well as professional literature and would seem a costly, time-consuming endeavor with no guarantee of any positive results.

Finally, and most important, denying the reality of the situation denies food animal clients a valued and trusted source of objective information at the time they need it most. Rather than commiserating about the raw deal the industry is getting from animal rights groups, the human medical community, and the media, it would seem to make more sense for Dr. Kennedy to help his clients find viable alternatives.

Among these, the concept of using these animals to produce bio-genetically engineered substances (as opposed to organs for transplants) looms as a viable possibility. Although such use carries its own animal rights implications, the negative human response is not nearly as strong as that elicited by the idea of raising animals for slaughter or the negative health benefits of meat. In fact, most emotional responses toward these products focus far more on their effects on humans rather than their effects on animals because the very value of these animals as producers earns them a quality of life far superior to that of most used for food production.

To be sure, such use of food animals would require Dr. Kennedy to develop new skills as well as the philosophy to go with them. However, so did the introduction of artificial insemination and ova transplants and he can still remember how inflexible and unrealistic he considered a former employer who dismissed these as a "passing fad."

Regardless of whether practitioners counsel their food animal clients to mount aggressive campaigns for a viable share of a shrinking market by maintaining the highest standards of food animal husbandry and management or to diversify, the fact remains that food animal veterinarians can't afford to become embroiled in messy confrontations about animal rights or support their clients' anti-animal rights attitudes out of a sense of loyalty or fear of change. They serve as far too valuable a source of information to both their clients and the public to try to recreate a bygone era when the future holds so many exciting personal and professional challenges.

Chapter 15
The Art of Treating Critical Illness and Injury

When critical illness or injury befalls an animal all the factors previously discussed come into play, and often dramatically so. Simultaneously, for many veterinarians the successful treatment of the critically ill or injured animal serves as the professional raison d'être. The instant the owner holding that limp body rushes into Dr. Collins's waiting room, the instant he sees that severely depressed prize Jersey, the adrenalin starts to flow and his mind fills with presumptive diagnoses, diagnostic procedures, and treatments. By the time he finishes his examination of the animal, all these thoughts and impressions have arranged them-selves into a coherent plan. In these situations, he feels challenged to use all of his knowledge much more than when he vaccinates a healthy animal or treats a routine milk fever or lameness.

Perhaps because critical illnesses and injuries cause us to summon such a vast amount of scientific and technological knowledge, the clients and their needs can get lost in the shuffle. "After all," Dr. Collins tells himself, "I'm involved in a life-and-death struggle here. I can't be bothered with useless chatter. Besides, I'm doing this *for them*." Is it any wonder he feels confused and angry when he discovers his clients don't share this view?

A general rule for client interaction may be stated thus:

The amount of client interaction must increase proportionately with the complexity of the problem, the cost of the treatment, and the expectations of the client and the clinician.

Although most practitioners readily would accept this as a sensible course to follow, in fact just the opposite often holds true. The more complex the case, the more we focus on its science and technology and the less on client issues. Ask practitioners to describe their idea of the perfect owner of a critically ill or injured animal and many will say it's someone who tells them to do everything possible and then leaves them alone to do it. Nonetheless, a review of cases in which communication breaks down to the point of legal action against the veterinarian or to collect fees reveals the obvious converse of the above: Clients become increasingly intolerant of what they consider a lack of quality interaction as the procedures on their animals become more complex and the expectations greater (Dinsmore and McConnell 1992, 201:383). And even as our science and technology enable us to cure more conditions than ever before, we also must bear in mind that it also enables us to maintain life in what some would consider a less than optimal state.

Initial Client Contact

If we imagine ourselves in the instant we first encounter a critically ill or injured animal, the idea of taking time to talk to the owner may seem alien to the point of malpractice. However, this initial contact serves two purposes.

- It provides us with necessary information about the animal.
- It serves as a means whereby we gain the owner's acceptance and commitment to the treatment process.

The most clinically perfect examination gains Dr. Collins nothing if he can't communicate his findings to the Gormans in a manner that enables them to comprehend the value of the proposed treatment for their dog, Ziggy. And if they don't comprehend the value of it, naturally the idea of paying for it won't appeal to them. Nonetheless, the idea of assuming center stage with the animal and shuttling the distraught owners off to the periphery may loom so strongly as a part of normal procedure, the veterinarian may need to make a specific effort to incorporate them into the treatment process.

The clinician's goal should be to balance and meet the needs of both the animal and the owner, either simultaneously or within a relatively short amount of time. This holds particularly true for clients who tell us to do everything possible, because a great discrepancy may exist between their "everything possible" and ours. And, as noted previously, such client statements may arise from guilt, which can yield to resentment over time.

Because of this, an assessment of the owners' relationship with the animal, their expectations of the treatment process, and the implications of those expectations plays a critical role in the successful treatment of serious conditions. Although these initial evaluations may be altered and/or refined over time, collecting such owner-related information should begin when the first contact is made. Admittedly, the idea of considering the owner's relationship with the animal may seem at least time-consuming if not irrelevant when faced with a seriously ill or injured animal, but in reality most practitioners make such assessments intuitively, if haphazardly. In addition to the tears and worried looks, Dr. Collins notices those owners who cringe and wring their hands every time he touches the animal, those who turn away at the sight of blood, or sneak looks at their watches or the clock on the wall. He remembers comments such as "Oh God, what else can go wrong this week!" or "I'll die if anything happens to Ziggy!" or "I'm missing the Super Bowl!" Unfortunately, we often perceive these displays as incidental or even distracting as we seek to focus all of our attention on the animal.

Because the urge to do something for the animal looms as the primary concern, it actually makes good sense to address the owner first. Compare the veterinarian who makes a conscious effort to block out everything the owner says while conducting the examination to the clinician who deliberately pauses at various points during the examination to address the owner directly. Granted, in critical situations the idea of life slowly ebbing away as we waste vital time talking serves as a most potent image to induce us to ignore the owner. However, even though we may see the loss of the animal as the worst thing that could happen, many clients consider the lack of communication the greater sin.

For those practitioners who cannot focus on the owner and the animal simultaneously or who find the owner a distraction for whatever reason, asking the client to stand off to one side or even leave the area does provide a viable option. However, doing so requires extreme care so clients do not feel they are being separated from their animals in a time of need or, worse, evicted. It would be far better for Dr. Collins to explain his need to concentrate fully on Ziggy for a few minutes with the idea of sharing his findings as soon as possible rather than making the Gormans feel ignored.

Regardless of whether Dr. Collins integrates the owners into his examination of the animal or speaks to them separately afterward, both the assessment of the owner and the discussion of the animal's condition should precede the commencement of any treatment. During this discussion he should accomplish the following:

- Describe the animal's condition in a manner the client can understand.
- Describe the treatment, including any options, and its immediate
  and long-range implications for the animal and owner alike.
- Determine if and how the client wants to treat the animal.

When initially discussing the animal's condition, bear in mind that
owners may respond fearfully in these situations. And, like animals,
their fear commonly takes one of three primary forms: freeze, fight, or
flee. Some owners stand rigidly throughout the entire examination and
nod dumbly whenever addressed. Others become contentious, most
commonly lashing out at themselves or others they perceive as responsible for the animal's condition, but also occasionally turning on the veterinarian. More than one examination and treatment room bears a
dent where a frightened client pounded the wall with his fist when told
of his animal's critical condition. Still others want to get away from the
area as quickly as possible.

Consequently in order to communicate effectively with these clients
we must first dispel their fears, and the best way to do that is to communicate effectively with them. Although this sounds like an impossible
proposition, remember that knowledge is power. The Gormans feel
impotent because things are happening that they don't understand and
they are frightened by the implications of these for both Ziggy and
themselves. The more information Dr. Collins can give them, the less
their fear. The less their fear, the more objectively they can listen to
what he tells them.

We also need to note that owners whose fear precipitates a flight
response may seem like the ideal clients to those practitioners who prefer to work in solitude, but that may not be true. Dr. Collins construes
the Gormans' flight as total commitment to a state-of-the-art treatment
process; when he talks to them hours later, however, he discovers they
want no such thing. In these situations, practitioners should ask owners
who do not want to remain with the animal to wait in another room and
then provide them with the necessary information as soon as possible.

Also bear in mind that the fear most likely exists because the owner
questions his or her ability to cope with some aspect of the animal's condition. It may be seeing the animal in pain. It may be the specter of
death. It may be guilt. It may be the ability to pay for even the most rudimentary care. It may be not knowing what lies ahead for them and the
animal. By addressing those fears immediately and objectively, clinicians can do much to relieve this tension and pave the way for client
cooperation.

We noted previously that preprinted estimate forms can do much to focus both the clients and clinician, and those designed to cover common emergency procedures prove particularly helpful. Those clients who remain with the animal during the examination may be given a clipboard with a copy of the estimate form, which they can follow as the practitioner describes his or her findings and proposed treatment. For example, when the physical examination reveals that Ziggy is in shock, Dr. Collins refers the Gormans to the section of the estimate sheet that lists the drugs and procedures used to treat this condition and notes those necessary for Ziggy. Because the unit price is listed opposite each entry, the Gormans can see how much the treatment will cost. Dr. Collins then reiterates this by giving them an estimate of the total cost for that part of the treatment.

Some practitioners find that treating complex cases in segments works best for both them and their clients. They focus on the animal's immediate problems and their necessary treatment, and describe the remainder in more general terms until after the first round of treatment is completed. Using this protocol, Dr. Collins discusses the shock component of Ziggy's problem in detail, but limits that of the animal's fractures to an estimate of the total cost of repair.

Client response at this point usually gives reliable information regarding their commitment to the process. The owner who says, "What will that involve?" or "Do you accept time payments?" communicates a much different orientation from the one who exclaims, "You must be joking!" If the Gormans choose to delve more deeply into other aspects of the treatment at that time, Dr. Collins won't feel guilty about not immediately initiating the first part of the treatment. Or, theoretically at least, he shouldn't.

However, cases do arise in which the clinician believes the animal suffers while owners struggle to assimilate all the implications of its condition or agonize over whether to treat it or not. Although a temptation may exist to force such owners to commit themselves one way or another "for the sake of the animal," such strong-arm tactics may backfire if the owner later regrets the decision. Some practitioners who find themselves in this position prefer to do whatever necessary to insure the animal's comfort with the idea they will not charge the client for this treatment if the owner opts for euthanasia of the critically ill or injured animal. To these clinicians, their peace of mind as well the desire to work with owners who feel comfortable with their choice—be it to treat or not—more than offset the cost.

Practitioners who meet with clients not present during the examination would follow this same procedure. In this situation, it works best if the meeting occurs privately in an examination room or, preferably, in a more comfortable lounge or office if one exists. Above all, owners of critically ill or injured animals never should be asked to sit in a waiting room full of happily chattering clients and healthy animals. Nor should any discussions with these owners occur in that setting.

Implications of the Owner-Animal Relationship

Just as clinicians often harbor specific ideas about when an animal should or should not be treated, so clients maintain their own criteria which may have nothing to do with the medical aspects of the case. Paramount among these is the owner's relationship with the animal. The stronger and more stable the owner's bond with the animal, the greater the owner's commitment to the animal and its recovery. The greater the owner's commitment to the animal, the greater the compliance. The greater the compliance, the greater the chance of success. The greater the success, the more readily owners justify the cost of any treatment and praise the clinician who formulated it. And finally, the more serious the problem, the greater the influence of all these relationship parameters.

At this point, recall the discussions of the different kinds of owner relationships and the role of love in the treatment process. An owner who possesses a strong, stable bond with an animal is *not* synonymous with hysterical anthropomorphically oriented Ms. Gorman agonizing over the fate of her beloved Ziggy. Although Ms. Gorman may indeed love Ziggy and possess both the desire and financial wherewithal to move heaven and earth to make him better, this does not necessarily translate into the long-term commitment often required for successful treatment of these cases.

At their best, anthropomorphically oriented owners will take a very intimate interest in their animals, allow the practitioner to go the extra mile, and follow even the most complex instructions to the letter. However, the anthropomorphic orientation also may undermine the treatment of critically ill or injured animals in two different ways. First, the tendency of these owners to see the animal's problem as their own may leave them in such a state of agitation that they barely can comprehend what the clinician tells them, let alone carry out any instructions at home. Although it would be wrong to doubt both the magnitude and sincerity of these owners' feelings, the fact remains their feelings may render them incapable of even the most basic aftercare. Ms. Gorman misses all the early signs of infection as well as contributes to its presence because she wraps Ziggy's injured legs in layers of colorful plastic so she wouldn't see his "horrible wounds" instead of checking the area daily as directed.

Second, anthropomorphically oriented owners may find it very difficult to comply with those instructions that they believe treat the animal as inferior. We noted how owners who feed table food often perceive therapeutic diets in this light, even those prescribed following heroic medical procedures to get the animal's kidneys, liver, or heart functioning acceptably again. Similarly, a request for the owner to maintain something so critical and yet simple as cleanliness may earn the practitioner an incredulous look: "Surely you intend to put Ziggy on some really strong antibiotics after all he's been through, don't you?"

At the opposite end of the spectrum, those who take the chattel approach also can add their own special dimensions to the treatment of critically ill or injured animals. Although we most commonly associate this orientation with those who reject treatment for the most superficial reasons, their emotional distance from the animal may make those who opt for treatment very reliable and compliant clients. The chattel-oriented herdsman who confronts a critical illness in a prize breeding animal may display a dogged determination to treat it successfully that evades those whose relationship with the animal carries a more emotional charge. However, more commonly we see those clients whose interaction with the animal is sufficiently limited or superficial that we cannot trust them to provide the magnitude and/or quality of monitoring and aftercare that usually attends the treatment of the critically ill or injured animal. The herdsman who puts such an animal back in with the herd or flock as soon as possible for his own convenience or the owner who intends to show or breed regardless of the animal's condition exemplify this orientation.

Owner Expectations

Once we ascertain the owner's relationship with the animal, we need to discuss the implications of treatment as well as the anticipated result of these for both animal and owner alike. We noted how estimate sheets provide an effective way for clinicians to describe the medical aspects of the case as well as the associated costs. However, there are other costs involved in the treatment of the critically ill or injured animal that also must be considered. The most immediate of these relates to the purpose of the practitioner's proposed course of action. We have repeatedly used the phrase "treatment process" to include the examination, history, and any diagnostic work-up as well as any treatment because this reflects the proper sequence we've all been taught. However, over the years that proper sequence has become more complex and more expensive. Where a thorough physical examination and history, complete blood count and profile, EKG, and radiographs once provided what most considered a solid diagnostic data base, practitioners now may feel the basic work-up includes endoscopic exams, sonar, and any one of a number of highly specialized in-house or outside tests.

Although no one can dispute the soundness of this from a medical point of view, the fact remains that we expect clients to pay for all this. And because we do, it behooves us to determine if they share our view of the purpose underlying the process. For example, discussions with Dr. Collins's clients reveal that a significant number believe that the only reason to know the cause of the problem is to cure it; if it can't be cured, knowing the cause becomes academic. These clients don't share his desire to know which particular virus undermined the immune response of the terminally ill cat, or the exact nature of the secondary infection that ultimately caused the cat's demise. Moreover some clients may be so strongly cure-oriented, they can't imagine that Dr. Collins would perform any test unless he specifically believed the animal could be cured. Consequently, no matter how strongly he may feel that any diagnostic procedure represents a necessary step in a necessary process that he *must* complete before treating the animal, he should explain both the nature of the test and the reason for it to the owners first. Few events in practice can elicit more confused and negative owner responses than the presentation of a bill for a work-up that proves there is no hope for an animal which the owners believed beyond hope when they first presented it. Although some owners may feel gratified to know they were right, others don't like the idea of paying the veterinarian to prove the obvious.

According to many clients, the only sin worse than the unauthorized work-up of a critically ill or injured animal occurs when such an animal dies during that procedure. Although these owners admit their responses may be irrational, most feel the animal would not have died had the veterinarian focused on supportive care and let the tests go for a while.

The message here is that familiar litany: Communicate with the client *before* beginning the treatment and make sure they understand not only what any procedures involve (including any possible risk to the animal) and the cost, but also the presumptive diagnosis the tests are being conducted to confirm. Practitioners lacking a presumptive diagnosis might want to consider conducting a more thorough physical examination and taking a more in-depth history before proposing a technological fishing expedition. That way when the client says, "I can't afford all that, Doctor. What do *you* think the problem is?" the veterinarian won't give the impression that he or she merely serves as a conduit between the animal and the technology.

Most clients do not object to any procedure for which they believe a legitimate purpose exists. Nor do they object to practitioners conducting diagnostic procedures on a terminally ill animal if these will provide information that may benefit other animals in the household or herd, or even animalkind in general. And most certainly, few balk at ascertaining whether a critically ill animal suffers from something that possesses public health significance. What most clients resent is not being told the purpose of the procedure in a manner that makes sense to them before it's performed. Granted the emotions that surround the presentation of the critically ill or injured animal may make this seem like the very worst time to discuss such issues. However, practitioners who don't do this who commence any form of treatment without the owner's understanding and permission should do so with the idea that, having made this choice for the owner, they then must assume the responsibility for any consequences of it—which may include the cost if the owner disagrees with their approach.

Many times at the moment of crisis and immediately following it, owners summon the wherewithal to face two probabilities:

- The animal will die.
- The animal will recover completely.

For most, coming to grips with the fact that the animal might die proves the far more emotionally exhausting task and, here again, some may use the "Do everything you can, Doc!" approach to project this probability away from themselves or at least far enough into the future to buy themselves time to come to grips with it. Similarly, some practitioners also get so involved with the idea of saving a life that they give little thought to what lies ahead for that life once it's been saved. Other owners who come to grips with the idea that the animal might die often see this as the major hurdle and, compared to death, perceive any kind of positive response on the animal's part as indicative of full recovery during this interval.

However, at some point the fear of death and losing the animal wanes and clients begin to ponder the long-term implications of the animal's condition. This may occur within the first twenty-four hours or maybe not for weeks or even months when other events in their lives cause them to see the animal's condition in a different light. At that point they will ask or often simply expect the veterinarian to answer the question, "What lies ahead for us and the animal?" Rather than expect clients to extrapolate the answer from a lot of medical jargon or to guess our thoughts, it makes sense to address this issue directly to insure that everyone is thinking the same thing.

For example, the clinician's positive comments during the treatment process may fuel the owners' belief that the animal will fully recover. Unfortunately, the clinician may be measuring the animal's response against a standard quite different from that of the owner. When Dr. Collins comments on Ziggy's "excellent progress," the Gormans interpret this to mean the animal's fractured limbs are progressing well toward the return of full function. In fact, Dr. Collins's remarks actually refer to the fact that Ziggy's wounds have remained free of infection, and his remarks have nothing to do with the dog regaining function at all.

Many times we view critically ill or injured animals as visitors to our domain where we oversee and control every aspect of their lives until we feel they reach a point at which the owners can continue the process at home. In this ideal situation, money is no object and these animals go home to an environment where a willing person capable of carrying out our instructions exists to attend to the animal's needs for however long necessary. In reality, we know that when these animals go home may be determined by financial rather than medical factors, and/or that they may go home to an environment where owner life-style and limitations may undermine the treatment process. Because of this, it is essential that the practitioner and the owner discuss and agree on the purpose of the treatment, the prognosis, any short-term and long-term care required, and whether the owner can consistently accomplish this. Although we may like to tell ourselves that noncompliance occurs because owners don't care, more often than not it occurs because they don't *know*. And because we consider ourselves the most knowledgeable relative to the animal's health, if we don't tell the owners, who will?

A little thought about all those nonmedical owner parameters that can undermine the treatment process should make it obvious why veterinarians might want to shy away from such discussions when faced with a critically ill or injured animal: Everything in our training prepares us to preserve a quality life for the animal, which many times we define in strictly medical terms. The idea that the owner's definition of a quality life might include factors that we see as totally unrelated to the medical aspects of the case strikes us as at least confusing if not downright blasphemous. How can the client not want to treat something so readily treatable as diabetes mellitus? What's the big deal about keeping an animal confined until the fracture heals?

Special Practitioner Considerations

It seems that every profession recognizes the existence of "20-80" or "10-10-80" rules and veterinary medicine is no different. Most practitioners suspect that 20 percent of their clients give them 80 percent of their headaches and surely every student has been consoled by the fact that we make 10 percent of our patients better, 10 percent worse, and a wonderfully reassuring 80 percent will probably get better no matter what we do. However, unfortunately that 10 percent for whom we could potentially do the most good also represents those for whom we could potentially do the most harm, and nowhere does this become so apparent as when dealing with the critically ill or injured. When we couple this with the belief that successfully treating such difficult cases—not giving vaccinations, providing behavioral counseling, or other preventive measures—was and is the goal of all our training, we can appreciate how practitioner emotions can run as high as the clients' at such times. Whether or not our feelings complicate the treatment process depends more on their relationship to the owner's feelings than the nature of the feelings themselves.

Veterinarians practicing in economically depressed areas commonly complain about clients who don't let them do what they want to do. Although a quick survey of the client base makes it apparent that these people lack the financial wherewithal as well as the life-style and other qualities that would lead them to request extraordinary care for their animals and successfully carry it to completion, some clinicians in these settings choose to believe that these people don't care. Although any practitioner can succumb to this temptation, new graduates are particularly susceptible because many times the greatest gap exists between their definition of "extraordinary care" and the owners'. This occurs because the veterinary colleges pride themselves in presenting the epitome of science and technology and students become accustomed to using it routinely; they share the belief of one very sincere senior who exclaimed incredulously, "How can you possibly practice without ultrasound!"

Regardless of the underlying reasons and their legitimacy, practitioners who feel they care more about their patients than the owners do can complicate the treatment of the critically ill or injured animal immensely. Recall the basic rule: The more complicated the animal's condition, the greater the need for quality communication and owner compliance. As soon as Dr. Collins judges an owner or owners as lesser in any way, he sets up a belief structure that may lead to a self-fulfilling prophecy with detrimental consequences for the animal. Because he believes the owners don't care about the animal and he takes pride in his animal-loving nature, he limits his contact with these people as much as possible. This may mean giving them only the barest details regarding any (inferior) treatment process he believes they subject him and the animal to due to their lack of caring. This lack of communication, in turn, causes them to question *his* caring and limit their communication with *him,* which makes it difficult if not impossible for them to accomplish any aftercare successfully. Simultaneously, Dr. Collins doesn't take quite as much care performing a treatment he considers lesser and interacts with the animal quite differently from the one whose owner gives him carte blanche. Reassuring comments such as "C'mon fella, I know you can make it," give way to "Poor old guy, nobody cares about you."

Remember that faith in the individual's ability to get well and in the clinician to perform his or her duties serves as the core of the healing process. When practitioners believe they care more than clients, and that clients "force" them to treat an animal in what they consider an inferior manner, that faith is undermined on all fronts. The practitioner and owner lose faith in each other, the clinician lacks faith in the treatment because it doesn't meet his or her standards as the best, and the animal may be consciously or subconsciously treated in a manner that confuses rather than reassures it. And it is this lack of faith, more than the failure of any medical procedure, that greatly reduces the probability of successfully treating the animal.

Clinicians also may encounter cases in which the client's feelings for the animal and the treatment exceed their own. In these situations the combination of the severity of the animal's condition and any owner or practitioner limitations results in a terminal prognosis, but the client refuses to give up and often imbues the veterinarian with a magnitude of faith worthy of any god. Unfortunately, even at his most godly, Dr. Colins as yet can't create a functioning liver or heart to replace one ravaged by time, disease, or trauma.

In these cases as well as those in which the veterinarian shares the owner's very deep feelings about the animal, the goal remains to maintain sufficient distance that we may perform our duties efficiently and serve as a source of objective information to the client. The art and science of veterinary practice, the emotion/caring and intellect of the practitioner, should share equal billing in any client encounter. When it tips too much in one direction, it disrupts the balance of the patient-client-practitioner relationship and undermines the treatment process.

A final practitioner consideration leads naturally into our discussion of death and euthanasia in the next two chapters: knowing when to quit. Of all the skills necessary for successful practice, none is so subtle yet powerful as the ability to recognize when the patient, owner, and/or the practitioner him- or herself has reached its, his, or her limits. Although sometimes by dint of personality and quality communication we can stretch the limits, inevitably we encounter cases whose limits we cannot exceed no matter how much we (and the owners) may care and try. As soon as practitioners become aware that the animal cannot live a quality life given the limitations imposed, it behooves them to share this observation with the client for several reasons:

- Clinicians will then know if the owner shares their definition of a quality life.
- It opens the door to a discussion of death and/or euthanasia.
- It enables the practitioner to interact with the client and patient in a meaningful way throughout the entire encounter.

Granted, trained as we are in the science and technology of saving lives, no one wants to admit that death looms on the horizon, let alone that we might play an active role in it. Nonetheless, to let such a case drag on because we and/or the client lack the courage to discuss its termination hardly constitutes a caring response. Just as the presentation of the critically ill or injured animal offers us the opportunity to bring all our science and technology into play, so it requires that we muster all of our practice art when that science and technology fail to produce a quality life for the owner and animal. At that point it is primarily the art of veterinary practice that we must rely on to carry the case to its conclusion in a caring and dignified manner.

Chapter 16
The Art of Death and Dying: The Patient and the Client

Schooled as we are in the preservation of life, few events can generate more emotional havoc for us than the death of a patient, be it by natural or unnatural causes. Regardless of science and technology, death remains an inevitability of life, and, given the shorter life span of most of our patients as well as the relative ease with which most of them give birth without our assistance, veterinarians in practice more likely will find themselves bidding old friends good-bye rather than welcoming new ones into the world. Moreover death remains the most profound human fear, which practically guarantees that practitioners and clients alike will bring a certain amount of emotional baggage into the process. Consequently, when we combine our lack of training in dealing with patient death with the inevitability of dying and death and the ever more complex and symbolic human-animal relationships encountered in practice, it comes as no surprise that this often most feared and traumatic event also can serve as one of the most significant encountered in practice.

For those who feel uncomfortable interacting with clients facing the loss of an animal, the following articles and texts may be of help:

"Helping People Adjust to the Death of a Pet," by J. E. Quackenbush and L. Glickman (*Health and Social Work* 9 [1984]:42–48).
"Helping Pet Owners with the Euthanasia Decision" and "Supporting Clients Who Are Grieving the Death of a Pet," both by Joan Guntzelman and Michael Riegger (*Veterinary Medicine* [January 1993]: 26–41).
"Humane Euthanasia and Companion Animal Death: Caring for the Animal, the Client, the Veterinarian," by Lynette Hart et al. (*Journal of the American Veterinary Medical Association* 197:1292–99).

"Pet Loss and Human Emotion," a brochure available from the American Veterinary Medical Association.

"Parent Care: Total Involvement in the Care of a Dying Child," by Martha Pearse Elliot in *Living with Death and Dying*, by Elisabeth Kübler-Ross (New York: Macmillan, 1981).

On Death and Dying, by Elisabeth Kübler-Ross (New York: Macmillan, 1969).

Of value to clients as well as practitioners:

When Your Pet Dies: How to Cope with Your Feelings, by Jamie Quacken-bush (New York: Pocket Books, 1985).

When a Pet Dies, by Fred Rogers (New York: Putnam, 1988).

The Tenth Good Thing About Barney, by Judith Viorst (New York: Macmillan, 1971).

Charlotte's Web, by E. B. White (New York: Harper and Row, 1952).

Although written for children, the Rogers, Viorst, and White books present the death of an animal in terms many adults find both eloquent and comforting.

Coming to Grips with Terminal Conditions

Physician Elisabeth Kübler-Ross first described the five-stage process dying patients and their loved ones go through as they come to grips with the inevitable (Ross 1966, 57:3; Kübler-Ross, 1969). Because the veterinarian may serve as the most accessible target for clients dealing with the impending or actual death of an animal, an understanding of how the various stages may manifest can help us understand what these people experience. The stages are:

1. Denial
2. Anger
3. Bargaining
4. Depression
5. Acceptance

Although the overall sequence remains essentially the same for most people, variations can and do occur. The ten-year-old who faces the loss of her favorite ewe may take a lot longer to accept this than her farmer father, who also may internalize the entire process to the extent that the child accuses him of not caring at all. Rather than following a neat progression from step one through step five, many people vacillate between stages before moving on to the next. When Dr. Weisburg first tells Mr. Clay about his animal's terminal condition, the owner insists it can't be true: "Just look at old Fuzzy," he demands, "he hardly looks sick at all." When Dr. Weisburg stands by his diagnosis, the owner becomes angry: "I'm taking Fuzzy to someone who knows what they're doing!" When the second opinion supports the first, he then takes the animal to a teaching hospital where he bargains for the latest science and technology to save his dog's life. Each bad day the dog experiences may send him either into a fit of rage or depression; each good one leads him to deny the animal's condition.

Other people get stuck at some stage in the process. Some clients will deny a patient's illness right up until the day the animal dies and then appear genuinely shocked by the event. Unfortunately, many times practitioners will reinforce denial for several reasons. First, they may be in a state of denial themselves regarding the animal's terminal condition: Dr. Weisburg knows Fuzzy suffers from widely metastasized osteosarcoma but he's such a wonderful dog, the veterinarian tells himself that surely something can be done for him. Clinicians also may view the client's denial as a sign of faith: When Mr. Clay tells Dr. Weisburg Fuzzy will surely recover, the veterinarian agrees because he doesn't want Mr. Clay to give up on an animal which needs his support more than ever. Third, clinicians may accept and even reinforce client denial to avoid what they consider the much more emotional and potentially problematic state of accepting the animal's impending death: Dr. Weisburg knows how attached Mr. Clay is to Fuzzy and dreads what will happen when it dawns on the owner that there's no hope for the dog.

Clients who get stuck in the anger stage can be very trying because nothing the clinician does can mollify them. Fortunately, their anger often leads them to take the dying animal to someone else so such responses are relatively short-lived. Some veterinarians may see this as passing the problem on to an unsuspecting colleague, but many times going to another practitioner enables the angry client to let go of this stage. Mr. Clay rants and rages at Dr. Weisburg for his diagnosis, but readily accepts the same from Dr. Hennesy, with whom he immediately begins the bargaining process.

Clients who get stuck in the bargaining stage can readily seduce practitioners steeped in science and technology who have not worked through their own feelings about death and dying patients. These owners intellectually may acknowledge the animal's terminal condition, but they hope to put off actual acceptance of this fact by immersing themselves in various activities to buy time. Whether we agree with this approach or not, it becomes problematic when these attempts result in the animal living a less-than-quality life. This becomes particularly tragic when the owner rationalizes that any kind of life is acceptable for the animal rather than accepting its terminal condition.

Depression regarding the animal's condition most commonly leads the client to opt for euthanasia. Unfortunately, many perceive this as the logical mental state for a person making this decision, but that isn't true at all. Depressed people believe themselves unable to control their own lives, and those who opt for euthanasia while in this stage see the act as more proof of their helplessness rather than as a caring response to a suffering animal. Sadly, well-meaning friends and even veterinarians may force the issue thinking it will end the depression more quickly.

Consider what happens when Dr. Weisburg pressures Ms. Begley to consider euthanizing her terminally ill cat. First, he overlooks the fact that Ms. Begley's depression exists because she has yet to accept her animal's terminal illness, let alone its death. Consequently, euthanizing the cat at this time will only add to her emotional burden. Second, because she feels helpless she may allow herself to be talked into euthanasia by him or other well-meaning friends. This, too, may serve only to make her feel more depressed rather than relieving her from that feeling. Third, after the animal is dead, Ms. Begley may trade in her depression for anger at Dr. Weisburg for euthanizing the animal prematurely; and she may blame him even if the pressure to do so came from others because he performed the deed. Because she never accepted the terminal nature of the animal's condition, she more readily can cling to the illusion that it might have recovered had she not given up on it. Needless to say, the emotions that feed the process at this point can become very strong and negative, and clients have been known never to relinquish those aimed at the veterinarian.

Clients who accept their animal's terminal condition pose few problems for practitioners unless they accept this reality and the veterinarian doesn't, which causes sufficient clinician emotion to warrant discussion in the next chapter. When clients reach acceptance, this often enables them to make any decisions regarding the dying animal's care or euthanasia with a certain calmness that practitioners who don't accept the animal's condition may see as cold and even callous. Conversely, and because some owners may vacillate between depression and acceptance, practitioners who believe a suffering animal should be euthanized should resist the temptation to do so unquestioningly when a previously depressed owner suddenly appears to agree. When Ms. Begley calls Dr. Weisburg after a week of tears and despondency and calmly announces, "You're right, I think we should put Fluffy to sleep," he should discuss all the pros and cons of such a choice rather than congratulate her for doing the right thing. It's far better to see this change in attitude as a first step in the right direction than to act prematurely and plunge the client back into a state of depression.

Coping with Death

Owners coping with the death of an animal go through the same five-step process that attended the acceptance of its dying condition. Although denial does occur, it's usually short-lived because the very nature of death makes denial a difficult mental state to perpetuate. Most clients will make comments like "I can't believe he's gone," but these tend to become less frequent over time. A sufficient number—including veterinarians whose animals have died—speak of still sensing the animal's presence in the household, sometimes vividly so. Although the idea of seeing fleeting images of the animal or feeling it jump up and lie down on the foot of the bed boggles the linear scientific mind, those who have these experiences find them most comforting. Consequently, it would seem to serve no valid purpose to challenge their reality.

More than any emotion associated with the grieving process, client anger once again creates the most negative results for the practitioner. Because once death occurs both denial and bargaining lose their meaning, Mr. Clay lashes out at the staff and faculty of the teaching hospital and tells anyone who will listen that their incompetency caused Fuzzy's untimely death, an opinion that never wavers over the years. Interestingly, some clients whose animals die in state-of-the-art facilities experience more anger, perhaps because the similarities between these facilities and human hospitals are much more difficult to ignore. This also may occur because the relationship between the client and any practitioner(s) may be less intimate at such facilities and this remoteness makes it easier for owners to make these clinicians the target of their anger when the animal dies.

Conversely, other clients may express much more anger toward the regular clinician following death and euthanasia. The Schillers opt for euthanasia and act so in control at the time that Dr. Weisburg never thinks to challenge their decision. Later they decide that fear led them to make this decision and that they abandoned the animal in its hour of greatest need. They then lash out at Dr. Weisburg, claiming he should have *insisted* that they try another drug or do those tests they said they didn't want to do. Although he once enjoyed a close relationship with them, they now detest him. Obviously, such client behavior comes as quite a shock to a practitioner who chose not to question the owners' decision because he didn't want to cause them any unnecessary discomfort.

Another troubling client response occurs when a normally reserved client cries or otherwise expresses vulnerability in the practitioner's presence. These clients may later turn on the veterinarian or ignore that person after the event. The executive whom the practitioner comforted for hours while he grieved over the loss of his animal who from that day on crossed the street rather than meet her and never set foot in her clinic again comes to mind here.

As these examples indicate, client anger can be difficult for the practitioner to accept. However, it does tend to be a more active and involved state, and that keeps alive the possibility that these people may move closer to acceptance as time goes on.

It would seem that bargaining plays little role once death occurs, but a report describing a business that mummifies animals (as well as people) would seem to indicate that some people prefer a compromise position between life and death. These owners don't deny the animal has died, but they want to preserve the physical remains in a state as close to that of a living being as possible. That same article also describes another company that manufactures caskets for pets with a sealed barrier to protect the remains and a domed lid to accommodate any personal belongings the owner might wish to bury with the animal ("Mummification," 1993, 6:11). Here again, owners who request such services don't deny the death of the animal but rather choose to strike a bargain by maintaining it in an intermediate state they find comforting. Because owners who take this route more commonly view their animals anthropomorphically, we can understand why they would want the animal's remains handled in a manner comparable to their own.

Many grief counselors see long-standing depression over the death of an animal as the most detrimental condition because those who experience it cut themselves off from others who might either distract or help them make that final step to acceptance. Unfortunately, veterinarians may not realize that the loss of an animal has resulted in their client's prolonged depression because it appears to occur more commonly in those who live alone and lose their only pet. Unless Dr. Weisburg makes a special effort to check on Ms. Begley following the death of her cat, he would have no way of knowing about her mental state. This is unfortunate because he may be the only person who knows about the death of the animal as well as the single owner's relationship to it. In these situations, a personal phone call from either the veterinarian or a staff member who knows the client works better than a card or letter because it provides the client with an opportunity to share his or her feelings about the loss.

Depression also may result because owners, rightly or wrongly, believe others do not understand why they feel so bad about the loss of an animal. For as much headway as studies of the human-animal bond have made over the years, the awareness of the power and effect of the bond remains a curiosity for most human health-care professionals. Consequently, even if owners do reveal the loss of the animal as the cause of their depression, they might do so to a physician or counselor who dismisses the idea as ridiculous, thereby adding to the owner's depression. Because of this, an increasing number of veterinarians keep the names of those both skilled in the art of grief counseling and aware of the human-animal bond in their referral file and do not hesitate to refer clients to them. If the depression appears profound, a follow-up call to verify that these people have gotten help is in order.

Sometimes depression occurs because the clients themselves believe it wrong to grieve for the animal. Although both men and women may believe this, men seem more likely to take this approach, perhaps because in our society some men see depression as more stoic and hence more masculine than grieving. These cases can prove particularly troublesome because these people withdraw from the situation: Mr. Clay doesn't want to discuss Fuzzy's death because that would mean admitting he cared, which he doesn't want to do. If the depression persists, these people also need the help of a mental health professional with knowledge of the human-animal bond. Unfortunately, suggesting this may precipitate a fear response. Those who take the freeze or flight fear responses revert to the denial phase of the loop again: "I am not depressed over the death of a dumb dog!" Those who take the fight route may lash out at the veterinarian as well as revert to the anger phase of the acceptance process: "Why do you keep insisting Fuzzy's death is bothering me? Why don't you mind your own business!" Although these all would seem like steps backward in the grieving process, sometimes they do suffice to free the owners from depression long enough to view the loss of the animal in a different light.

Most commonly, practitioners notice clients experiencing depression secondary to the loss of an animal when they see the owner to treat another animal. Interestingly, the depression experienced by food animal owners may exceed that of companion animal owners at that time.

When the Schillers' cat dies, their close relationship with their other cat and dog helps them through the grieving process. However, when John Moore loses his top producer, who coincidentally happened to be an unacknowledged personal favorite, he feels obligated to put her death in what he considers acceptable business terms: "I don't know how I can keep the herd going without her," he says dejectedly. Unfortunately, if the farmer can't accept the loss on both levels—that is, as the loss of a good friend as well as a business asset—then he can involve himself in a self-fulfilling prophecy. Because of his depression, he doesn't pay as much attention to the herd, illness becomes more common, production falls off, expenses increase and income decreases, and the future of the herd becomes uncertain. Unfortunately, if the idea of a grown man grieving over a poodle strikes many as ludicrous, the idea of him grieving over a cow or sheep strikes many as insane.

A second food animal-related depression may occur in children raised in farm environments where acceptance of death occurs almost as a matter of routine who find their inability to share their grief over the loss of an animal overwhelming. The twelve-year-old who disappears the day his 4-H project goes off to slaughter and responds mechanically to his proud father's report of the price it commanded would seem to send a strong message, yet those insensitive to this possibility will miss it. Adults who are used to companion animal relationships may experience similar depression: The farmer's Chicago bride or the new hired hand from Los Angeles may become overwhelmed with emotions that others present don't even acknowledge as real when the old cow dies. Unfortunately, if the veterinarian also doesn't acknowledge these feelings as real, these people wind up questioning their own values—and even their sanity—as well as those of others even as they struggle to come to grips with the animal's death.

Clients who accept the death of an animal radiate that same calmness of those who have accepted terminal illness or the termination of their relationship with the animal. There may be tears and sadness, but there is an underlying strength in these people that doesn't exist in the other stages. Ironically, practitioners may experience this most dramatically when clients reach that stage before they do and they find themselves leaning on the owners for support:

"I'm so sorry, Ms. Begley," says Dr. Weisburg dejectedly. "I wish I could have done more for Fluffy."

"I know you did your best," replies Ms. Begley, giving her veterinarian a reassuring pat on the arm.

Any clinician who has received such support from a client knows how much it can do to speed the transition from depression to acceptance.

Because of this, it makes sense to make some comment that recognizes some positive aspect of the grieving client's relationship with the animal. Sometimes this may mean noting how these people excelled in their care of their animal, be it by going the extra mile medically or supporting the animal emotionally under trying circumstances. Other times, focusing on the relationship prior to the illness or trauma helps the owners replace thoughts of death and dying with fond memories of the past. Other times an unembarrassed hug says it all.

Patient Considerations

It goes without saying that dying animals should be treated with respect, and this should include respect for their bond and behavioral needs as well as their physical needs. We noted in our discussion of codependencies and separation anxieties that some animals' attachment to their territories and/or owners may be so strong that these may complicate recovery during hospitalization (Chapter 6). Similarly, these relationships may complicate these animals' deaths. Theoretically we can say that if we separate highly dependent Fuzzy from Mr. Clay it would hasten the terminally ill animal's demise, which we may see as positive if Mr. Clay can't bring himself to euthanize the animal. However, if the animal is responsive enough to recognize its surroundings as hostile, this hardly constitutes a caring approach. Furthermore, many owners do not accept any logic that defines the animal as too ill to have visitors; most believe that it is exactly under these conditions that the animal needs them the most. If the clinician refuses them access to the animal and it dies, many will believe their absence contributed to the animal's death.

Nor can we fault their logic. Dr. Weisburg may engross himself completely in his daily physical examination and evaluation of Fuzzy's treatment regime because of the animal's critical condition. When he puts his stethoscope to Fuzzy's chest, he blocks out everything but the sound of heart and lungs: Fuzzy the dog ceases to exist. When he evaluates Fuzzy's current state, he compares today's test results to yesterday's and those of the day before. He might ask his technician how the dog is doing, but he interprets the response as it affects the animal's medical parameters.

However, when Mr. Clay visits Fuzzy there is no poking or prodding. Mr. Clay's every action focuses on the dog as a whole and making the animal feel comfortable. He strokes all of Fuzzy's favorite spots, and tells the dog all those special things people tell their animals. Although

Mr. Clay listens attentively to Dr. Weisburg's report of Fuzzy's condition, he places equal or more value on the results of his own bond-based examination of the dog.

Whether we believe in the validity of this or not, it does occur and it is not a behavior limited to anthropomorphically oriented owners. Recall those good dairy farmers who love their cows: They place as much stock in their intuitive feelings about their animals as they do in the veterinarian's findings, and often these feelings will determine whether they keep treating the animal or opt to put it down. When Mr. Clay visits his sister's farm, he's awed that she gets to keep her sick animals at home where she can interact with them routinely and give them a word of encouragement. True, both the veterinarian and the farmer may say economics rather than good medicine mandate this approach, but to those owners who feel isolated from their hospitalized animals it seems like a much more caring way to do things.

Because of this, many owners who relate to their terminally ill animals in this manner and choose not to euthanize them may prefer to have their animals die at home. With the advent of the hospice movement, they see this as a caring and viable alternative to hospitalization. However, animals sent home to die should not be left to their own and their owner's devices any more than those dying in a hospital. Clients should be carefully instructed regarding the importance of keeping the animal clean and comfortable. They should know that the animal might lose bladder and bowel function at some time and that recumbent animals need to be repositioned periodically. Above all the client should know what to expect when the animal dies. Many times people maintain the same hope for their animals they maintain for themselves: The animal will die peacefully in its sleep, at worst following a period of decline with few signs of obvious physical or emotional suffering. And some animals do die this way, but others may experience a prolonged demise during which each system shuts down, one by one, not unlike the shutting down of a sophisticated factory over a period of hours or even days.

Of all the signs associated with death, agonal breathing and vocalization prove the most nerve-racking for owners and they should be forewarned of these possibilities. The vocalization of cats, in particular, may shock unsuspecting owners because these cries possess a quality unlike any other which more than one client and veterinarian has described as "otherworldly." Because these may last for hours and the animals are oblivious to their surroundings—including their owners, who often frantically try to comfort them—the need to prepare clients for this possibility cannot be overstated. Above all, rather than condemning owners who choose to take their animals home to die, practitioners should offer their full support so clients who discover they cannot meet the physical and emotional demands of coping with a dying animal will feel comfortable requesting hospitalization or euthanasia if they reach that point.

The art of feeding and medicating the dying patient may differ significantly from its science. The science mandates that we treat the animal with the idea of saving its life right up to the last minute even as the likelihood of doing that approaches nil. The art proposes we do whatever we can to make the last days as comfortable as possible for both the animal and its owner. For the anorectic animal this may mean offering special foods the owner knows the animal likes even if these might tax its digestive organs. It means using painkillers and sedatives, often as much or more for the owner than the animal, based on the rationale that the animal needs the owner's emotional support more than anything at that time. If Mr. Clay believes Fuzzy experiences pain or is unable to sleep, he will transfer his anxiety regarding this to the dog. If his belief becomes sufficiently strong, he may reach for human medications in hopes these will alleviate the symptoms. Because of this, it makes more sense for Dr. Weisburg to prescribe these medications and clearly describe any negative as well as positive effects these may have on the animal. This isn't done with the idea of frightening Mr. Clay into changing his mind, but rather because terminally ill animals often maintain such a delicate balance that even a seemingly innocuous medication may precipitate exaggerated results.

If the animal is difficult to medicate, some owners will opt to stop all medications rather than force the issue. Every time Mr. Clay tries to open Fuzzy's mouth, the dog struggles and tries to get away, which leaves him gasping for breath. In his owner's mind, Fuzzy never comes so close to death as when engaged in this struggle and the idea that his beloved pet could succumb under those circumstances is more than he can bear. Nor does he find Dr. Weisburg's suggestion that they put Fuzzy on all injectables a viable alternative: The idea of daily taking his dying dog to the veterinary clinic for such medication or sticking needles into Fuzzy at home does not impress Mr. Clay as a quality life.

The Special Needs of Euthanasia

The many different aspects of euthanasia could easily fill an entire book, so we can only touch on a few areas that prove the most troublesome for practitioners. Three criteria relative to the client and the patient take precedence:

- Clients must believe the choice was theirs and that it was the right one.
- Clients must be informed of the mechanics of the act itself.
- Everything must be done to insure the comfort of the animal.

Veterinarians whom clients believe pressured them to request euthanasia rarely are perceived as caring after the fact, regardless how hopeless an animal's condition. Remember that death serves as the greatest fear for many people and they may transfer this fear to their animals. If they also believe their animals possess rights which include a right to life, then the act of euthanasia may take on enormous implications for the owner.

For those veterinarians who share this view, theoretically no problem exists: They simply keep treating the animal as if it could recover right up until the day it dies. However, what if the animal is suffering? Under these circumstances many practitioners will suggest adding analgesics and sedatives to the treatment regime even if these might hasten the animal's demise. A surprising number of clients will agree to this because they don't want to hold their animals hostage to their beliefs. However, some can't even accept this responsibility. Instead they'll make comments such as, "If you think Fuzzy is suffering, I want you to do what you think best." In other words, they want the veterinarian to make the choice that they can't and preferably not tell them about it.

Morally and legally, surely the thinnest of lines exists between this treatment and euthanasia, but few of these owners see it that way. They want the veterinarian to do it, but most won't admit this until months or even years later, if then. Whether or not the veterinarian can fulfill these clients' wishes depends on the veterinarian and his or her knowledge of the client and the animal as well as any related personal beliefs.

Even if they don't wish to be present, owners who opt for euthanasia should be told how this will be accomplished to dispel any unspoken fears they may harbor about the act itself. "I'll inject the solution right into Fuzzy's IV catheter," Dr. Weisburg tells Mr. Clay. "And then he'll fall asleep and it will be over in a matter of seconds." Other times, comparing the procedure to one familiar to the owner helps alleviate their fears: "We'll use the same technique we used to get blood for those tests only this time we'll inject a drug that acts like a very strong anesthetic.

First it will put Fluffy to sleep, and then it will stop her vital functions."
Clients who have favorite technicians also appreciate knowing that person will assist at this time.

It goes without saying that when clients choose to remain with their animals during euthanasia, they should be told exactly what will happen, including what may go wrong. No one can always guarantee a perfect venipuncture, especially on a terminally ill animal whose owner sobs in the corner of the room. Rectum and bladder do let go; animals who normally resist handling or try to bite don't suddenly become well-behaved.

Owners extremely attached to their pets may feel an obligation to remain with them even though they don't want to do this. The entire experience can become a nightmare for them, especially if they are not allowed to, or cannot, hold the animal during the process; they stand in the corner, obviously distressed, their fists clenched, tears streaming down their faces. When owners appear obviously upset during the preliminary discussion, taking them into a different room and explaining that it's not unloving not to stay with the animal if they don't want to may help these people a great deal.

"You know how much Fluffy likes Beth," Dr. Weisburg reminds Ms. Begley referring to the technician holding the cat in the next room. "You can say good-bye to Fluffy now, and then wait here and I'll come get you when it's over. That way Fluffy won't get upset seeing you so upset. She can just relax with Beth like she always does."

These are more than kind words meant to get a troublesome client out of the way. Human emotions definitely affect animals, and owners assign emotional meanings to animal behaviors whether or not science agrees with these interpretations. Owners aware of this option may still choose to remain, but most will then make every attempt to respond calmly to avoid needlessly upsetting their animals.

Finally, every attempt should be made to use the best possible equipment and drugs for euthanasia even though some practitioners maintain exactly the opposite on the grounds that it doesn't matter. The idea of using a bargain syringe or deal-of-the-century euthanasia solution in the owner's presence surely repulses every practitioner. However, sometimes we find the idea of performing the act sufficiently distasteful that we choose not to give it our full attention until the last minute. Dr. Weisburg reaches into the drawer and finds only those syringes he hates, but the technician already holds the animal, the owner looks on expectantly, and an emergency awaits him in the treatment room. Or he gets to the farm and realizes he only has the euthanasia solution that gives uneven results, and barely enough of that.

Regardless of whether the owner chooses to remain during the euthanasia or not, if any doubt exists about the equipment or the skills of the handler or any other aspect of the euthanasia, the solution is simple and inviolate: *Don't do it.* Clients almost invariably will forgive a practitioner who performs any act they believe in the best interests of their animals, even if it means waiting a few minutes or even hours under trying circumstances. Granted, veterinarians can and do finesse less than ideal situations on occasion, but the one time they don't will remain indelibly imprinted in their own minds as well as that of the client and anyone else present who will repeat the tale again and again. Even though clinicians may choose to believe these people do this out of ghoulish interest, inevitably the aspect of the debacle that strikes the most powerful and negative response in others is the same one that so affects the veterinarian: the poor animal. Those who realize it was avoidable can only feel a thousand times worse. The worst can happen to anyone under the best of circumstances, but there is no reason for it to result from the use of substandard equipment or drugs.

Although it can be very difficult, practitioners should bear in mind that everything that occurs when an animal dies possesses the potential to form a much more potent and vivid memory than anything that occurred during the animal's life. Owners who feel they were separated from the animal during that time may feel as guilty as those who believe they overlooked critical signs of illness or opted for euthanasia too soon. More than anything else, what owners experience when their animals die will influence their relationship with animals in the future. If they feel sufficiently troubled by what happened, they may choose never to own another animal. If they believe that their animal's death, regardless of the circumstances, was accomplished with dignity and respect for the animal's needs as well as their own, then the sadness eventually will fade and memories of the animal's life will replace those of their last days or hours together.

Chapter 17
The Art of Death and Dying:
The Practitioner

When asked how he deals with euthanasia, a veterinary faculty member replied that he always waits until there are no students around so he can be alone with his thoughts and the animal at that time. He also noted that at such times he consoles himself with the knowledge that he did everything possible to save the animal, and he makes every attempt to attend the necropsy so he can learn the maximum amount from that case.

For many in private practice, the idea that the pain of every euthanasia could be tempered by the knowledge that one had done everything possible as well as by the knowledge gained from a full necropsy seems nothing short of heavenly. In the private practitioner's world, when euthanasia occurs is just as likely to be determined by various client limits as those of medical science; and because of the emotional components of the human-animal relationship and the cure rather than cause orientation of many owners, clinicians may do relatively few necropsies. When we add those animals which owners want euthanized because they "didn't work out" for one reason or another, the lack of closure can prove particularly trying for the clinician. If the veterinarian works in an area serviced by shelters and/or other practitioners who adhere to a no-kill policy for moral reasons, the additional emotional burden placed on the clinician who then becomes "immoral" by definition can become enormous.

Food animal practitioners often experience the best of worlds possible in private practice when it comes to dealing with death. First, they may be protected from emotional involvement by both their own and their clients' chattel orientations. Even those food animal practitioners who claim not to adhere to a chattel approach find it much easier to separate animal welfare from animal rights and define themselves as agents only of the former. Second, a concern for the health of others in the herd or flock makes owners of food animal more amenable to the idea of necropsy. Compare this to the companion animal practitioner who often must deal with sobbing owners, discuss the pros and cons of burial and cremation (and now perhaps help the owner choose a casket or weigh the advantages and disadvantages of mummification), and never know for sure what caused the animal's illness and subsequent death.

Because so many highly subjective, nonscientific factors can assault the practitioner when patients are dying or die, and because clients still expect us to function as the most knowledgeable persons under those circumstances even if our training in these areas may approach nil, this chapter will take a closer look at death and dying from the practitioner's view.

In addition to the references cited in the previous chapter, the following are particularly beneficial because they specifically address practitioners and their needs at these times:

"Pet Loss: A Survey of the Attitudes and Feelings of Practicing Veterinarians," by B. Fogle and D. Abrahamson (*Anthrozoös* [1990] 3:151–54).

"Grief and Stress from So Many Animal Deaths," by Lynette Hart and B. Benjamin Hart (*Companion Animal Practice* 1[1987]:20–21).

"How to Handle a Client in Tears," by Priscilla Stockner (*Trends* [January 1986]: 61–63).

Preventive Measures

As we noted in the discussion of practitioner orientations, the art of practice depends on the practitioner's ability to strike a balance between the needs of the patient, client, and clinician him- or herself. Because nothing brings out bizarre client behavior more than the fear of impending or actual death, the more veterinarians can do to prepare owners for this possibility, the less traumatic the experience will be for themselves as well as their clients.

Numerous practice management experts recommend giving new clients a brochure that describes the services offered by the practice. However, many practitioners delete any reference to death-related services or provide only the most limited mention of them in these publications believing it negates the positive image they wish to convey. Thus clients may read of the state-of-the-art death-defying science and technology offered by Dr. Fiedler's River Valley Veterinary Hospital, but nothing about his crematorium, working relationship with the nearby pet cemetery, or full necropsy facilities.

What Dr. Fiedler considers his upbeat policy costs him on two fronts. First, he contributes to his clients' ignorance when he fails to present the often practitioner- as well as client-healing necropsy option, which few companion animal owners (and some food animal owners) even recognize as real, as a routine aspect of veterinary practice. Second, he denies his clients the opportunity to consider these death-related options under nonthreatening circumstances. Compare responding to the owner of the healthy pup asking about necropsy and cremation after reading the description of these services and their benefits in a brochure to trying to explain these same options to the distraught client at the time of the animal's death. Whether death comes as a result of sudden trauma or following protracted illness, at that time many owners feel their animals' bodies have been through enough. Couple this with their mental image of a necropsy as something closer to a butchering than a human autopsy and we can appreciate why they would not want to subject their to animals this procedure, let alone pay for it. Granted practitioners rightfully may question these client interpretations, but most veterinarians (and clients) find it at least unseemly if not ghoulish for a clinician to pressure owners for a necropsy if they express any negative feelings about it whatsoever. Consequently, it makes sense to raise the issue in a positive manner with the owners of healthy animals so they can ask their questions and work through their feelings in a nonthreatening environment. When and if the time comes to face these death-related options, clients already will possess a working knowledge of what these options involve.

Brief discussions of disposal of the remains should include those offered by the practice as well as those offered by others with whom the practice maintains a working relationship. If local laws permit, many people much prefer to bury their animals on their own property, yet few may realize they have this option. For many, the very act of preparing the grave and burying the animal in what owners consider familiar surroundings can play a critical role in the grieving and healing process. Practices that use mass graves provided by local town governments should describe these as such to clients. That way when the journalism senior at the local college who envisions himself a budding investigative reporter writes that front page exposé—complete with photos of dead and decaying bodies—about the "despicable practice," clients who opted for this service won't feel shocked or betrayed. For example, Dr. Fiedler might say to the new pup's owner, "The town provides a common grave for animals behind the police department that's little more than a deep hole where they layer the bodies with a covering of dirt. It's not attractive by any means, which is why a lot of owners prefer cremation or bury their animals at home or at the Peaceful Meadows Pet Cemetery."

The brochure also should state any policy the practitioner maintains regarding euthanasia. This may include the basics, such as the need for owners to sign a release and a brief description of the method used, as well as any other pertinent issues such as:

- the owner's option to be present during the process
- any requirements that owners of animals brought in for euthanasia be interviewed by a clinician
- existence of any no-kill policy

Naturally, no service should be offered that violates the standards or sensitivities of the veterinarian or the laws of the area. Those practitioners who can barely deal with euthanasia themselves should not feel obligated to perform these in the presence of the owners. This only makes a bad situation worse and increases the probability that the clinician will make a technical error or relate poorly to clients at a time when they may need quality support the most. However, any practitioner who feels this way should apprise clients of this policy beforehand and refer them to another clinician capable of performing this service for them.

Geriatric Examinations

Much has been written about the value of specifically addressing the problems of older animals, but most of this focuses on the medical aspects of this life stage. However, such examinations also provide an excellent opportunity for practitioners to broach the subject of death and dying with their clients. Unfortunately, many practitioners dread doing this because they fear that clients will perceive them as pessimistic, or perhaps because of their own fears regarding death and dying. However, knowledge is power and in reality most clients prefer discussing these subjects when their animals appear healthy so they can ask questions, mull over the various aspects involved, and discuss any options with other family members. Some practitioners prefer to make this a separate "nonmedical" examination and tell owners they needn't bring the animal if they feel it will inhibit their discussion of these troublesome but necessary subjects in any way, an option many clients appreciate. Additionally, some meet with clients in their offices rather than an examination room to provide a more informal and intimate environment for this discussion.

What topics should practitioners cover during these sessions? We noted in our discussion of the critically ill or injured animal that many times owners see serious problems as possessing two possible outcomes: The animal will die or it will recover completely. During this meeting, the veterinarian can ask the client to seriously consider his or her limits, not with the idea of passing judgment, but to help the client gain a clear idea of how far he or she wants to and can go when and if the animal becomes ill. When Dr. Fiedler raises this issue with the O'Dells, who own a healthy eleven-year-old beagle, they note that they both work and spend a great deal of time away from home so any long-term nursing care would be out of the question for them. Other clients might mention financial limitations, while others say they want the best possible care right up to the end, including referrals to specialists if necessary.

This doesn't mean clients can't change their minds. In fact, many who profess to possess no limits at the time of their discussion with the veterinarian—often fearing the veterinarian will think ill of them for considering time or money a factor—will then go home and mull over these issues and discuss them with others. Although not all of them will formulate a clear plan, the very fact that the veterinarian raised the issue and frankly discussed any options enables them to view the subject with far more objectivity than most can muster when faced with a dying animal. Furthermore, this gives the veterinarian an opportunity to present options that might enable them to treat the animal longer.

Compare Dr. Fiedler's describing his optional payment and hospitalization/day-care plans to the O'Dells during such a meeting to his bringing these up at the time of serious illness when the O'Dells are considering euthanasia. Many clients find it difficult to objectively evaluate their alternatives under these circumstances and complain of feeling pressured by the veterinarian to make a decision. At its very worst, we see situations like the one described by one very angry client: "When no one told me about any options until I said I wanted the animal put down, I felt like they didn't give a damn about me. No matter what they say, they'll never convince me they were more interested in that dog than the money they'd make treating him!"

Most certainly, the issue of euthanasia also should be raised during geriatric counseling sessions. Ideally this merely means reiterating the material in the client brochure. At that time, clients who voice strong sentiments regarding this option tend to fall into two opposite categories:

- Those who say they couldn't consider euthanasia under any circumstances
- Those who do not want the animal subjected to life-sustaining procedures that do not result in what they consider a quality life

A note to this effect can be made in the client record at the time, although neither pronouncement should be considered inviolate. Clients who said they could never euthanize an animal may feel quite differently after they watch it deteriorate from a nonresponsive, degenerative disease; others who believed they could euthanize may experience a bond with a particular animal that possesses so much symbolism that they can't bear to part with the animal under any circumstances. Nonetheless, even if people change their minds, such interviews do serve to inform them of their options in a relatively benign setting and help limit the negative emotions associated with the actual event for the veterinarian every bit as much as for the owner. Veterinarians also should reiterate their own views regarding euthanasia so clients can seek the services of another practitioner if these views differ substantially from their own.

Dealing with the Dying Animal

As we would expect, practitioners go through the same five-stage process that owners do as they strive to accept the dying animal's condition. However, because veterinarians confront this reality more often than most clients, and from a different perspective, the sequence merits discussion. Moreover, many times practitioners fully cognizant of this process in owners fail to recognize that they experience it themselves. Dr. Fiedler believes that losing a patient goes with the job to the point that he doesn't even mention the trauma case that fails to respond to treatment. Nonetheless, his wife and children know from past experience that his angry outburst at dinner that evening most likely relates to a dying animal. As time goes on, practitioners may face so many dying animals that they zip through the five-stage process relatively quickly. However, no matter how experienced we become, a particular case always possesses the potential to get us stuck in one stage of that process or another.

Three practice situations lend themselves to denial more than others. First, clinicians are as apt to deny terminal illness in a favorite patient as the animal's owners. When Seymour, the Whitmans' cat and Dr. Fiedler's first patient the day he opened his practice, develops chronic renal problems that one day fail to respond to treatment, Dr. Fiedler refuses to accept this. He questions the test results as well as the technician who collected the samples; he wonders whether the owners medicated the animal properly; he checks the drugs to make sure he prescribed the right dosage. In short, he does everything in his power to convince himself that the animal's lack of response is not related to irreversible kidney failure, but rather to a rectifiable problem.

Second, practitioners may refuse to accept impending death that results from what they consider the owner's refusal to treat a treatable condition. When Dr. Fiedler diagnoses a fracture he knows will respond well to pinning, he can't believe it when the owners refuse treatment and ask him to put the ewe down. Even though they appear quite adamant, he asks them to think about it some more and give him a call later in the day.

Third and most troubling, clinicians may deny deterioration that occurs as a result of conditions they do not acknowledge as real. Recall the case of the highly dependent Siamese cat admitted for routine OHE, which then proceeded to fade away as a result of the combined assault of hospitalization and separation from its owner. Because Dr. Fiedler is convinced everything about the surgery went perfectly and considers his hospital a state-of-the-art facility, he refuses to accept the fact that the cat is dying.

Surely every practitioner can see how each one of these examples possesses the potential to precipitate an angry response. Although most clinicians feel angry at themselves for their inability to make the animal well, unfortunately they may aim their anger at others. When Seymour fails to respond, Dr. Fiedler lashes out at his technician when she stops to replace another patient's soiled bedding on her way to give Seymour his medication: "No wonder he's not getting any better!" he rages. That evening as he waits to hear from the ewe's owners, he berates his wife for letting the children make so much noise while he's trying to work. When the breeder tells him the cat will die if he doesn't let her take it home, he angrily accuses her of practicing veterinary medicine without a license.

Just as client anger can precipitate a lot of problems for practitioners, practitioner anger can precipitate a lot of problems for clients and others, including the veterinarian. Dr. Fiedler's angry outbursts eventually lead yet another good technician to seek employment in more stable surroundings even as his wife questions the quality of her relationship with him. And while few veterinarians feel that client anger provides them with a viable reason for legal action, a significant number of clients may view angry practitioners as a cause for litigation. When Dr. Fiedler shouts at her that he will *not* send her cat home, the breeder shouts back, "If that animal dies in this hospital, you'll hear from my lawyer!"

Just as we noted that clients may use modern technology to bargain their way out of accepting an animal's terminal condition, so do clinicians. This poses few problems if the client shares that view: If neither Seymour's owners nor Dr. Fiedler can accept the cat's failure to respond as anything more than its need for a different or expanded treatment, then client and clinician can continue working as a team. If the client doesn't share this view, this doesn't necessarily mean the practitioner also must give up on the patient, but he or she must handle the situation very carefully.

For example, suppose the Whitmans decide they don't want to try any more treatments, but Dr. Fiedler reads a journal article about an experimental protocol that has shown promise in some cases like Seymour's. Should he try to convince the owners to try this? The answer to that depends on the answers to two other questions:

- Why don't the owners want to treat the animal?
- Why does the veterinarian want to treat it?

If consultation with the Whitmans reveals that the primary reason they don't want to try another treatment is because they can't afford it, Dr. Fiedler might offer to accept monthly payments or even treat Seymour at a reduced rate because of the experimental nature of the proposed treatment. Some veterinarians also will lower their fees for strictly emotional reasons: Seymour carries such an emotional charge, Dr. Fiedler can't bear to give up on the animal for something he sees as so materialistic and inconsequential as money. Although some would question the business sense of such a choice, those practitioners who take this route rarely see this as a factor.

However, if the Whitmans tell Dr. Fiedler they don't want to try another treatment because Seymour now runs from them fearing more medication or because distress over the cat's condition is aggravating Ms. Whitman's own medical problems, then trying to bargain with the owners for more time would not seem to be a caring practitioner response.

Obviously, veterinarians who perceive themselves as the ultimate authority on what is best for the animal and see this as separate from the owners' needs probably wouldn't even think to communicate with clients in this manner. If Dr. Fiedler assumed the god role with the Whitmans he simply would tell them what he intended to do; if they resisted, he would either insinuate or state outright that they didn't care about Seymour. However, most clients resent being treated in this manner, and those who believe the practitioner usurped the responsibility for all choices regarding the animal's treatment from them (except for payment), often hold that clinician personally responsible for all consequences. Although this may enhance the god practitioner's status when the animal recovers, when the critically ill animal dies at the end of a long string of treatments, these clients will blame—and often eagerly blame—the practitioner for this, too.

Finally, if the practitioner's fear of death rather than the quality of life of the patient and client serves as the primary motivator, urging owners to continue treatment can create serious problems. Throughout this text we noted how owners who feel pressured to treat their animals in a manner with which they disagree may consciously or subconsciously sabotage the treatment. This poses few if any problems for the hospitalized patient, but when the Whitmans must come home from work every night and clean up vomit or diarrhea and drag Seymour out from under the bed to medicate him, then wake up to the sound of him vomiting during the night, we can appreciate that these "normal side effects" of the treatment could greatly undermine their relationship with the cat to the point that they decide to skip the medication every once in a while.

Some owners remain charitable toward the clinician who places them in this position and, ironically, commonly express pity for the practitioner's lack of sensitivity, the one quality the majority of these veterinarians would claim above all others. Other owners may resent what they consider the veterinarian's unwarranted interference, a view they may keep to themselves or share with others. In either case, like those practitioners who set themselves up as the authority of what is best for the animal unmindful of the owners' needs, these clinicians set themselves up for much more negative client responses when the animal dies.

Although depression related to a dying animal can strike any practitioner, new veterinary graduates succumb to it most frequently. Following graduation, Dr. Morris takes a position in a rural clinic with the idea that she will bring quality state-of-the-art medicine to the area. When previously unacknowledged client limitations as well as the clinic's limited facilities repeatedly thwart her attempts to successfully treat what she considers serious but treatable conditions, she succumbs to depression.

New graduates as well as experienced practitioners who either know for sure or intuitively sense that they've overlooked some critical factor in the dying animal's diagnosis and/or treatment may also experience depression. When Dr. Fiedler watches that Siamese cat fade, the idea that the owner might be right depresses him more than if he were losing the animal to a virulent infection.

The only problem conferred by acceptance is the same one experienced by clients: Sometimes we can comprehend an animal's dying condition intellectually before we do so emotionally. Remember that people may vacillate between various stages before finally accepting a particular situation, and practitioners are no more immune to this than their clients. If Dr. Fiedler accepts that all Seymour's test results indicate a continued decline but he personally does not agree with that conclusion, he would be better off sharing his mixed feelings with the Whitmans than presenting the test results as definitive evidence that it's time to accept that Seymour is beyond hope. Not only can clients pick up on these practitioner inconsistencies, many veterinarians tell tales of animals who beat what various test results indicated were unbeatable odds. Although clinicians should never give clients false hope, neither should they discount their own strong intuitive feelings or those of the client, either. As always, however, these feelings must be communicated with the client when they arise, not after the fact in an attempt to placate an angry or confused owner.

Dealing with Death

As we noted in our discussion of client responses, human responses toward death tend to be more dramatic than those toward the dying patient. This holds particularly true for practitioners schooled in the death-defying tradition because under those circumstances, every death becomes a failure in one way or another. For those practitioners who have chosen not to work through their own feelings about death, the sense of inadequacy can be overwhelming when a patient dies.

Consider the case of Dr. Fiedler and the ewe with the broken leg. Because of his beliefs about animal rights, he feels that every treatable case should be treated regardless of the species. Although morally a consistent view, it completely denies the reality in which the ewe's owners live. When they call to tell him they don't want the animal treated and have sent her off to slaughter, his shock quickly converts to rage and he accuses them of heartless cruelty. Many client responses come to mind, but this retort brought one practitioner up short: "How can you call *me* cruel when your inability to accept reality meant that animal had to spend the whole day in that condition?"

Like clients, veterinarians who lose patients have been known to yell, pound counters, and throw things, while others opt for the freeze response and internalize their anger, and still others flee the scene. Whichever approach we take, these all represent variations of the fear response, a logical reaction to this greatest of human fears.

Whereas owners may bargain with death via the disposal of the remains, veterinarians may try to soften death's sting by attributing it to something other than themselves. During this phase, the clients often come in for more than their share of the blame. Dr. Fiedler tells himself Seymour would have lived at least a month longer had the Whitmans been more conscientious; the ewe never would have died if there were laws to prevent such cruel behavior. As owner life-styles become increasingly complex, he also can blame the owners' lack of time, money, and all the other owner limitations previously discussed for the animal's demise.

Veterinarians who work for others in what they consider under-equipped facilities may blame these for the animal's death during the bargaining phase: "If only we had ultrasound, I could have picked up that problem sooner." "If only I had access to a fully equipped lab like I did at school, this never would have happened."

If practitioners perceive the issues raised during this phase as remediable and then set out to accomplish this, they may pass quickly through depression to acceptance of the animal's death: "I messed up because I didn't find out exactly what Seymour was doing at home and how it affected the Whitmans," notes Dr. Fiedler, "but the next time I see an animal with problems like that, I'm going to be sure I spend a lot more time talking to the owners." Meanwhile the practitioner in the under-equipped facility may decide her dream of bringing state-of-the-art science and technology to the boondocks isn't realistic and apply for a residency in a large teaching hospital.

However, if practitioners see themselves as failures in any way, then the death of the animal can cause profound depression and can serve as a major contributing factor to burnout (Chapter 18). Most certainly those veterinarians who see their function strictly in terms of defying death and preserving life fail every time an animal dies. Fortunately, few practitioners take such a narrow view. Rather, most of us maintain an often arbitrary and highly subjective criteria for what we consider a good death. If a particular situation fulfills that criteria, we can accept it sooner than if it does not. Thus, even though saddened by Seymour's death, if Dr. Fiedler feels that he, the animal, and the owners fulfilled that enigmatic medical criterion known as "doing enough" or "going the extra mile" then he can accept the outcome. When we believe this true, most of us can not only accept death but also perform euthanasia with a clear conscience.

However, if by our definitions the owner, animal, or we ourselves did not do enough, then practitioners may plunge themselves into a black hole of depression in which the phrase "I should have" echoes again and again. If this occurs often, practitioners owe it to themselves, their families, their clients, and their patients to take a very serious look at their criteria for a good death and determine whether these are, or ever can be, compatible with that particular practice setting. If Dr. Fiedler's criteria include access to all the science and technology available to him as a veterinary student and fulfillment of an animal rights philosophy that perceives all animals as equal, he most likely will experience far more bad deaths than good ones in his mixed practice in an economically depressed area. Practitioners who discover this initially may believe that the solution to the problem means changing everyone else's beliefs to coincide with their own. However, this usually proves such a time-consuming and relatively unrewarding endeavor it serves only to increase rather than diminish the depression.

Many times acceptance of death comes so gradually for busy practitioners that they don't even acknowledge its existence. More commonly, they recognize it more as a lack of depression when they think of that particular patient. When neighbors of the Whitmans mention how Seymour used to chase their dog, Dr. Fiedler finds himself laughing and adding his own fond memories of the cat. Initially, he may not even remember that the cat is dead, but when he does there will be a fleeting sense of loss and maybe even still a little pain, but it quickly gives way to the memories of the positive interactions he shared with the animal and its owners.

Using Rituals to Cope with Euthanasia

Human behavioral scientists increasingly acknowledge the beneficial role rituals play in our lives, and no act receives more ritualistic attention in all cultures than death. Consequently, it seems most tragic that the death-defying (or perhaps more correctly death-denying) attitude of medical education many times denies students the opportunity to appreciate death—regardless of how it occurs—as a consequence of life, and to formulate their own philosophies and any necessary comforting rituals to go with these. Even worse, new graduates may find themselves "eased" into doing "real" veterinary work by being assigned all the euthanasias when they take a position working for someone else. Many times employers do this because they want to relieve themselves of this emotional burden, although few will admit this to the new employee. More commonly they imply that the act is so inconsequential that, like giving a dose of vaccine, even a new graduate can do it.

However, for the average graduate who may possess little first-hand experience with death by medically acceptable causes let alone euthanasia, performing euthanasias is not a simple matter in the least. It would make more sense to prepare new graduates for this by allowing them to build their confidence, first by treating responsive cases with their few negative client-related problems, and then terminally ill animals with their more complex owner components, before allowing them to perform euthanasias. Only after they work through their own feelings about when and if they can justify euthanasia and if they can do it in the owner's presence should they be permitted to do this.

Arnold Arluke describes the way one group of shelter workers deal with euthanasia in "Coping with Euthanasia: A Case Study of Shelter Culture," an article that should be required reading for every veterinary student and every practitioner hiring a new graduate or technician. In it, Arluke describes how workers gradually introduce new employees to the reality of euthanasia and how they make their peace with it. Unlike many veterinarians, these workers do not expect a new employee to begin doing euthanasias immediately and without training, but rather see it as a very special art and skill different from that required for their other duties. In short, they acknowledge the enormity of the act and incorporate this into a meaningful ritual for the new employee rather than running away from it and even denigrating it, as some veterinarians do. For them, euthanasia isn't the most insignificant act: It's the most significant one (Arluke 1991, 198:1176–80).

For many practitioners, crying clients rank as even more troublesome than a cow down in a back field at midnight during a snowstorm or a vicious Shar Pei with generalized pyoderma and multiple antibiotic allergies. However, clients overwhelmingly agree that the practitioner who doesn't feel self-conscious about shedding a tear makes it much easier for them to express their own sadness, too. This particular ritual also appears to make good physiological as well as psychological sense. Studies done by William H. Fry, director of the Dry Eye and Research Center at St. Paul Ramsey Medical Center, indicate that tears of sadness differ chemically from those produced in response to irritants, and these differences represent the waste products of negative emotion. He and others postulate that crying serves as an effective way to rid the body of these wastes more quickly ("Tears" 1992, 10:4). Similarly, because one of the signs of depression is the inability to cry, those who feel no need to inhibit their tears at the time of euthanasia stand a better chance of warding off depression regarding the event after the fact.

Even if practitioners can't cry with their clients, doing something so simple as placing a box of tissues within easy reach of clients communicates acceptance of tears under these circumstances and makes it easier for owners to express their grief without embarrassment.

Among the other rituals used by practitioners, one comes from Native American culture: asking the animal's permission to euthanize it with dignity and without pain, and then thanking it for its cooperation and wishing it well when the act is completed. Obviously such a ritual can only comfort those who believe such human-animal communication possible, but a surprising number of veterinarians (as well as clients) fall into this category. Some, like the faculty member, prefer to perform euthanasias alone so they can follow their thoughts and feelings wherever they may lead without embarrassment. Others prefer the assistance of a particular technician with whom they feel comfortable sharing their thoughts and emotions at the time. Many find follow-up phone calls or notes to owners as helpful to them as their clients.

A final comforting message for those practitioners who find themselves doing more than their share of euthanasias for fearful colleagues and those with no-kill policies. In his book, *All I Really Need to Know I Learned in Kindergarten*, minister Robert Fulghum writes that routinely facing death and all its trappings as part of his work greatly affects his view of life. In addition to listing activities he no longer worries about that others consider important, Fulghum mentions that he no longer kills spiders, either. He doesn't claim any great moral virtue for this choice, but rather simply notes that there is neither the time nor the need to do this (Fulghum 1986, 123).

Any clinician who routinely confronts rather than avoids death as a part of practice immediately can identify with Fulghum's philosophy. Unlike those who espouse animal rights and decry the owner's right to euthanize an animal for any reason that violates the clinicians' own beliefs or those who seek to avoid the reality of death and their role in it by decrying the animal rights movement and hiding behind chattel views, those who accept the reality of euthanasia and formulate the intimate rites and rituals necessary to comfort themselves, their patients, and clients come to see both life and death in a completely different way. It is knowing that they have faced this particular gorgon and lived that gives them a certain peace and tolerance. They see themselves as stewards, exercising dominion over rather than seeking to dominate the animal kingdom with their own beliefs; and they see that dominion spanning the animal's life from birth to death regardless of the circumstances. They have neither the time nor the need to pass judgment on others, any more than they have the time or need to squash a spider simply because it's there.

Regardless of what thought processes or rituals practitioners use to help them cope, a good death embodies a quality best summed up in a sentiment typed on a three-by-five-inch card that one practitioner keeps in the drawer of her examination table: "Sometimes the ultimate act of love is knowing when to let go." Sometimes practitioners may believe death comes too soon or not soon enough, but those who see meeting the needs of both their patients and their clients as a privilege as well as a responsibility can learn as much or more about life and love when they face the reality of death in veterinary practice.

Chapter 18
Burnout

A discussion of burnout logically follows a discussion of the subjective aspects of critical illness and injury, death, and euthanasia because many practitioners cite these as major causes of burnout. Whereas veterinarians who find the technological aspects of practice too demanding or boring tend to come to this conclusion relatively soon after graduation from veterinary school and make changes, those who find the subjective factors troublesome commonly tolerate these much longer. Depending on the year of graduation, the lack of or limited exposure to these factors during the practitioner's education initially may lead to denial of the effect of these parameters. When she first entered practice, Dr. Moore approached each case as a medical challenge. She examined a dog with polyuria and polydipsia and saw her role as diagnosing and treating a possible case of canine diabetes in adherence to the standards set down in various texts, classes, and seminars. She initially dismissed the little kinks and curves put into this linear process by the dog—an aggressive male poodle named Skippy with chronic ear and skin problems—and the owners, the McKenzies, who both worked swingshifts and inherited the less than pleasant animal when Mr. McKenzie's mother died the previous year. When the Jackson brothers asked for what she considered the bare minimum treatment for their herd, which they considered more than adequate, she also ignored all those unresolved feelings about animal rights she had subordinated during her education because she didn't want to antagonize faculty by bringing up the issue.

In addition to the lack of previous exposure to these nonmedical aspects of practice making it tolerable if not necessarily easy to dismiss them initially, a second and paradoxical reason leads veterinarians to endure the burden of emotional stress much longer: Those experiencing it can always find colleagues who share their views. At any given veterinary meeting, practitioners are as likely to talk about long hours capped with emergency-call duty, exhaustion, high debts, low salaries, and deteriorating (or nonexistent) social or family life as any medical or surgical procedure. This, in turn, makes it possible to perpetuate the belief that these things go with the territory of veterinary practice. When Dr. Moore mentions her feelings of frustration when dealing with the McKenzies and Skippy, sympathetic nods and comments like, "I must have ten of those!" and "Aren't those cases the absolute worst!" greet her from all directions.

Psychologists Elliot Aronson and Ayala Pines note that individuals who experience burnout almost invariably are those who are the most enthusiastic and idealistic about their work, and naturally exude a certain optimism (Aronson and Pines, 1992). When Dr. Moore first enters private practice, she sees those almost daily euthanasias and all the negative feelings they elicit as a problem she easily can remedy once she becomes settled into the practice and the community: Surely if she gives presentations on animal rights to the grange, 4-H, Rotary Club, and other organizations in the area, that will end the abuses.

Further help denying the reality and consequences of failure to deal with these subjective factors comes from other personality traits of those susceptible to burnout. Childhood images as "the little helper," "the rescuer," "the smart one," and "good" form the core of the idealist professional's personality (Elkins and Kearney 1992, 200:604). When we overlay those with the mystique of "the most knowledgeable person" regarding animals and their welfare conferred by our education and regarding their rights as expected by the general public, the bright idealists initially may dismiss any negative feelings as a necessary cross to bear: "If I don't care for all these animals and their owners," asks Dr. Moore as she pours herself another glass of wine, "who will?"

The problem with all of these approaches is that none of them do anything to resolve the underlying causes of burnout. Dismissing the frustration caused by Skippy's behavior and the McKenzie's life-style doesn't make these conditions (or their negative effects) disappear any more than yielding to it will guarantee it won't occur when dealing with other patients and clients. Commiserating with other practitioners also usually offers little in the way of solutions. Following such sessions, Dr. Moore leaves with whatever reassurance she gains from knowing she's not alone as she seeks to make sense of these aspects of practice, but this does nothing to help her make sense of these parameters. While the idea that others fare as badly or even worse may console her for a while, that quickly fades as she faces the same problems again. Similarly, her enthusiasm and idealism quickly make her a favorite clinician, her work load increases, and she never finds the time to get out into the community and educate the public. Consequently, she can't stop the flow of euthanasias that result from treatable medical and/or behavioral problems; when she makes those farm calls she sees the same abuses she saw before only they begin to bother her more. Finally, her image of herself as a self-sacrificing martyr also reinforces rather than resolves the problem: The more she suffers, the more holy she becomes.

Signs of Burnout

Although practitioners may deny the need to address the subjective factors of practice for a while, those who continue to do so eventually begin to experience the signs of burnout:

- a sense of malaise
- emotional, physical, and psychological fatigue
- feelings of helplessness

Consider the case of Dr. Moore, the once enthusiastic young graduate determined to insure a quality life for every animal in her practice area if not the world. By the time she makes her monthly payment for her educational and car loans, pays her rent and various professional expenses (insurance, journal subscriptions, license, DEA registration, dues to various organizations), what remains of her salary barely covers the essentials; the idea of someday buying a house where she can have the animals she longs for, let alone raise a family, seems next to impossible. Because many in the community do consider her on a par with a physician, a stream of Girl Scouts, high school band boosters, and neighbors representing numerous charitable organizations solicit donations of both time and money which she feels obligated to make and which further drain her limited resources. As the new employee, she inherits the euthanasias and the majority of the call duty. Because she can't afford to get away, the two one-day continuing education meetings a year that her employer pays for serve as her vacation. She spends her day "off" in a flurry of activity as she tries to catch up on all the things she let go during the previous week; her two weeks of vacation time consist of more of the same plus a few days visiting her folks.

All of these factors form a common backdrop for the daily life of many new graduates, and we can see how these hardly create a supportive environment for someone coping with a less than vet-school-perfect practice as well as coming to grips with all the subjective aspects of practice for the first time. Just thinking about all those idealistic, hardworking Dr. Moores coming home to their stacks of bills and journals elicits feelings of emotional, physical, and psychological fatigue. More than a few veterinarians can recall nights spent lying exhausted in bed, minds swirling with professional and personal doubts: Why didn't the Chambers tell me they couldn't afford that treatment? Why did they wait until it was over to yell at me about the cost? Who can I call at the university to ask about the Bancrofts' cat? How can the Langs let those sheep live in such conditions? How can the boss ask me to work two weekends in a row? How can I ever afford a new muffler for the car if it doesn't pass inspection? Dear God, am I doomed to spend the rest of my life in this town alone?

Naturally, being the good little trouper and seeing so much that needs to be done to help the animals in her community, Dr. Moore finds some way to subordinate all her doubts and she immerses herself in her work. Over the months and years and mostly by trial and error, she learns about the emotional, physical, mental, financial, and other limits of her clients and the critical role the bond and behavior play in the treatment process. Because she's so conscientious, her reputation grows more rapidly than her salary; and because she remains the junior clinician in a two-person practice, she still gets all the euthanasias, most of the holiday work, and whatever other undesirable duties her employer wants to pass on to someone else. After all, that's why he hired her: to keep from burning out himself.

Initially Dr. Moore's optimistic nature enables her to convince herself that this all constitutes an orientation period and once she gets the routine down, she won't feel so pressured. However, the euthanasias keep coming, new technological and medical advances fill practically every page in the growing stack of unread journals, each client and animal combination presents her with new subjective factors she never even acknowledged as real let alone learned to address. By her fifth year in practice with five more years of loan payments and a boss who seems more than content to let her do more and more while he does less and less, feelings of helplessness begin vying with those of fatigue.

Interestingly, at this point veterinarians may attempt to retreat to the education womb psychologically, as it were, by taking a more chattel-oriented approach to patients and objectifying clients in an effort to protect themselves from emotional assaults which they feel powerless to control. Elkins and Kearney describe the resulting progression as the four D's (1992, 200:604):

- disengagement
- distancing
- dulling
- deadness

During the disengagement phase, Dr. Moore decides she can't allow herself to care so much about her patients and clients. She vows not to spend her evenings pondering troublesome cases, reading journals, or speaking about responsible pet ownership to Girl Scouts, 4-H groups or anyone who will listen; instead, she'll curl up with a good mystery and a glass of wine. As the work load continues or increases, she tries to place even more distance between herself and her patients and clients. When a client mentions how difficult it is to medicate his dog, she dismisses this with an "I'm sure you'll think of something." When she visits the farm and sees the poor quality hay the farmer is feeding, she tells herself it's none of her business. Now when she reads her book or watches television, it takes two glasses of wine to take her mind off work. Spring comes and with it all the increased activity on the farm and in small animal practice, and distancing gives way to dullness as Dr. Moore attempts to cope. With so much to do and so little time, she focuses all of her diminishing energy on the cases that don't respond and ignores the rest. She reduces Skippy to "a diabetes" and his owners to little more than a vehicle which brings the dog to the clinic; she treats the down cow and ignores the early signs of respiratory problems in the calves in the next pen. She barely notices the pups and kittens in for routine vaccinations or the healthy cavorting lambs which used to make her laugh: She doesn't have time for them.

Finally, and not surprisingly because she has cut herself off from all the positive aspects of practice, a feeling of deadness overwhelms Dr. Moore. She goes about her duties like a robot, putting in her time, fueled primarily by the desire to get home, have a few drinks, fall into bed, and hopefully not be scared out of her wits by a call from yet another client with yet another avoidable "emergency" at midnight. Each day strikes her as being pretty much like the day before and she sees an endless stream of them stretching out in front of her with no respite in sight. She'll never get enough sleep; she'll never get her debts paid off; she'll never have a real vacation where she can lie on the beach and do nothing; she'll never have a home and someone to share it with.

At this point it bears noting that, as lonely and depressing as Dr. Moore's life appears, those married veterinarians with or without children who experience burnout fare no better. Although theoretically the single veterinarian may feel more isolated, the circumstances underlying burnout often lay bare those communications problems between couples that go unnoticed or ignored when leisure time and the money to enjoy it exist. As burnout begins to consume the veterinarian, the spouse and any children may become one more burden to bear instead of a source of renewal and support.

Similarly, even though burning-out employees often think their employers live the ideal life, more often than not those employers who knowingly or unwittingly create burnout conditions for their employees suffer from burnout themselves. Consider Dr. Moore's boss, Dr. Beckman. Dr. Beckman hired Dr. Moore because he was tired after being on call twenty-four hours a day, seven days a week for almost twenty years. True, he and several other practitioners in the county shared call duty, but he was well known in the community, many clients considered him a personal friend, and he felt that no matter where he went in town he was on call one way or another. As an established pillar of the community and family man, he accumulated a lot of social obligations that struck him as being more and more obligatory and less and less enjoyable the older he got. When he added all the changes occurring in practice thanks to the burgeoning technology, the increased public awareness of the animal rights movement and the bond, to say nothing of all the new government regulations, it seemed practice was becoming increasingly complex just when he thought he earned the right to slow down and enjoy the fruits of his labors.

Confronting Burnout

The majority of the articles and texts written on the subject of burnout and job stress agree that the first step to resolving the problem involves recognizing it as a function of the work situation and one's relationship to it rather than as a personal failure (Aronson and Pines, 1992; Brady 1992, 15: 31–33; Fletcher 1991; Gross 1993, 26:10; Underwood 1992, 23:86–88; Williams 1991, 34:26–29). Dr. Moore does not feel exhausted and disenchanted because she is a lousy veterinarian; she feels that way because she's a very good one who feels thwarted at every turn. If she weren't a compassionate and qualified practitioner, she wouldn't have all those clients telling their friends to seek her services. Nor would the Girl Scouts and 4-H groups want her to speak to them, judge their fairs, and attend their picnics. She wouldn't feel obligated to become involved in professional and other organizations to enhance the image of the veterinary profession in her community and the state. She wouldn't spend all those hours finding homes for abandoned animals and salavageable euthanasias and working with the local humane society trying to figure out some way to stop them. Regardless of what the veterinarian who experiences burnout may choose to believe, few in the community or among their colleagues would describe them as failures.

Once clinicians accept that the burnout doesn't result from some irreversible, tragic personal flaw, the next step involves accepting responsibility for resolving the problem. Ironically, even though most veterinarians who find themselves in this position excel at assuming responsibility for their patients and clients, they experience great difficulty assuming it for their own lives. "What can I do?" moans Dr. Moore. "I can't afford to quit."

At this point practitioners often make a bad situation worse by trying to project the problem away from themselves. Even if Dr. Moore could make a case for the fact that her boss is a chauvinistic, penny-pinching, barely qualified dolt, that his facility borders on the primitive, and that her education did next to nothing to prepare her for many of the most troubling aspects of practice, none of these realizations does anything to solve the problem. In fact, because these position her as a hapless victim of circumstance, they serve only to reinforce her feelings of helplessness.

Compare that approach to what happens when Dr. Moore sees resolving the problem as her goal. In this situation she assumes an active rather than passive role which immediately helps alleviate those feelings of disengagement and distancing. However, we also can appreciate that the longer she has experienced these states and the more these incorporate elements of dullness and deadness, the more difficult it may be for her to overcome her inertia and actually do something besides blame others for her problem. Mental health professionals usually recommend counseling for those in this position, but, unfortunately, more than a few veterinarians resist for several reasons:

- They can't afford it.
- They feel embarrassed that, as professionals, they can't solve their own problems.
- They don't believe any counselor can comprehend what they're experiencing.

Although an element of truth may undoubtedly underlie all of these concerns, those in this position do need someone they can talk to who won't reinforce the villain/victim mind-set that so often characterizes those experiencing burnout. If funds are limited, a good friend or even a casual acquaintance can function as a sounding board. Interestingly, many practitioners who have experienced burnout recommend *not* using colleagues in this capacity because fellow clinicians may reinforce the burning-out practitioner's blame-placing out of sympathy, particularly if they consider their own work situations less than ideal. Conversely, those who enjoy their work may serve only to depress the burning-out clinician more: "Sure, I could be happy too if I had a job, a salary, and a boss like Jim's!" grouses Dr. Moore after a former classmate takes her out to dinner in a failed attempt to cheer her up. Because of this, those outside the profession who can see the larger issue—the need for the practitioner to assume some control over the situation rather than assign blame for it—may provide greater help at this time.

The Messiah Trap

Once the veterinarian assumes the responsibility for resolving the problem, the next step involves realistically evaluating what changes can and cannot be made. Unfortunately, even though burnout results more from the work situation than professional inadequacies on the clinician's part, the veterinarian's feelings about his or her work definitely contribute to the problem at this stage. Although many would like to believe that if they had more money and more free time all their problems would magically disappear, that may not be true if they see themselves as the savior of all animals, the sole hope of legions of clients and patients in dire need of help.

Before physical, mental, and emotional exhaustion led Dr. Moore to disengage herself, practically every minute of her day was filled with what she considered important and necessary veterinary work. She was the first new practitioner in the area in almost twenty years and Dr. Beckman found preventive medicine boring and the bond and behavior confusing at best. Dr. Moore's food animal clients listened eagerly when she discussed the value of good nutrition, ventilation, and drainage; all that extra time spent with the owners of new pups and kittens paid off in fewer behavioral problems and more solid relationships. If any doubt existed in Dr. Moore's mind about the validity of her work, there was always a client or staff member to remind her: "You're so wonderful with the animals! What would we do without you?" Had someone told her that others felt the same way about her employer at one time, she would not have believed it.

Although different individuals use different terminology to describe the orientation that results from this combination of client devotion and public acclaim, the phrase "messiah trap" best sums up the tremendous emotional hold it can have on practitioners in this position. Dr. Moore knew months if not years ago that she could never be content working in that practice because of very real, albeit often undefinable, philosophical differences with her employer. It was these, not the lack of facilities, the low salary, or the long hours that created the greatest stress. To escape this awareness, she immersed herself in her work, losing herself (and her troubling thoughts) in the company of animals as she had so many times during her life. As her reputation grew, she assumed the responsibility for more and more clients and animals even as she retreated further and further from assuming responsibility for her own life. Now she tells herself she can't quit because all those animals and people need her. As one burned-out practitioner put it, "That would be like Jesus saying, 'I don't feel like getting crucified today. You folks are on your own.'"

As bizarre as this may sound to an outside observer, those who have been enmeshed in the messiah trap know just how insidiously seductive it can be. Moreover, there are more than enough clients, staff members, employers, and colleagues willing to reinforce this orientation because the messiahs often do a tremendous amount of good work and do much to advance the image of the profession. Until they begin to burn out, that is. At that point, a sense of hopelessness as well as betrayal may inundate them. Not only must Dr. Moore cope with the realization that her burden will never lighten as long as she pursues her current course, she also must deal with the fact that so many nice people appear more than content to allow her to destroy herself physically, mentally, and emotionally to do this. These realizations, in turn, often lead to two recurrent, highly volatile thoughts:

- How can those people do that to me?
- What will happen to the animals if I stop doing what I'm doing?

It takes no great insight to see that neither of these contributes anything beneficial to the process of coping with burnout any more than they lead the person to realistically evaluate any changes possible to relieve the stress. Consequently, those in this position first must free themselves from the messiah trap, which means facing what appears to be a very harsh and cruel reality to those idealists who most often find themselves in this position. A few insights offered by those who survived this process include:

- Reality Number 1: You can't save them all. No one can, regardless of how good the facilities, how smart the clinician, and how many hours in the day.
- Reality Number 2: Regardless of what you tell yourself, if you're unhappy you're not doing a good job.
- Reality Number 3: You might not be spending all that time at work because you're so dedicated; you might be doing it because you're inefficient.
- Reality Number 4: If you were to drop dead tomorrow, even your most dedicated clients and their animals would survive and even find a new messiah if that's what they want.

Putting out the Fire

Once practitioners free themselves from any messianic feelings and their resultant obligations, they can turn their attention to solving the problem of burnout. For example, when Dr. Moore objectively views her situation, she realizes that she can never be happy working for or with someone whose basic philosophy of practice so differs from her own. That, in turn, leads her to consider pursuing an advanced degree and teaching in a more idealistic veterinary school environment or striking out on her own. Given limited financial resources and the emphasis she places on the need for state-of-the-art equipment to practice quality veterinary medicine, she may decide academia offers the environment most compatible with her needs. On the other hand, if she enjoys the intimate one-to-one contact with her clients and patients and yearns for the freedom to do things her own way, then the idea of owning her own practice will hold the greater appeal.

Smoldering practitioners barely able to scrape by on their salaries might think it impossible to even consider owning a practice, but those determined to do so have come up with an amazing array of financial alternatives. Moreover, just thinking about solving the problem often enables these practitioners to see their situations in a new light. As soon as the idea of being on her own takes hold, instead of commiserating with other potential or real burnouts at meetings, Dr. Moore spends her time listening for news of those retiring or considering taking on a partner with the idea of ultimately selling the practice to that person. She puts the journals on hold for a while and reads some basic business books about how to start or buy a practice. She conducts informal mar-

keting surveys to determine if her area could support a house-call practice or one offering some other service not currently available. As the
idea takes on more form, she discusses it with friends or relatives who
offer suggestions regarding financial and other alternatives she didn't
even know existed, let alone ever considered. Even though it may take
her several years to finally get out on her own, the very process of thinking about it displaces the paralysis that perpetuates burnout.

Meanwhile employers like Dr. Beckman experiencing burnout face
different alternatives. If he finds the business aspects of practice overwhelming, he might consider selling the practice and going back to
school or to work for someone else. If he discovers he prefers to work
alone, the idea of letting Dr. Moore go and scaling back the practice or
selling her that part (large or small animal, or equine) that he finds
least rewarding might appeal to him. If he enjoys the professional stimulation of working with another clinician, he may consider adding
another practitioner to relieve some of the pressure on Dr. Moore. Or
he may decide to offer her a partnership. Like Dr. Moore, as long as he
focuses on those changes he can make rather than considering himself
a failure and seeking someone or something on which to blame this,
these will serve as a source of renewal.

In addition to working toward an obtainable goal, clinicians also need
to alleviate stress in their current situations. Ironically many employees
tolerate what they consider intolerable conditions, fearing they will be
fired when, in fact, that is often the last thing in their employers' minds.
Remember, those who burn out most commonly do so because they are
very good at what they do, and this often means they generate a fair
amount of income and goodwill for their employers. Consequently,
although some employers may agree to any demands with less grace
than others, most really don't want to lose these practitioners, any more
than they want them to be unhappy and miserable and alienating
clients. By the same token, employers may fail to communicate with
their employees about remediable situations, fearing the latter might
take it the wrong way. In these situations we see a workplace in which
employer and employee both hope the other will *guess* what's bothering
them and rectify the problem. However, unless they actually communicate with each other regarding their concerns, changes rarely occur.

What kinds of demands can employees experiencing burnout make
to lessen the stress? Although more money tops many a list, this often
results because so many see money as a symbol of success. However,
because money can carry such an emotional charge for employer and
employee alike, sometimes it's easier for both to deal in another form of

currency: time. For example, once Dr. Moore sheds her messiah identity and decides she wants to own her own practice, time to pursue this
interest means as much to her as money. She tells Dr. Beckman she will
give him a forty-hour work week which she considers fair based on her
experience and salary. If he sputters about all that call duty and weekend coverage, she offers to continue doing it and take compensatory
time off during the week. Above all, she makes her demands with a full
awareness that the worst that could happen would be that he fires her.
However, considering what her life has become, that would hardly be
any worse than what could happen if she continues working under the
present conditions. This, in turn, gives her the confidence to present
her case in an objective, professional manner.

Veterinarians who cringe at the idea of taking an approach they feel
could cost them their jobs should bear two things in mind. First, if they
don't do something, burnout could cost them their jobs anyway, plus a
lot more. Second, if they choose not to make changes out of fear, even
accepting responsibility for that choice will help alleviate some of the
pressure. Remember: More stress comes from doing nothing than from
doing the wrong thing.

Whatever demands practitioners feel their employers must meet, the
advantage of calmly and objectively pursuing these cannot be overemphasized. Far too often those in the throes of burnout allow a situation to reach crisis proportions in an effort to force themselves to overcome their fears and confront at least some of the underlying causes
head-on to relieve the pressure. After a night on call, losing a cow due to
sheer owner negligence, and euthanizing two aggressive dogs, Dr.
Moore loses it and screams at her boss about everything and anything
before she breaks down in tears and runs from the clinic, slamming the
door behind her. Although she may feel better after a good cry, it does
nothing to change the situation.

Compare that to her presenting her demands calmly to Dr. Beckman
during a time set aside specifically for that purpose. In the former case
Dr. Beckman easily could dismiss everything Dr. Moore tells him as the
ravings of a distraught employee having a bad day. In the latter, she provides him with an opportunity to consider her concerns as well as his
own options in an objective and professional manner.

Once again, not enough can be said about the value of quality communication for those seeking to relieve job-related stress. In retrospect,
almost every practitioner who experienced burnout commented that
no confrontation with an employer or employee ever turned out to be
as bad as he or she anticipated. Even those who quit or were fired, or
fired someone in the heat of the moment said they felt relieved that it

was over because, once it was, they no longer had to worry about what *could* happen when and if the confrontation occurred.

One clinician noted that when he compared those who experienced burnout to those who didn't, the one thing that struck him was that those who didn't knew how to say no, whereas the burnouts always felt obligated to say yes. Another said she thought that burnout didn't result so much from saying yes all the time as it did from believing she *had* to; if she didn't say yes, others would think she didn't care. However, all agreed that what traps practitioners in the downward spiral of burnout more than anything is the inability to make choices. Because of that, it seems wise to further examine the role choice plays in the art of veterinary practice.

Chapter 19
The Art of Making Choices

Whether we speak of owners who don't see things the way we do, animal rights, alternative approaches to medicine, coping with death and euthanasia, or burnout, confronting those subjective elements whose mastery constitutes the art of practice can seem mind-boggling at first. For those trained to perceive things in terms of not only right and wrong answers but also the selection of that one right answer from a limited collection of multiple choices, the idea that each of these issues could conceivably encompass an infinite number of right (as well as wrong) answers violates not only the way we've been taught to think, but also what we've been taught to think about.

Consider this worst-case scenario which begins with Dr. Ogilvie wavering on the brink of burnout. Even as he faces all the choices inherent in confronting that condition (including an unstable working relationship with his employer), he encounters Ms. Pritchard—a fixed-income senior citizen whose multiple medical problems rank on a par with those of her highly dependent, fourteen-year-old, biting Chihuahua, Salsa. After Dr. Ogilvie finishes with Ms. Pritchard and Salsa, he examines a lame horse belonging to a ten-year-old whose parents couldn't care less about the animal. When Dr. Ogilvie arrives, he finds the child and a blank check waiting for him in the barn with the horse. On his way home, he passes two farms and a trailer where he knows animals receive substandard treatment. When he arrives home, he opens his mailbox and finds at least one journal, numerous flyers for new drugs, books, and other veterinary paraphernalia as well as those from animal rights groups and national and local conservation and humane organizations. There are five messages on his answering machine: two from clients with urgent questions, two requests for him to speak to local organizations, and one from his mother wondering why he never writes.

In any one of these components of Dr. Ogilvie's less than ideal but hardly unique day, he faces so many probable courses of action we can see why he feels tempted simply to play it by ear and hope for the best. However, that approach leads to several familiar disadvantages.

- He more likely will forget any details of an improvised approach that works because these resulted from spur-of-the-moment decisions.
- He may wind up reacting to the situation rather than acting in a positive manner.
- His reaction rather than purposeful action may communicate lack of knowledge and/or caring to others.

In order to avoid these complications, many practitioners find it helpful to simplify the process by categorizing all alternatives as reflecting one of four possible choices:

- Accept the situation as it exists, including any negative feelings.
- Accept the situation, but eliminate the negative feelings.
- Change someone or something.
- Terminate the relationship.

By evaluating problems in this manner, we can eliminate those time-consuming and energy-draining results that arise when we react rather than act purposely, as well as all the negative effects associated with considering so many different probabilities that we never get around to making any choice at all. Additionally, utilizing these four possible response categories may help clients struggling to make choices regarding their animal's medical and/or behavioral problems. Surely all practitioners have found themselves in situations in which the clock ticks while owners summon a hundred reasons why they should treat the animal, interspersed with a hundred reasons why they should not. As we noted previously, assuming the god role can end this agony but the client's unwillingness to make choices may carry over into the treatment process. Consequently, Dr. Ogilvie may succeed in forcing Ms. Pritchard to try a different medication on Salsa, but then Ms. Pritchard blames Dr. Ogilvie (and calls him up!) every time she encounters even the slightest problem with the new approach.

Accept the Situation as It Exists, Including Any Negative Feelings

Although the idea of accepting situations that evoke negative feelings seems less than ideal, situations do arise in practice in which this approach serves as a viable alternative. For example, it bothers Dr. Ogilvie that Salsa growls and snaps and must be muzzled and restrained for even the most simple procedure. However, he discussed every way he knew to alter the dog's behavior and referred Ms. Pritchard to a behaviorist, all to no avail. Ms. Pritchard doesn't see Salsa's "nipping" as a problem and therefore never consistently responds to the animal in a way necessary to change the behavior. As Dr. Ogilvie finds himself becoming more and more frustrated with the client to the point of anger, he opts to accept Salsa's biting as well as his negative feelings about it rather than alienate the owner.

Within the medical arena, situations also arise in which the veterinarian and the client disagree about the nature of the problem and/or its treatment. Dr. Ogilvie sees what he considers Joe Cromwell's substandard husbandry practices (poor quality feed, faulty drainage and/or ventilation, heavy-handed handling, uneven surfaces or exposed hazards that could injure animals) and he mentions these time and time again to no avail. Every time he sees the animal with the recurrent lameness or eye problem, he recommends a more aggressive approach to cure it once and for all, and time and time again the owner benignly ignores the recommendation. Although theoretically he could force the issue legally or assume full responsibility for rectifying the problem himself, like most busy practitioners he opts to accept the situation and his negative feelings rather than become involved in an ideological battle with the client.

Similarly, practitioners do encounter (hopefully few) clients and animals they just don't like. Although sometimes we can give specific reasons for this ("She's drunk all the time," "He never listens to me," "That dog growls for no reason at all," "That mare bites"), other times it boils down to that highly subjective, unscientific element called "chemistry." On some primitive level, Dr. Ogilvie looks at these clients and animals and doesn't like them; *then* he comes up with the reasons to justify this intuitive feeling. Barring the presence of a definition that would enable him to make concrete changes to resolve the negative feelings, he simply accepts them.

Finally, practitioners may take this approach to the troublesome issues of alternatives therapies, animal rights, euthanasia, and burnout. Dr. Ogilvie tells himself he really should take the time to work out his feelings and a personal philosophy regarding these issues, but he barely has time to perform all his veterinary duties. He accepts all the negative feelings these subjects evoke, telling himself these constitute a normal part of the practice of veterinary medicine.

The advantage of this approach is that it enables practitioners to let go of troubling situations they believe beyond their control. Note that the first word in this choice is *accept.* As we know from our discussion of death and dying, acceptance results from a sequence that includes denial, anger, bargaining, and depression. Until Dr. Ogilvie accepts Salsa's biting, Joe Cromwell's substandard treatment of his livestock, that he just doesn't like some clients and animals, and his erratic responses to alternative therapies, animal rights, and euthanasia, he most likely will experience at least some of that sequence every time he encounters or even thinks about these issues. During one examination of Salsa, he tries to convince himself that Salsa is basically a nice dog, but he can't see it because he's having a bad day. When the dog snaps at him as usual, he decides that's not true. "That dog's an idiot!" he thinks angrily. "And his owner's an idiot for letting him act like that!" Then he remembers his oath and begins to bargain: Maybe if he explained things clearly to Ms. Pritchard or used a different approach. Then he remembers all the different approaches he tried during the past years, and depression sets in. Rather than unknowingly going through that sequence every time he sees Ms. Pritchard and the dog, accepting the situation and his negative feelings about it saves him a lot of time and energy. However, note that choosing this option does not mean Dr. Ogilvie condones the dog's negative behavior: What he accepts is that he can't change the behavior because the owner doesn't consider it a problem.

Similarly, although perhaps not what many would consider the optimal response, practitioners who accept their negative feelings about alternative therapies, animal rights, euthanasia, and burnout do gain a certain peace from knowing this represents a choice they made rather than the result of circumstances beyond their control. This, in turn, frees them from at least some of the feelings of frustration and hopelessness that can arise when confrontations with those holding different views occur.

The disadvantage of this approach is that it can become a convenient dumping ground for those who don't want to initiate changes because they lack either the expertise or interest in the problem to do so. As we would imagine from our previous discussions, the majority of the cases that fall prey to this involve behavioral or bond problems. Dr. Ogilvie's client records boast a population of aggressive large and small animals for which the sum total of his attempt to address the problem consists of a bold-faced "Watch!!" or "Muzzle!!" at the top of the record. "I *hate* examining and treating animals like that," he complains. "But it goes with the territory." In this situation, the practitioner's acceptance of the problem permits him to disengage himself from an entire aspect of practice.

We already noted that this serves as a valid approach if the owner shares it. It makes no sense for Dr. Ogilvie to lie awake nights trying to figure out how to correct Salsa's biting if Ms. Pritchard doesn't see it as a problem. But what if the owner doesn't like the problem behavior? What if former teacher Joe Cromwell doesn't even realize he has ventilation problems in his barn, let alone their negative effects on his flock and how to remedy them, and Dr. Ogilvie never offers this information in a way the client can comprehend? Similarly, what if Dr. Ogilvie accepts his negative feelings about alternative therapies, animal rights, euthanasia, and burnout because he believes no other options exist? In these situations, accepting the negative feelings serves to prolong rather than resolve a remediable problem. Consequently, before choosing this option, it makes sense to consider the remaining three choices.

Accept the Situation, but Eliminate the Negative Feelings

Eliminating negative feelings about what we consider negative situations proves the most difficult in those cases in which we assume the god role or become involved in what we consider matters of principle. "How can I possibly feel good about Ms. Pritchard's refusal to train Salsa or Cromwell's abuse of his animals, let alone killing treatable animals while working for slave wages in a substandard facility?" fumes Dr. Ogilvie. However, such clinician responses miss the point of this option because they assume that changing negative feelings means seeing the negative situation in a positive light. Although sometimes it is possible to do that, more often those who successfully use this approach neutralize their negative feelings. In other words, they remove the emotional charge from the situation altogether. Thus rather than convince himself to perceive biting Chihuahuas or abused animals and their owners in a positive light, Dr. Ogilvie merely accepts that these conditions constitute those animals' and those clients' normal states and works within those limits to the best of his ability.

Interestingly, many practitioners who take this approach in an effort to save their own sanity when confronted with situations that continually thwart their attempts to effect change discover that doing so may precipitate positive change in others. This occurs because negative emotional responses tend to elicit other negative emotional responses. Dr. Ogilvie's frustrations with Salsa and Ms. Pritchard alter the way he responds to them; he takes less care with the examination and maybe even gives the dog's paw an unnecessarily hard squeeze when Salsa resists having his nails clipped. Not only does this reinforce Salsa's tendency to resist Dr. Ogilvie, the clinician's handling of the dog makes the owner more defensive, too. However, when Dr. Ogilvie chooses to see Salsa's problems and his relationship to Ms. Pritchard in a neutral light, he stops supplying negative emotion to this interaction. Consequently, no need exists for the negative emotion that the client and animal summoned in response to his.

A change from a negative to a neutral response works particularly well in realms such as alternative therapies, animal rights, and euthanasia if practitioners feel they have no control over the situation. If they believe they lack the time to formulate their own opinions regarding any acceptable answer or solution to these problems, or feel they can't because they work for someone whose beliefs they must parrot as part of the practice's philosophy, then accepting this state as normal and neutralizing any negative feelings can eliminate a lot of emotional and physical stress. Because such situations and their resultant negative feelings do much to contribute to burnout, neutralizing them can do much to neutralize the negative effects of burnout, too.

"How can changing my feelings put more hours in the day?" asks Dr. Ogilvie skeptically.

Practitioners need only keep track of how much time they spend inwardly or outwardly ranting about various situations over which they believe they lack control to see how much they would gain if they let these feelings go. For some, it turns out to be an impressive amount.

What about changing negative feelings to positive ones? Such magic can and does occur all the time to those open to it. Recall the different client limits and ways animals respond based on their species, individual personality, and the situation. For those practitioners who don't recognize these differences as real, every day may present more than its share of interactions that leave the clinician feeling frustrated, angry, and inept. However, when we learn to accept client limits as both real and valid for those people, we can see them and their animals in a whole new light. When Dr. Ogilvie expects Ms. Pritchard to respond like a healthy thirty-two-year-old and Salsa to act like Dr. Ogilvie's own well-trained greyhound, both owner and dog repeatedly fail to meet the veterinarian's standards. However, when Dr. Ogilvie realizes the magnitude of Ms. Pritchard's own medical problems as well as the complexity of her relationship with Salsa, he finds himself admiring both the owner and the power of the human-animal bond. This translates in a subtle but perceptible difference in the way he responds to the dog, which takes some of the pressure off the animal, too. When Dr. Ogilvie learns that Joe Cromwell spends every waking hour that he's not working his farm reading about husbandry and attending classes and seminars on the subject, the practitioner's scorn changes to admiration and a desire to help his client any way he can. When Dr. Ogilvie realizes only he can make the changes necessary to resolve burnout, he stops blaming others (and all the negative feelings that go with that) and sees each day as an exciting opportunity to consider other options rather than yet another endurance test.

The obvious advantage of this choice lies in its ability to eliminate or at least neutralize negative feelings about those situations we feel powerless to change, and thereby eliminate all the negative effects of these feelings. Once Dr. Ogilvie neutrally if not positively accepts Ms. Pritchard and Salsa as they are, he no longer cringes every time their names appear in the appointment book; he no longer sees the animal's unresolved medical or behavioral problems as a negative statement about his ability. He realizes his views of alternative medical approaches and animal rights run contrary to those of some of his clients and his employer, but he accepts their views as normal for them and feels no need to engage them in debate as a matter of principle. He still doesn't like euthanizing animals but he accepts that reality and doesn't allow his negative feelings about it to make a difficult situation more difficult for the owner and animal.

As in the previous choice, the disadvantage of this option arises from its attraction for those who want to avoid confronting certain aspects of practice rather than face them. Rather than working through their own feelings and changing them because they believe it will best serve their own, the client's, and/or the patient's needs, they dismiss the matter as inconsequential and define that as a neutralizing or even positive emotional change. For example, some may take this approach rather than admit they lack the knowledge and don't want to gain it to effect change in others. Once again, behavioral and bond problems fall victim to this approach far more commonly than medical ones. Rather than learn about treating aggressive animals and the ramifications of dependent owner-animal relationships, Dr. Ogilvie dismisses Ms. Pritchard and Salsa with "The way it is, is the way it is." Behavioral problems fall in the realms of behaviorists and owner problems into that of psychologists and psychiatrists; they're no concern of his.

Compare Dr. Ogilvie accepting Ms. Pritchard's and Salsa's relationship or his employer's antagonistic views toward the use of alternative therapies and animal rights as normal for them to his saying, "I'm not going to let their stupid ideas bother me." Regardless of what he might want to believe, in the latter case these issues *will* bother him because he hasn't *accepted* them and their effects: He merely attempts to deny their existence. And as we know from our discussion of death and dying, the distance between denial and acceptance can be long and filled with negative emotion. Once again, whether acceptance works depends on whether practitioners see it as a conscious choice or a convenient escape.

Change Someone or Something

Many times practitioners and clients faced with problems see making an active change as their only choice rather than one of four options. We see the sick or injured animal and immediately want to do something to resolve the problem; we don't want to waste time thinking about what the owner thinks about the animal or the problem, or even the consequences (costs, aftercare, prognosis) of our actions. For practitioners, making changes in the animal most closely fits our education definition of purpose: We see an animal with a problem; we do whatever we need to do to make it better.

We noted in our discussion of alternatives therapies (Chapter 13) that this often highly reinforced desire to do something may lead practitioners to prescribe antibiotics for viral infections and other placebos, as well as to delve into the area of nontraditional treatments when traditional medicine leaves us with nothing to do. Although such responses might seem to fly in the face of our training, in reality they permit us to fulfill that "do something" focus of our education and the definition of the purpose of veterinary medicine it espouses. Recall the surgeon's "A chance to cut is a chance to cure," a sentiment with similar corollaries in medicine. Although we may intellectually rationalize a wait-and-see or do-nothing approach, most of us find these less satisfying. A good practitioner, we tell ourselves, would find *something* to do.

Making changes can most certainly benefit those situations amenable to change. Moreover, routinely taking this approach can save time. Joe Cromwell looks at Dr. Ogilvie incredulously when the veterinarian raises the options of accepting the cow with the recurrent lameness as normal or shipping her off to slaughter. How can a veterinarian waste time talking about such foolishness when he should be treating the animal?

Within the personal arena, those situations that give rise to negative emotions which the clinician cannot accept or change also respond well to definitive action. Practitioners who become upset when clients raise the subject of animal rights or alternative therapies may decide to gain enough information regarding these issues that conflicting ideas no longer threaten them. When Dr. Ogilvie objectively considers all sides of the animal rights issue, he formulates a personal philosophy that enables him to respond calmly even to those most rabidly antagonistic to his view. Practitioners who can neither accept nor change all the negative emotions elicited by euthanasia may refuse to perform all euthanasias or only perform those that fulfill their criteria for acceptability.

However, although we may save time by opting to make some change first, doing so poses its own risks. In treating an animal, this option will only save time if the owner agrees with both the need for treatment and the form that treatment takes. When we put doing something for the animal above communicating with the owner, we immediately complicate the treatment process. As soon as we do that, we set ourselves up to discover after the fact—and to our embarrassment if not the owner's rage—that the client didn't want to make those changes and maybe not any at all. The owner who only shows up for a rabies vaccination every three years and winds up with a bag full of ear wash, medicated shampoo and conditioner, vitamins, and an appointment for some routine blood work "just in case" comes to mind here. As far as the owner was concerned, the dog had no problem save the need for the rabies vaccination. Following the examination, he still believes the dog has no problem; however, now he also believes the veterinarian has a definite problem.

Consequently, before making any changes we need to ascertain if the clients want to make those changes and if these are realistic given any client, patient, and clinician limits. A critical point to bear in mind regarding change is one well known and accepted by philosophers, but often anathema to those in science and medicine: The only individual we can guarantee change in is ourselves. We like to believe that with a word, drug, or surgical procedure we can cause all kinds of wonderful changes to occur in our clients and patients, but as we've seen throughout our discussion of the art of practice, whether those changes actually happens depends more on them than us. Even when we and our clients believe us capable of achieving such an exalted state, these successes possess the potential to lure us into the messiah trap with all its problems even as we cure the otitis or foot rot.

Because of this, we can see why it makes sense to work through all the options with the owner before yielding to the temptation to make changes, because this involves the owner in the treatment process from the beginning. When Dr. Ogilvie says, "I want you to give these tablets [or strip that quarter or soak that foot]," his words as well as any medication serve primarily as a catalyst. Whether these will precipitate any reaction—let alone the one the veterinarian desires—depends on whether the necessary owner and patient components exist for it to do so. If not, if the client lacks the time, money, commitment, or ability to medicate the animal, Dr. Ogilvie will fail in his attempt to change them, that is, make the animal better as quickly as possible. If he sees the problem strictly in terms of medicine, he may try a different drug when the animal fails to respond to the first. If he sees it as a bond and/or behavioral problem as well as a medical one, he may recommend changes in those areas at the same time or before he treats the medical problem. He shows Joe Cromwell how to restrain the animal and soak the foot or strip the quarter before he dispenses the medication. If the client says he can't do that because he has a bad back, then Dr. Ogilvie might opt to treat the animal himself if the owner agrees. If the client says he can't do it because he's afraid of the animal, that leads Dr. Ogilvie to consider another group of possibilities. In the latter case especially, we can see the advantage of taking the owner through all four options first. Even though some consider the first two options "mind games" compared to the third, and the termination option blasphemous, what a person thinks and feels about the animal, its condition, and any proposed treatment will affect its recovery every bit as much as any drug prescribed or surgical procedure performed by the practitioner.

Terminate the Relationship

Terminating a relationship can take many forms in veterinary practice, and clinicians may find themselves involved in terminations that include:

- Owners and animals
- Veterinarians and animals
- Owners and veterinarians
- Clients and their beliefs
- Employers and employees
- Veterinarians and their careers
- Veterinarians and their beliefs

Terminations between owners and animals may mean euthanasia or finding a new home for the animal. Occasionally clients may terminate a relationship because their animals don't like the veterinarian even though the clients do. (Some farmers note that their cows prefer being palpated by women and stay around the barn to greet these practitioners, but run off when their male colleagues appear. Rather than chase the cows, these clients request the women even though they themselves believe the men equally qualified.)

Both practitioners and clients will terminate their relationships with each other for a multitude of reasons. Veterinarians may refer clients whose animals display medical or behavioral problems the clinician cannot resolve and the owner cannot accept for whatever reason. The most negative and unfortunately also the most common terminations between owners and practitioners, however, fall under the heading of lack of communication, and the same holds true for terminations that occur between employers and employees. In these situations the termination reflects the flight fear response more than a conscious choice. Veterinarians may sever their relationship with practice or the entire field of veterinary medicine for the same reason, but also as the result of a conscious choice to do so following objective analysis of the other options. Finally, all of us maintain the ability to terminate our relationships with any beliefs that no longer work for us, although more than a few see this as the most difficult change to accomplish.

Even though our education leads us to want to make changes, it also conditions us to view the termination option as pessimistic, insensitive, and equivalent to giving up: How can anyone dedicated to the saving of lives even consider stopping treatment or euthanasia? However, just as we noted that the more serious the problem, the more we need to communicate with the owner, so the more serious the problem, the greater the need for an open discussion of this option.

How come? Two reasons support this view. First, the more serious the problem, the greater the commitment needed to resolve it. An animal suffering from serious illness or injury which will require extensive nursing care needs—and deserves—someone committed to that process. Similarly, that animal and its owner deserve the full commitment of the clinician treating the case. Likewise, when serious problems arise between veterinarians and their colleagues or when serious doubts arise about one's abilities to perform one's duties well, a sense of commitment to resolving the conflict can make a tremendous difference.

When practitioners face the probability of terminating the relationship—be it to put the animal down, refer the client to another practitioner, quit the job, fire an associate, get out of practice altogether, or give up one's beliefs about animal rights—and can say with certainty that this is *not* what they want to do, this awareness gives rise to a commitment much greater than that available from any other source. As soon as Dr. Ogilvie realizes Joe Cromwell wouldn't think of putting down his animal, he can proceed with treatment confidently, knowing the owner is committed to the animal and its recovery.

We already know all the problems that can arise when practitioners simply assume clients share their view that an animal should be treated. However, another less dramatic but equally problematic situation can occur if practitioners don't ask owners to confront the termination option directly. Suppose Mr. Cromwell agrees to treat the animal, but in the back of his mind he continually toys with the option of putting it down. Now not only must Dr. Ogilvie guess his client's feelings on this matter, he also must cope with the client considering that possibility every time the animal (or he) has a bad day, as well as with the negative effects of any inconsistent treatment secondary to this lack of commitment.

On a more intimate level, we see those practitioners who forever threaten to quit or fire someone whenever the emotional pressure reaches a critical level. Others may work in environments where their beliefs about alternative therapies, animal rights, and/or euthanasia constantly put them in adversarial positions. Like the colleagues who scream threats at each other but never make any meaningful changes, emotional responses to challenges to our beliefs do little to end the agony. Rather these approaches function like an aesthetically acceptable incision just big enough to let sufficient pus drain out of an abscess to provide temporary relief: They don't solve the problem and may ultimately serve to undermine the health of the individual and any relationship more. Facing the termination option makes it easier for those in these situations to act in a meaningful manner rather than react haphazardly and emotionally.

Second, facing this option may cause clients to see the problem in a completely different light and, in an era in which people assign more and more symbolism to animals, such considerations may uncover completely different problems than those for which the animal was presented. For example, discussing the termination option with owners of animals with chronic medical or persistent behavioral problems may reveal that the owner or some Significant Other in the household doesn't like the animal and sees its treatment as a waste of time and/or money. If Joe Cromwell treats the cow on a schedule built around the absence of his antagonistic roommate rather than the needs of the animal, or if the roommate participates in the treatment reluctantly and erratically, obviously this will undermine the animal's recovery.

Clinicians who suggest owners consider termination along with the other three options provide clients like Mr. Cromwell with the opportunity to think the unthinkable in an emotionally neutral, supportive environment. In such situations, these clients may opt to terminate the relationship with the animal for its own sake as well as their own.

However, the realization that their relationship with other people could result in conditions sufficiently detrimental to the animal that they compel the veterinarian to raise this option may lead these people to make other changes. When Joe Cromwell realizes his roommate's negative feelings about animals contribute to the sick animal's problem, he decides he'd be better off living alone.

Similarly, when our beliefs consistently result in negative feelings, objectively confronting the termination option can provide valuable insights. Sadly, however, many times people cling to beliefs that no longer work for them because they see changing them as a violation of principle. Dr. Ogilvie knows his beliefs about animal rights represent a relatively narrow urbanized view, but he carried placards protesting some of the very activities he's come to see in a new light since he started working in the rural practice: What will his animal rights friends say if he changes his beliefs? Several animals show dramatic improvement after massage therapy, a subject his employer has held in contempt for years: What will he say if Dr. Ogilvie begins recommending this approach?

In these situations, sometimes simply recognizing that fear serves as the primary motivator can do much to alleviate the stress associated with the situation regardless of what we ultimately decide to do. The realization that his beliefs about animal rights result as much from peer pressure and habit as any conscious thought reflecting changes in his own experience and awareness may give Dr. Ogilvie the incentive to reevaluate his ideas. On the other hand, if those who support his existing beliefs serve as a dominant social as well as intellectual force in his life, he may choose to cling to his beliefs because he spends most of his time with these people. Although this won't eliminate the incongruity he experiences in his daily work, the awareness that he could change but chooses not to makes this more tolerable.

By taking what often may seem like an infinite number of probabilities and reducing them to these four options, we can remove much of the confusion from our own and our clients' lives. Although initially we may find ourselves sharing Reinhold Niebuhr's prayer for the serenity to accept the unchangeable, the courage to change what we should, and the wisdom to know the difference, once we discover the advantages of making such conscious choices and allowing others to do likewise, that serenity, courage, and wisdom will become a natural part of our practice philosophy.

Chapter 20
Creating a Workable Practice Philosophy

For those accustomed to taking a linear approach to the practice of veterinary medicine, the preceding chapters conceivably raised more questions than they answered and left a yearning for some good old-fashioned concrete facts. As one practitioner put it, "I see my job as answering 'what?' and 'how?' I leave the 'why?' to the philosophers." In fact, one need only mention the p-word (philosophy) among some veterinarians to precipitate sighs and groans, nervous coughs and foot shuffling, and a sometimes not-so-subtle migration toward the nearest exit. Nonetheless, and whether we admit it or not, everything we do in practice results from a personal philosophy, a set of beliefs about ourselves, our patients, and clients, and what constitutes the practice of quality veterinary medicine. Although we may lose some sleep pondering the what and how of our patients' medical problems, the very nature of these plus our training compel most of us to make some sort of response. Even if we do nothing, the majority of medical problems we see follow their own physiological timetables and will resolve themselves one way or another.

However, the subjective whys of practice don't treat us so kindly. When we lie awake pondering why the Carlsons won't treat the treatable animal, why the Heberts let their terminally ill pet languish, why the Jackson brothers take such poor care of their herd, why the Roccos refuse to leave their dog overnight, or why the Charests allow their animals to bite and kick, we're as apt to summon an infinite number of answers as none at all. Moreover, unlike medical problems, these issues won't go away. Even if all these animals were to disappear, we all realize their owners most likely would treat the next batch the same way.

Given that reality, either we may make a conscious effort to examine our beliefs regarding all the subjective issues previously discussed so we may achieve or at least actively pursue the fulfillment of a personally rewarding philosophy in our work, or we may function as passive players or even spectators and judge these aspects of practice as "good" or "bad" with little awareness of either the source or the validity of those pronouncements. If that doesn't serve as a sufficient incentive to undertake this unscientific task, bear in mind that these issues represent the most common—and emotional—client concerns in any given interaction. Consequently, acknowledging their reality, validity, and variability as well as our own orientations forms the foundation of quality client communication.

An Ideal Integrated Education

Numerous individuals and studies point to the increasing need to integrate subjective concerns into veterinary education (Beaver 1991, 198:1241–42; Self et al. 1991, 198:782–87 and 199:569–73; Stone et al. 1992, 201:1849–53; Thornburg 1992, 201:1352–54). However, at the same time new science and technology assaults us from all sides and most of us can't find the time to assimilate all that, let alone anything else. In spite of that and as more than one disenchanted practitioner or victim of burnout can attest, the inability to respond confidently to these aspects of practice looms as the far greater and more troubling reality than the selection of the right drug or surgical procedure.

However, is it possible to teach another a philosophy of practice? To some extent, no, because much unlike science few right and wrong answers exist. Throughout the preceding pages various concepts did keep recurring but more as threads in a tapestry, weaving some scenes that may have seemed familiar and others that may have irritated or even struck the reader as totally incomprehensible and wrong. However, the art of practice and its underlying philosophy is unique to every individual as well as capable of constant change and refinement, and consequently all any text can do is provide an environment in which previously unrecognized or avoided issues may be confronted as objectively as possible. Because our practice philosophies reflect our most intimate beliefs, we need to create them ourselves; we can't accept the views of others as a matter of course or habit because these might not work for us as individuals or in our particular practices.

Because so many successful practitioners do maintain philosophies which are then reflected in their work, some benefit and more than a little enjoyment may be had by imagining an ideal veterinary curricu-

lum which incorporates all the subjective aspects from these practitioners' point of view. Although this may seem little more than a flight of
fancy, doing so enables us to target our own areas of weakness which, in
turn, makes it easier to make any changes necessary to alleviate those
deficiencies. For students, such an exercise provides a real-world overlay
that might permit the evaluation of course work in a different light. For
faculty and administrators, perhaps a new look at a seemingly impossible old problem will trigger new solutions.

But how can we make such changes—or even imagine doing so—in a
world where science and technology appear to take up every minute of
our time? Consider the following Ideal University College of Veterinary
Medicine scenario that results from informal conversations with many
practitioners. During the first semester of the freshman year, students
take a course on the practical aspects of behavior and the bond.
Additionally, they do volunteer work in area animal shelters where they
gain a real-world view of the animal overpopulation problem, animal
abuse, and euthanasia. By coupling this with classes on the bond and
behavior where students can share their feelings about their experiences, they begin to formulate their own beliefs about these troubling
aspects of practice as well as those about animal rights.

At the end of the first semester, each student adopts one intact cat
and dog of opposite sexes which they live with under real-world conditions; the animals remain at home and the students must train, medicate, and otherwise fulfill the criteria for a healthy and well-behaved
animal the same way we expect our clients to. Throughout their education, students keep journals recording their feelings about these animals as well as about how their classwork relates to them. Although the
college provides reduced student rates for all veterinary services provided, a running tab is kept so students know exactly how much any procedure or treatment would cost a client under the same circumstances,
and students note in their journals their feelings about if and how their
own financial situations affect the treatment process. During the senior
year, students spay and castrate their own animals.

For those in private practice, many of the advantages of such an experience are obvious. First, those students who give in to their emotions
when they choose their animals very quickly discover the practical implications of applying the basic principles of behavior when selecting an
animal, as well as the practical ramifications of the human-animal bond.
When they come home after a grueling day in class and find the shredded drapes and read the nasty note from the landlord or neighbor
about the dog's incessant whining or barking, they feel the knot in their
own stomachs and the fear so common to owners confronting this situ-

ation. Because of this, when their clients mention similar concerns, they more likely will offer help rather than dismiss the problem as inconsequential. If the students' animals fall ill, they will experience this from an owner's as well as a veterinarian's viewpoint: worrying about what the animal is doing in their absence, wondering how to get all the doses of medication in as directed, dreading wrapping the cat in a towel and prying its mouth open.

In addition to functioning as a living-learning laboratory of the bond and behavior, these animals also provide students with readily available input related to virtually every course in the veterinary curriculum. The words and line drawings of anatomy come to life when these same structures are observed and palpated. Procedures so routine and easily dismissed as fecals and vaccinations take on new meaning when students look at their own animals. Not only do they perceive these activities in terms of the principles of parasitology and immunology, they realize how their animals fit into a neighborhood population where other owners might not care as much as they do. Because of this, preventive medicine and client education also become real concerns. That surprisingly large number of students who have never seen an animal in heat experience this and all its physiological, behavioral, and bond implications firsthand, and reproductive physiology becomes far more than just another subject to tick off the list of requirements.

At Ideal U., courses in medicine, surgery, pharmacology, and anesthesiology take on a whole new dimension, the answer to the philosophical question "What does this mean to me and my animal?" which is paramount in the client's mind. This occurs because these students know *their* animals' health depends on their knowledge and skill. Although we might argue that that awareness always exists, we need only eavesdrop on student conversations to realize the primary concern for most remains as always: the grade.

During the senior year, all the components of veterinary education merge at Ideal U. when students castrate and spay their own animals. In those perhaps agonizingly long moments, they learn what it means to work with living tissue if their education has been limited to models and computer simulations prior to then. Equally important, they learn what every successful practitioner knows—what it means to be responsible not only for a life, but all that the owner invests in that life, regardless of whether we believe in the wisdom or even the reality of those investments. Whether we speak of the economic investment of a chattel-oriented farmer or the emotional investment of the most highly anthropomorphically oriented pet owner, these investments comprise an inextricable part of that animal every bit as critical as its vital organs.

Do we allow these to influence our treatment of the animal? How? Via these two simple surgeries, students will discover whether they do or not and, if they do, how they do. What they learn from that experience, too, will influence how they interact with clients in the future.

At Ideal U., always seeking to answer the question, "What does this mean to me and my animal?" helps students develop their communication skills even as they maintain their educational perspective. That question does not lend itself readily to the answer, "So I can pass this course and graduate [or get my CE credits]." When students can answer this question at the end of every course or seminar, they can more readily incorporate that information into practice.

But how can we provide students with this knowledge when their teachers often must follow stringent criteria for the achievement of academic credentials that often leave little, if any, time for experience in private practice? One practitioner suggested that each course offered at Ideal U. include a session during which randomly picked graduates tell students how that class benefits them in practice. However, most practitioners believed that such a summons would leave them quaking in their boots. Comments such as "I'd feel obligated to bone up for weeks before I'd ever stand in front of one of Dr. R.'s classes," and "I'd sweat bullets thinking Dr. B. was going to ask me something I hadn't thought about in years" reflected commonly held opinions. More than a few practitioners said they wouldn't mind meeting with students alone, but . . . More communications problems.

Many practitioners wished they'd had more experience speaking to various target groups as a means of learning to convert scientific terminology into everyday language as well as to interact with the different kinds of people who make up the client base. Because of this, most felt that public interaction should be part of the curriculum at Ideal U. and that it could take the form of career days, guided tours through the college, presentations to schools and various organizations, and pet-visitation programs to nursing homes, among others. Although most interviewed dreaded the thought, all agreed that essay tests which required students to describe various scientific concepts in everyday terms would benefit those going into practice—provided these concepts were taught in everyday as well as scientific terms initially. At the same time, most felt that undergraduate requirements in both speech and writing would facilitate this aspect of education as well as benefit those who planned to enter private practice.

Finally, the Ideal U. curriculum includes sessions in both small and large animal medicine during which all faculty members briefly present their personal philosophies of veterinary practice—including their views on the use of alternative therapies, animal rights, and euthana-sia—and then answer students' questions regarding how they came to hold these beliefs and how these influence their approach to patients and clients. Not only does this expose students to the broad range of opinions that exists within the teaching community as well as the thought processes behind them, it serves as an incentive for faculty to consider these issues more objectively, too. Such sessions could also confirm an as yet unconfirmed suspicion that food animal faculty know a great deal about these subjective factors, but because they tend to clas-sify the bond as a small animal issue they don't share their valuable insights with students and others. For example, many food animal prac-titioners routinely incorporate economic factors and the client's ability to handle the animal into the treatment process, whereas these may only become factors in small animal practice when clients thwart the "ideal" medical approach. Unfortunately and most ironically, rather than recognizing how this sensitivity to the owner's needs can enhance the treatment of the animal, it is sometimes used as proof that those treating food animals care *less.*

Right, Wrong, and Different

As we consider the rich variety of subjective challenges offered by clients and patients in even the smallest practice in an effort to create a work-able philosophy, another recurrent theme bears repeating one last time: Different is not necessarily wrong. After an intensive education that focuses on the *right* answers to test questions and the *best* way to do things, it can come as quite a shock to enter a practice or an area where clients may maintain quite different views about what constitutes right and best for themselves, let alone their animals. When we come to accept the validity of their views as well as our own, we recognize yet another one of those amazing paradoxes of veterinary practice: The more sure we are of our own beliefs, the more accepting we are of those whose beliefs differ from ours.

"No way!" protests Dr. Ogilvie, thinking of that collection of placards in the back of his closet.

Nonetheless, it turns out to be true. Consider those aspects of your-self about which you feel the most sure: your name, address, names of any children and pets, where you work. If someone were to challenge the reality of these facts, most of us could readily ignore the challenge or, at worst, consider the challenger a minor irritant because we feel so secure in that knowledge. However, if we do not feel secure, then the other's challenge begins to grate.

This raises the interesting possibility that those differences in opinion that bother us most might do so because they are more *like* than different from our own. If someone insists that Dr. Ogilvie's name is really Dr. Stein, he can easily dismiss this with a laugh or perhaps feel sympathy for the challenger's obvious confusion. However, suppose a neighbor tells him that she believes humans have the right to do whatever they want to animals. Now Dr. Ogilvie becomes furious and yells that no human has that right and he's going to do everything in his power to get laws passed to make sure that doesn't happen.

We can think of formulating a personal philosophy as formulating a world view. If we believe the world is flat and take a linear approach, our concept of the distance between two points is quite different from that which we maintain if we believe the world is round. In the former case, the further apart the two points (or people or ideas) move, the more distance between them. However, in the latter case, the greater the distance between the two points (or people or ideas), the closer they become. So even though Dr. Ogilvie and his neighbor occupy positions at opposite ends of the linear animal rights spectrum, perhaps what really grates is the subconscious awareness that, outside those linear limits, their orientations are more alike than different: both of them desire to control animals and what happens to them, albeit in what they perceive as quite opposite ways. To use an analogy from music, our beliefs possess the potential to create harmony or disharmony with those of others not unlike two notes played simultaneously on a piano. Most people agree that a C and C-sharp offend the ear a great deal more than a C and a G played at the same time.

Because of this, we can appreciate why many cultures and theologies share beliefs in common with Christianity's "Make friends with your enemies" because our enemies may represent the people—and the beliefs—from which we can learn the most. Pay attention to those concepts and examples in the preceding pages that generated the most uneasiness, and most certainly those that evoked anger. True, the author and those clients and practitioners whose input forms the basis of this book could be absolutely wrong, but it might be that their wrong is closer to your right than you want to admit.

Above all, remember that whether we speak of human orientations toward animals, human limitations or special needs, money, alternative therapies, animal rights, euthanasia, or any other of the subjective matters of practice, acceptance of our beliefs regarding these issues frees us from feelings of denial, anger, bargaining, and depression when we encounter those whose beliefs differ from our own. That is not to say we need to provide service for clients whose beliefs differ from our own: It is to say we can refer them to others without anger or guilt when they fail to see things our way.

Philosophical Tools

Although the idea of formulating a personal philosophy of practice may appear overwhelming, in reality we all already possess one and it's simply a matter of evaluating it, keeping what works, and eliminating what doesn't. Where did this philosophy come from? For most of us, it results from conversations with clients and colleagues, personal experience, and input from those whose opinions we value for one reason or another.

To understand how this works, consider the references (listed at the end of this book) which provided the background material as well as specific documentation for this text. This eclectic collection literally boggles the scientifically trained mind, and yet a certain logic underlies it. In addition to articles from some of the most prestigious journals, we see those from unscientific sources such as *Time, Newsweek, Glamour*, and the *New York Times Magazine* discussing the same material. These were deliberately chosen to contrast and compare the general public's view with that of the professional scientist(s). Because the majority of our clients dwell outside the scientific community, this provides valuable clues regarding what these people are thinking and how best to communicate with them. Regardless of what subject we consider, the ability to take people from what they know and understand to what they do not serves as the most efficient and effective means of communication and education. If we dismiss the mass media's handling of a particular subject as irrelevant or stupid, we similarly dismiss those who rely on these sources of information as irrelevant and stupid, too.

Although this may make us feel superior, it does nothing to educate these people and will hardly make them think kindly of us, particularly if the only option we offer uses our language instead of their own. We need only imagine how we would feel if an expert scoffed at the news articles on the trade deficit and then launched into a discourse on micro- and macroeconomic theory to realize how our clients feel when we opt to give them the/our truth in scientific terms. Because of this, an excellent way to fine-tune practice philosophy relative to client needs involves little more than leafing through *Reader's Digest, Good House-keeping*, and other publications written for the general public rather than the latest journal as we wait in the dentist's office.

Similarly, personal philosophies often find support in a wide variety of books that superficially may appear to have little or nothing to do with veterinary medicine at all. Readers of Antoine de Saint Exupéry's *Little Prince* ([1943] 1971) get a completely different view of process and "matters of consequence" from the businessman the Little Prince meets; and surely all of us eventually learn what the Little Prince learns—that we are forever responsible for those we tame, and that those who allow us to tame them the most are those who cause us to weep the most when we lose them.

From Machiavelli's *The Prince* ([1537] 1961), we learn that fear and love cannot coexist but we will choose the fear-based response because it's the safer of the two. How often those in practice can trace a break-down in communication to taking the safer rather than the more intimate caring approach with others! William Jordan's *Divorce among the Gulls* (1991), Edward Wilson's *Diversity of Life* (1992), and Donald Griffin's *Animal Thinking* (1984) and *Animal Minds* (1992) provide three different views of the animal kingdom and our relationship to it which may reinforce or challenge our own views. Any feelings of superiority that infiltrate our views of animal rights falter when Henry Beston (1956) reminds us of the hubris as well as the ignorance that leads us to believe we can measure animals against ourselves and consider them lesser or even brothers.

Then there's Lewis Thomas's rare combination of scientific and medical knowledge, writing skill, and delight in the natural world that has resulted in a series of books (some of them his collected essays from the *New England Journal of Medicine*) that also provide valuable insights, not the least of which is that he feels no embarrassment whatsoever about imagining himself thinking or feeling like a moth or a cat, an anathema in animal science. Rather than threatening, reading his books is like going into a neighbor's yard to play. His background in science and human medicine provides a common knowledge base, but because he feels no need to play by our rules, his views can be most refreshing and intriguing.

Sometimes we need to get away from the science of medicine or see it from a completely different perspective before we can relax enough to realize what it means to us, our clients, and our patients on the most intimate level. As human medicine finally penetrates the mind-body barrier, the implications for the human-animal bond, the animal rights movement, and the practice of veterinary medicine are enormous. We can enter this new world through scientific texts such as *Psychoneuroim-munology* (Ader et al. 1991), read of one person's discovery of these same concepts as he evolves from a patient diagnosed as beyond medical help to adjunct professor of medicine at UCLA (Cousins 1979; 1989), or get an overview of similar material form Bill Moyers's *Healing and the Mind* (1993) in either book or video form. Similarly oncologist Bernard Siegal's books (1986; 1989) and the Rodale Press's compilation of mind-body research (Padus 1992) not only apprise us of these changes in scientific thinking but also of what our clients are reading about these same subjects because all of these texts were written for—and are eagerly read by—the general public.

In such ways, we can take complex issues and break them down into nonthreatening and even enjoyable components that we can then evaluate in terms of our own, our patients', and our clients' needs. Whether we accept or reject the science is immaterial. The goal is to create a belief structure that makes sense to us as individuals so we can react consistently and objectively to those whose views differ substantially from our own.

Nor should we disregard the ability of seemingly unrelated books, television shows, movies, social events, music (all kinds), and walking alone or with a good friend in the woods or on the beach to serve as reliable sources of input for a workable practice philosophy. Unlike the science of veterinary practice which depends on a highly defined data base, the components that comprise its art reflect some of the most timeless and universal human qualities. Consequently, when we seek to formulate or change our philosophies we can find our answers practically anywhere.

Practice Philosophy and Client Education

Of all the recurring themes in the art of veterinary practice none recurs more frequently than that of communication. It makes no difference how great our knowledge of medicine and surgery or how much we care about our patients and clients if we can't communicate this to them in a way they can understand. Simultaneously, it is our responsibility to educate as we communicate so we may prevent problems in the future even as we cure them in the present. While developing communication skills helps us establish the common ground on which we and our clients can work comfortably for the benefit of the animal, via education we seek to take clients from their known to the unknown in a nonthreatening way. Because of this, it makes sense to incorporate our beliefs about client education into our practice philosophies. Although this might seem like just one more thing to worry about, in reality quality education flows naturally once we see clients and their relationships with their animals as integral parts of the treatment process rather than as extra appendages or supernumerary teats. When we add an awareness of both the power and the many effects of the bond and couple that with an awareness that knowledge can make even the most reluctant owner compliant, we find it much easier to share information with our clients.

No words more eloquently describe the art of client education than those of Lao-tzu:

> Good teachers are best when students barely know they exist
> Not so good when students always obey and acclaim them
> Worst when students despise them.
> Of good teachers, when their work is done and their aims fulfilled
> The student will say, *"I did this myself."*

When we interact with our clients we can dole out our knowledge in little packets and assume our roles as superior beings; and we may be worshiped and adored by our clients when things go right and despised when they go wrong. However, when we assume an equal role in the treatment process with the owner and animal to the point that we work as one rather than separate units, a special kind of magic unknown in any other profession occurs, one that exceeds Lao-tzu's ideal. Talk to any practitioners who have worked side by side with an animal and a client on a problem that seemed to laugh in the face of medical science and technology. Ask those practitioners how they felt when they dragged into the ward or drove into that barnyard dreading to face the owner of the animal given up for lost, only to be greeted by a now alert creature who somehow beat the odds, and an exhausted but jubilant owner who shouts:

"We did it, Doc! We did it!"

It doesn't get much better than that.

References

Adams, John. 1993. "Assuring a Residue-Free Food Supply: Milk." *Journal of the American Veterinary Medical Association* 202:1723–25.

Ader, Robert, David L. Felten, and Nicholas Cohen. 1991. *Psychoneuroimmunology*. San Diego, Calif.: Academic Press, Inc.

Ader, Robert, and Anthony Suchman. 1985. "CNS-Immune System Interactions: Conditioning Phenomena (Conditioned Responses to Placebos)." *Behavioral and Brain Sciences* 8:379–426.

Adler, Valerie. 1989. "Little Control = Lots of Stress." *Psychology Today* 23:18–19.

"AIDS Patients Can Acquire Some Infections from Animals." 1990. *Journal of the American Veterinary Medical Association* 197:1268.

"ALF Claims Research Raid; U.S. Committee Passes Protection Bill." 1992. *DVM* (May):4.

"All They Are Sayin' Is Give Pigs a Chance (Animal Rights Movement in Berkeley, California and Other University Towns)." 1989. *U.S. News and World Report* 106:15.

Allen, Karen, and Jim Blascovich. 1990. "Dogs and Their Women: A Psychosociological Study of Social Support." *Abstracts of Presentations.* Delta Society Ninth Annual Conference, Houston, Texas.

"Alternative Medicine: The Scientific Method Separates Help from Hype." 1993. *Mayo Clinic Health Letter* 11:6–8.

American Medical Association Council on Ethical and Judicial Affairs. 1992. "Decisions Near the End of Life." *Journal of the American Medical Association* 287:2229 (5).

American Psychiatric Association. 1987. "Passive Aggressive Personality Disorder." In *Diagnostic and Statistical Manual of Mental Disorders* (DSM-III-R), 356–58. Washington, D.C.: American Psychiatric Association.

American Veterinary Medical Association. 1991. *Companion Animal Guidelines.* Schaumburg, Ill.: American Veterinary Medical Association.

———. 1993. *The Veterinarian's Role in Animal Welfare.* Schaumburg, Ill.: American Veterinary Medical Association.

———. 1993a. *AVMA Model Program to Assist Clinically Impaired Individuals.* Schaumburg, Ill.: American Veterinary Medical Association.

———. 1993b. *The Impaired Veterinarian: A Resource Manual.* Schaumburg, Ill.: The American Veterinary Medical Association.

———. 1993c. *Pet Loss and Human Emotion.* Schaumburg, Ill.: The American Veterinary Medical Association.

————. 1993d. *Principals of Veterinary Ethics.* Schaumburg, Ill.: The American Veterinary Medical Association.

Andrews, Edwin J., B. Taylor Bennett, J. Derrell Clark, Katherine A. Haupt, Peter J. Pascoe, Gordon W. Robinson, and John R. Boyce. 1993. "Report of the AVMA Panel on Euthanasia." *Journal of the American Veterinary Medical Association* 202:229–49.

Antelyes, Jacob. 1986. "Animal Rights in Perspective." *Journal of the American Veterinary Medical Association* 189:757–59.

Arkow, Phil. 1987. "Animal Control, Animal Welfare, and the Veterinarian." *Journal of the American Veterinary Medical Association* 191:937–42.

————. 1994. "Child Abuse, Animal Abuse, and the Veterinarian." *Journal of the American Veterinary Medical Association* 204:1004–7.

Arluke, Arnold. 1991. "Coping with Euthanasia: A Case Study of Shelter Culture." *Journal of the American Veterinary Medical Association* 198:1176–80.

Arntz, A., et al. 1990. "Predictions of Dental Pain: The Fear of Any Expected Evil Is Worse Than the Evil Itself." *Behavioral Research and Therapy* 28:29–41.

Aronson, Elliot, and Ayala Pines. 1992. *Burnout.* New York: The Free Press.

Ascione, Frank R. 1991. "Generalization of Children's Attitudes about the Humane Treatment of Animals to Human-directed Empathy: An Intervention Study." *Abstracts of Presentations.* Delta Society Tenth Annual Conference, Portland, Oregon.

Bach, Edward. 1933. *The Twelve Healers and Other Remedies.* Essex, England: C. W. Daniel.

Bacon, Francis. [1537] 1980. In *Bartlett's Familiar Quotations.* 15th ed. Boston: Little, Brown and Company.

Bancroft, Kris. 1990. "Pets in the American Family." *People, Animals, Environment* (Fall):13–15.

Barnard, Julian. 1979. *The Guide to the Bach Flower Remedies.* Essex, England: C. W. Daniel.

Bath, Donald L., Frank N. Dickinson, H. Allen Tucker, and Robert D. Appleman. 1985. *Dairy Cattle: Principles, Practices, Problems, Profits.* Philadelphia: Lea and Febiger.

Beardsley, Timothy M. 1988. "Benevolent Bradykinins: New Compounds Might Get to the Root of Pain." *Scientific American* 259:41.

Beaver, Bonnie V. 1991. "The Role of the Veterinary Colleges in Addressing the Surplus Dog and Cat Population." *Journal of the American Veterinary Medical Association* 198:1241–43.

————. 1992. *Feline Behavior: A Guide for Veterinarians.* Philadelphia: W. B. Saunders.

Beck, Alan, and Aaron Katcher. 1983. *Between Pets and People: The Importance of Animal Companion Companionship.* New York: Putnam.

Begley, Sharon. 1988. "Can Water 'Remember'? Homeopathy Finds Scientific Support." *Newsweek* (July 25):66.

————. 1991. "Barnyard Bioengineers." *Newsweek* (September 9):55.

————. 1993. "Charlotte Said It Best: Some Pig." *Newsweek* (October 25):68–69.

Beil, Laura. 1988. "Nature Douses Dilution Experiment." *Science News* 134:69.

Belongia, Edward A., Michael T. Osterholm, John T. Soler, Savid A. Ammend, Jane E. Brown, and Kristina L. MacDonald. 1993."Transmission of *Escherichia coli* 0157:H7 Infection in Minnesota Child Day-care Facilities." *Journal of the American Medical Association* 269:883 (6).

Bergler, Reinhold. 1992. "The Contribution of Dogs to Avoiding and Overcoming Everyday Stress Factors." *Abstracts of Presentations*. Sixth International Conference on Human-Animal Interactions, Montreal, Canada.

Berlfein, Judy. 1988. "An Ill Nature (Research on Links Between Disease and Personality Types)." *Psychology Today* 22:16.

Berntzen, D., and K. G. Gotestam. 1987. "Effects of On-Demand Versus Fixed-Interval Schedules in the Treating of Chronic Pain with Analgesic Compounds." *Journal of Consulting and Clinical Psychology* 55:213–17.

Berry, Robert. 1983. "Stress and Safety Down on the Farm." *Psychology Today* 17:21.

Beston, Henry. 1956. *The Outermost House*. New York: Viking Press.

Birbeck, Anthony. 1991. "A European Perspective on Farm Animal Welfare." *Journal of the American Veterinary Medical Association* 198:1377–79.

Blix, Susanne, and Gregory Brack. 1988. "The Effects of a Suspected Case of Munchausen's Syndrome by Proxy on a Pediatric Nursing Staff." *General Hospital Psychiatry* 10:402–9.

Borasch, Douglas S. 1992. "The Mainstreaming of Alternative Medicine." *The New York Times Magazine* (October 4):86.

Bower, Bruce. 1987. "Depression and Cancer: A Fatal Link." *Science News* 132:244.

———. 1988a. "Pessimism Linked to Poor Health." *Science News* 134:54.

———. 1988b. "Emotion-immunity Link Found in HIV Infection." *Science News* 134:116.

Boyce, John R. 1993. "Farm Animal Welfare: Progress on Several Fronts." *Journal of the American Veterinary Medical Association* 203:356-57.

Brady, J. E. 1992. "Are You Beginning to Burn Out?" *Working Mother* 15:31–33.

Brumbaugh, Gordon. 1993. "Scientific Basis for Nonapproved Use of Drugs in Veterinary Practice." *Journal of the American Veterinary Medical Association* 202:1693–96.

Burke, James. 1985. *The Day the Universe Changed*. Boston: Little, Brown, and Company.

Bush, Alan H. 1992. "The Perils of Perfectionism." *Journal of the American Veterinary Medical Association* 210:1184–85.

Bustad, L. K. 1981. *Animals, Aging and the Aged*. Minneapolis: University of Minnesota Press.

———. 1990. "Recent Discoveries about Our Relationships with the Natural World." *People, Animals, Environment* (Fall):10–12.

Campbell, William. 1986. *Owner's Guide to Better Behavior in Dogs and Cats*. Goleta, Calif.: American Veterinary Publications.

———. 1992. *Behavioral Problems in Dogs*. Goleta, Calif.: American Veterinary Publications.

Campos, R. G. 1989. "Soothing Pain-Elicited Distress in Infants with Swaddling and Pacifier." *Child Development* 60:781–92.

Caras, Roger. 1993. "One Generation Away from Humanity." *Journal of the American Veterinary Medical Association* 202:910–12.

Case, D. B. 1988. "Survey of Expectations among Clients of Three Small Animal Clinics." *Journal of the American Veterinary Medical Association* 192:498–502.

Cassel, Christine K., and Diane E. Meier. 1990. "Morals and Moralism in the Debate over Euthanasia and Suicide." *The New England Journal of Medicine* 323:750–53.

Catanzaro, Thomas E. 1988. "A Survey on the Question of How Well Veterinarians are Prepared to Predict Their Clients' Human-Animal Bond." *Journal of the American Veterinary Medical Association* 192:1707–12.

Center for Information Management. 1988. *The Veterinary Services Market for Companion Animals 1988.* Schaumburg, Ill.: The American Veterinary Medical Association.

———. 1992. *The Veterinary Service Market for Companion Animals 1992.* Schaumburg, Ill.: The American Veterinary Medical Association.

Centers for Disease Control. 1992. "Outbreak of Salmonella Enteritidis Infection Associated with Consumption of Raw Shell Eggs." *Journal of the American Medical Association* 267:3263 (2).

———. 1993. "Update: Multistate Outbreak of *Escherichia coli* 0157:H7 Infections from Hamburgers—Western United States 1992-1993." *Journal of the American Medical Association* 269:2194 (2).

Charles, Charles Associates. 1983. *The Veterinary Services Market.* Overland Park, Kans.: Charles, Charles Associates.

Charles, M. M. 1992. "Welcome to the Age of Overwork." *Fortune* 126:64–67.

Charmin, Robert C. 1992. *At Risk: Can the Doctor-Patient Relationship Survive in a High-Tech World?* Dublin, N.H.: William L. Bauhan, Publisher.

Clark, Janet Bennett. 1993. "Alternative Medicine Is Catching On." *Kiplinger's Personal Finance Magazine* (January):98.

Clavin, Thomas. 1991. "The Thrill of Insubordination (Managing a Passive-Aggressive Employee)." *Working Woman* 16:70–73.

Cleland, Janice. 1993. "Extra-label Drug Use—Veterinary Practitioner Views: Companion Animals." *Journal of the American Veterinary Medical Association* 202:1642–44.

Coates, C. David. 1989. *Old McDonald's Factory Farm.* New York: Continuum.

Cogan, R., and D. Cogan, W. Waltz, and M. McCue. 1987. "Effects of Laughter and Relaxation on Discomfort Thresholds." *Journal of Behavioral Medicine* 10:139–44.

Colen, B. D. 1989. "It's Hard to Know What's Worse: The Hurting or the Drugs That Treat It." *Health* 21:34.

"Comforting Words (Reassuring Tapes Played to Anesthetized Women Undergoing Hysterectomy Reduced Need for Post-operative Medication)." 1991. *Harvard Health Letter* 6:1.

Committee on the Use of Animals in Medicine. Report. 1991. *Science, Medicine, and Animals.* Washington, D.C.: National Academy Press.

Coniff, Richard. 1990. "Fuzzy-wuzzy Thinking about Animal Rights." *Audubon* 92:120–32.

Cooper, Cary L., and Roy Payne. 1991. *Personalities and Stress: Individual Differences in the Stress Process.* New York: John Wiley and Sons.

Cousins, Norman. 1974. *Celebration of Life: A Dialogue on Immortality and Infinity.* New York: Harper and Row.

———. 1979. *Anatomy of an Illness.* New York: W. W. Norton.

———. 1989. *Head First: The Biology of Hope.* New York: Dutton.

Cowley, Geoffrey. 1993 "Seeking the Cause of a Killer (Meat Link to Prostatic Cancer)." *Newsweek* (October 18):77.

Crow, Steven. 1985. "Usefulness of Prognosis: Qualitative versus Quantitative Designations." *Journal of the American Veterinary Medical Association* 187:700–703.

Dinsmore, Jack, and David McConnell. 1992. "Communicate to Avoid Malpractice Claims." *Journal of the American Veterinary Medical Association* 201:383–87.

"Do You Need Meat?" 1992. *Glamour* 90:124.

"Does Pet Ownership Reduce Your Risk for Heart Disease?" 1992. *InterActions* 10:11–13.

Donoghue, Susan. 1992. "Nutritional Support of Hospitalized Animals." *Journal of the American Veterinary Medical Association* 200:612–15.

Dyer, Kirsti A., and Austin H. Kutcher. 1992. "Reshaping our Views of Death and Dying (Educating Medical Students About Death)." *Journal of the American Medical Association* 267:1265 (3).

Elkins, A. D., and J. R. Elkins. 1987. "Professional Burnout among U.S. Veterinarians: How Serious a Problem?" *Veterinary Medicine* 82: 1245–50.

Elkins, A. D., and Michael Kearney. 1992. "Professional Burnout among Female Veterinarians in the United States." *Journal of the American Veterinary Medical Association* 200:604–8.

Elliot, Martha Pearse. 1981. "Parent Care: Total Involvement in the Care of a Dying Child." In *Living with Death and Dying* by Elisabeth Kübler-Ross. New York: Macmillan, 95–159.

Evans, A. Thomas, Richard Broadstone, James Stapleton, Toni M. Hooks, Sharon Marie Johnston, and Judith R. McNeil. 1993. "Comparison of Pentobarbital Alone and Pentobarbital in Combination with Lidocaine for Euthanasia in Dogs." *Journal of the American Veterinary Medical Association* 203:663–64.

Evans, Job Michael. 1985. *The Evans Guide for Counseling Dog Owners.* New York: Howell Book House.

"Finding a Way to Mind Your Pain (Research Shows That Deliberately Suppressing Pain Worsens It)." *Science News* 143:156.

Fine, Aubrey. 1992. "The Flight to Inner Freedom: Helping Children Develop Healthy Self-Esteem Utilizing Birds as an Aspect of Treatment." *Abstracts of Presentations.* Sixth International Conference on Human-Animal Interactions, Montreal, Canada.

Fletcher, Ben. 1991. *Work, Stress, Disease and Life Expectancy.* New York: John Wiley & Sons.

Fogle, B., and Abrahamson, D. 1990. "Pet Loss: A Survey of the Attitudes and Feelings of Practicing Veterinarians." *Anthrozoös* 3:151–54.

Fox, Michael. 1983. "Veterinary Politics, Science, and Empathy." *Modern Veterinary Practice* (April): 266–70.

Fraser, A. F., and D. M. Broom. 1990. *Farm Animal Behavior and Welfare.* London: Bailliere Tindall.

Frazier, Anitra. 1990. *The New Natural Cat.* New York: Plume.

Freese, Wayne R. 1993. "Responsibilities of Food Animal Practitioners Regarding Extra-label Use of Drugs." *Journal of the American Veterinary Medical Association* 202:1733–34.

Friedmann, E. 1990. "The Value of Pets for Health and Recovery."*Proceedings of the First European Congress of the British Small Animal Veterinary Association,* 8–17.

Friedmann, E., A. H. Katcher, S. A. Thomas, J. J. Lynch, and P. R. Messent. 1983. "Social Interaction and Blood Pressure: Influence of Animal Companions." *Journal of Nervous and Mental Disease* 171:461–65.

Fritz, Robert, and Brian Smith. 1982. *The Power of Choice.* Charlestown, N.H.: Fainshaw Press.

Fulghum, Robert. 1986. *All I Really Need to Know I Learned in Kindergarten.* New York: Ballentine Books.

Gallagher, David. 1993. "New Studies Confirm Fee Level Is Key to Success."*Veterinary Advisory Report* 7:1.

Gill, Dawn, and Diana Stone. 1992."The Veterinarian's Role in the AIDS Crisis." *Journal of the Veterinary Medical Association* 201:1683–84.

Glasser, Stephen P., Pamela I. Clark, Raymond J. Lipicky, James M. Hubbard, and Salim Yusuf. 1991. "Exposing Patients with Chronic Angina to Placebo Periods in Drug Trials." *Journal of the American Medical Association* 265:1550 (5).

Glickman, Larry T. 1992. "Implications of the Human/Animal Bond for Human Health and Veterinary Practice." *Journal of the American Veterinary Medical Association* 201:848–51.

Goldberg, Joan Rachel. 1987. "Crying It Out." *Health* 19:64–66.

Gonser, Patricia. 1989. "Life Events Changes, Stress-Related Illness, Injury and Hospitalization in Six Through Eleven Year Olds and Stress-Related Illness and Behavioral Changes in Companion Animals. " *Abstracts of Presentations.* Delta Society Eighth Annual Conference, Parsippany, New Jersey.

Gorczyca, Ken. 1992. "Pets and the Immunocompromised Patient." *Syntex Journal Rounds* 4–6.

Gorham, Mary Ellen. 1992. "DVMs Can Heighten Awareness, Difference of Animal Rights and Welfare." *DVM* (February):32.

Gorman, James. 1992. "Take a Little Deadly Nightshade and You'll Feel Better." *The New York Times Magazine* (September 30):22.

Grant, E. 1987. "It Only Hurts When I Don't Laugh." *Psychology Today* 21:21.

Gregory, Greg. 1989. "Placebo Effect: Power of Suggestion." *Current Health* 15:23(3)

Griffin, Donald. 1984. *Animal Thinking.* Cambridge, Mass.: Harvard University Press.

———. 1992. *Animal Minds.* Chicago: University of Chicago Press.

Gross, Edith. 1993. "When Doctors Sweat (Stress Factors Vary for Male and Female Physicians.)" *Psychology Today* 26:10.

Grossarth-Maticek, R. 1980. "Psychosocial Predictors of Cancer and Internal Disease: An Overview." *Psychotherapy and Psychosomatics* 33:120–28.

Guntzelman, Joan, and Michael H. Riegger. 1993a. "Helping Pet Owners with the Euthanasia Decision." *Veterinary Medicine* (January) 26–34.

———. 1993b. "Supporting Clients Who are Grieving the Death of a Pet." *Veterinary Medicine* (January):35–41.

Gutfield, Greg, Melissa Meyer, and Maureen Sangiorgio. 1991. "Surgery Soother: Supportive Voices May Aid Recovery." *Prevention* 43:18.

Hannah, Harold. 1992a. "The Standard of Care—Some Legal Considerations." *Journal of the American Veterinary Medical Association* 200:610–11.

———. 1992b. "Some Legal Implications in Biotechnology." *Journal of the American Veterinary Medical Association* 200:1634–35.

———. 1992c. "Examining Veterinarians for Physical and Mental Fitness." *Journal of the American Veterinary Medical Association* 201:1002–3.

———. 1993. Negligence in Diagnosis." *Journal of the American Veterinary Medical Association* 202:1066–67.

Hansen, Bernie, and Elizabeth Hardie. 1993. "Prescription Use of Analgesics in Dogs and Cats in a Veterinary Teaching Hospital: 258 Cases (1983–1989)." *Journal of the American Veterinary Medical Association* 202:1485–94.

Hart, Benjamin. 1985a. "Animal Behavior and the Fever Response: Theoretical

Considerations." *Journal of the American Veterinary Medical Association* 187:998–1001.

———. 1985b. *Behavior of Domestic Animals.* New York: W. H. Freeman and Company.

Hart, Lynette. 1992. "The Lifestyles of People Who Live With Companion Animals." *Abstracts of Presentations.* Sixth International Conference on Human-Animal Interactions, Montreal, Canada.

Hart, Lynette, and Benjamin Hart. 1987. "Grief and Stress from So Many Animal Deaths." *Companion Animal Practice* 1:20–21.

Hart, Lynette, Benjamin L. Hart, and Bonnie Mader. 1990. "Humane Euthanasia and Companion Animal Death: Caring for the Animal, the Client, the Veterinarian." *Journal of the American Veterinary Medical Association* 197:1292–99.

"The Health Benefits of Pets." 1988. *Abstracts of the NIH Technology Assessment Workshop—Health Benefits of Pets. September 10–11, 1987.* U.S. Government Printing Office, 1988-216–107.

Herrick, John. 1992. "Conventional and Nonconventional Medicine." *Journal of the American Veterinary Medical Association* 201:854–55.

———. 1993. "Integrated Resource Management." *Journal of the American Veterinary Medical Association* 203:501–2.

Holcomb, Ralph. 1992. "Mitigating Depression in Elderly Men Through Animal Exposure." *Abstracts of Presentations.* Sixth International Conference on Human-Animal Interactions, Montreal, Canada.

Holgrieve, Amy. 1992. "Shielding Clients from Injury Protects Against Malpractice Claims." *Journal of the American Veterinary Medical Association* 201:1681–82.

Houpt, K. A., and T. Wolski. 1982. *Domestic Animal Behavior for Veterinarians and Animal Scientists.* Ames: Iowa State University Press.

Hunter, Beatrice Trum. 1991. "A Newly Emerging Foodborn Disease." *Consumer's Research Magazine* 74:8 (2).

Jasper, James, and Dorothy Nelkin. 1992. *The Animal Rights Crusade: The Growth of a Moral Protest.* New York: Free Press.

Jimenez, Sherry. 1992. "Soothing Hands for Labor." *American Baby* 54:B8 (5).

Johnson, Darrel E. 1993. "Extra-label Drug Use—Veterinary Practitioner Views: Food Animals." *Journal of the American Veterinary Medical Association* 202:1645–47.

Johnson, Janna. 1991. "The Veterinarian's Responsibility Assessing and Managing Acute Pain in Dogs and Cats." *The Compendium* 13:804–7.

Johnson, Samuel. [1759] 1980. In *Bartlett's Familiar Quotations* 15th ed. Boston: Little, Brown and Company.

Jordan, William. 1991. *Divorce among the Gulls.* New York: Harper Collins.

Kaneene, J. B., and Rose Ann Miller. 1992. "Description and Evaluation of the Influence of Veterinary Presence on the Use of Antibiotics and Sulfonimides in Dairy Herds." *Journal of the American Veterinary Medical Association* 201:68–76.

Kaplan, Sherrie, and Sheldon Greenfield. 1989. "Assessing the Effects of Physician-Patient Interactions on the Outcomes of Chronic Disease." *Journal of Medical Care* 27:S110–S127.

Katcher, Aaron. 1990. "The Visual Dialogue with Nature: How Attending to Animals and Green Spaces Influences Health and Emotional Balance." *People, Animals, Environment* (Fall):19–20.

Katcher, A. H., and A. Beck. 1983. *New Perspectives on Our Lives with Companion Animals*. Philadelphia: University of Pennsylvania Press.

Katcher, Aaron, Erika Friedmann, Melissa Goodman, and Laura Goodman. 1983. "Men, Women, and Dogs." *California Veterinarian* (February):14–16.

Kehoe, P., and E. M. Blass. 1986. "Behaviorally Functional Opioid Systems in Infant Rats: Evidence for Pharmacological, Physiological and Psychological Mediation of Pain and Stress." *Behavioral Neuroscience* 100:624–30.

Kennedy, John F. 1962. Address at the University of California at Berkeley, March 23, 1962. In *Bartlett's Familiar Quotations* 15th ed. Boston: Little, Brown and Company.

Kitchen, Hyram, Arthur L. Aronson, James L. Bittle, Charles W. McPherson, David B. Morton, Stephen P. Pakes, Bernard Rollin, Andrew N. Rowan, Jeri A. Sechzer, Jack E. Vanderlip, James A. Will, Ann Schola Clark, and Joe S. Gloyd. 1987. "Panel Report on the Colloquium on the Recognition and Alleviation of Animal Pain and Distress." *Journal of the American Veterinary Medical Association* 191:1186–91.

Krener, P., and R. Adelman. 1988. "Parent Salvage and Parent Sabotage in the Care of Chronically Ill Children." *American Journal of the Diseases of Childhood* 142:945–51.

Kronfeld, D. S., and C. P. Parr. 1987. "Ecologic and Symbiotic Approaches to Animal Welfare, Animal Rights, and Human Responsibility." *Journal of the American Veterinary Medical Association* 191:660–64.

Kübler-Ross, Elisabeth. 1969. *On Death and Dying*. New York: Macmillan.

Lance, Susan E., Gay Y. Miller, Dan Hancock, Paul C. Bartlett, and Lawrence E. Heider. 1992. "Salmonella Infections in Neonatal Dairy Calves." *Journal of the American Veterinary Medical Association* 201:864–68.

Lautner, Beth. 1993. "Assuring a Residue-Free Pork Supply." *Journal of the American Veterinary Medical Association* 202:1727–29.

Lavin, Michael R. 1991. "Placebo Effects on Mind and Body." *Journal of the American Veterinary Medical Association* 265:1753–55.

Lawrence, Elizabeth Atwood. 1991. "Relevance of Social Science to Veterinary Medicine." *Journal of the American Veterinary Medical Association* 199:1018–20.

Levine, J. D., N. C. Gordon, H. L. Fields, and L. Howard. 1978. "The Mechanisms of Placebo Analgesia." *Lancet* 2:654–57.

Libow, J. A., and H. A. Schreier. 1986. "Three Forms of Factitious Illness in Children: When Is It Munchausen Syndrome by Proxy?" *American Journal of Orthopsychiatry* 57:602–10.

Litt, M. D. 1988. "Self-efficacy and Perceived Control: Cognitive Mediators of Pain Tolerance." *Journal of Personality and Social Psychology* 54:149–60.

Loew, Franklin. 1993. "Eating Habits." Letter to the editor. *Journal of the American Veterinary Medical Association* 203: 614.

Long, Patricia. 1986. "Medical Mesmerism: Once Considered Mere Trickery, Hypnosis Is Emerging as a Valuable Technique for Controlling Pain and Anxiety." *Psychology Today* 20:28.

Lynch, James J. 1977. *The Broken Heart and the Medical Consequences of Loneliness*. New York: Basic Books.

———. 1985. *The Language of the Heart: The Human Body in Dialogue*. New York: Basic Books.

———. 1987. "Man's Best Friendly Medicine." *Creative Living* 16:16–21.

Machiavelli, Niccolò. [1537] 1961. *The Prince*. New York: Viking Penguin.

MacKay, Clayton. 1993. "Veterinary Practitioner's Role in Pet Overpopulation." *Journal of the American Veterinary Medical Association* 202:918–21.

Makar, Adel F., and Paula J. Squierl. 1990. "Munchausen Syndrome by Proxy: Father as a Perpetrator." *Pediatrics* 85:370–73.

Marieb, Elaine N. 1991. *Essentials of Human Anatomy and Physiology.* New York: Benjamin/Cummings.

McCullough, William T. 1989. "The Effects of Pet Ownership on the Psychological Well-Being of Physically Disabled Children." *Abstracts of Presentations.* Delta Society Eighth Annual Conference, Parsippany, New Jersey.

McGuire, Tona, and Kenneth Feldman. 1989. "Psychologic Morbidity of Children Subjected to Munchausen Syndrome by Proxy." *Pediatrics* 83:289–92.

Meadow, R. 1977. "Munchausen Syndrome by Proxy." *Lancet* 2:343–45.

———. 1985. "Management of Munchausen Syndrome by Proxy." *Archives of the Diseases of Childhood* 60:385–93.

Meer, Jeff. 1984. "Who Will Heal the Healers?" *Psychology Today* 18:85.

Melson, Gail F. 1990. "Fostering Inter-Connectedness with Animals and Nature: The Developmental Benefits for Children." *People, Animals, Environment* (Fall):15–17.

Michaels, Bonnie, and Elizabeth McCarty. 1992. *Solving the Work/Family Puzzle.* Homewood, Ill.: Business One Irwin.

Milani, Myrna M. 1993. *The Body Language and Emotion of Cats.* New York: Quill.

———. 1993. *The Body Language and Emotion of Dogs.* New York: Quill.

Miller, Laurence. 1986. "Boy, Did That Hurt! Or Did It? (Research on Pain Perception)." *Psychology Today* 20:23.

Miller, Melody, and Dan Lago. 1989. "The Well-Being of Older Women: The Importance of Pet and Human Relationships." *Abstracts of Presentations.* Delta Society Eighth Annual Conference, Parsippany, New Jersey.

Monagia, Katie. 1992. "Are Animals Equal?" *Scholastic Update* 125:19–22.

Morris, Desmond. 1991. *The Animal Contract.* New York: Warner Books.

Moyers, Bill. 1993. *Healing and the Mind.* New York: Doubleday.

"Mummification among Options for Handling Animal Remains." 1993. *Veterinary Product News* 6:11.

Nassar, R., and J. Fluke. 1991. "Pet Population Dynamics and Community Planning for Animal Welfare and Animal Control." *Journal of the American Veterinary Medical Association* 198:1160–64.

Newman, Jennifer. 1992. "Homeopathy: Diluted or Deluded?" *American Health* (April):47.

Niebuhr, Reinhold. [1934] 1980. "The Serenity Prayer." In *Bartlett's Familiar Quotations* 15th ed. Boston: Little, Brown and Company.

Norris, Margaret P., and Bonnie V. Beaver. 1993. "Application of Behavioral Therapy Techniques to the Treatment of Obesity in Companion Animals." *Journal of the American Veterinary Medical Association* 202:728–30.

Osborn, Carl. 1991. "The Veterinarian's Oath: Are You Keeping Your Promise?" *Journal of the American Veterinary Medical Association* 198:1906–8.

Padus, Emrika. 1992. *The Complete Guide to Your Emotions and Your Health.* Emmaus, Pa.: Rodale Press.

Parker, Robert, Barbel Holtman, and Paul F. White. 1991. "Patient-Controlled Analgesia: Does a Concurrent Opiod Infusion Improve Pain Management After Surgery?" *Journal of the American Medical Association* 266:1947 (6).

Pederson, Niels C. 1991. *Feline Husbandry: Diseases and Management in the Multi-*

ple Cat Environment. Goleta, Calif.: American Veterinary Publications.

Perkins, A. G. 1993. "The Costs of Inflexible Job Arrangements." *Harvard Business Review* 71:9–10.

Pert, C., M. R. Ruff, R. J. Webber, and M. Herkenham. 1985. "Neuropeptides and Their Receptors: A Psychosomatic Network." *Journal of Immunology* 135: 820S–2S.

Pesut, N., and D. F. Kowalczyk. 1983. "Considerations on the Use of Placebos in Veterinary Medicine." *Journal of the American Veterinary Medical Association* 182:675–79.

"Pets Provide Comfort for Patients with AIDS, ARC." 1989. *Psychiatric News* 24:5.

Philips, H. C. 1987. "The Effects of Behavioral Treatment on Chronic Pain." *Behavior and Research Therapy* 25:365–77.

Podolsky, Doug. 1991. "Big Claims, No Proof." *U.S. News and World Report* (September 23):77.

Poresky, Robert H. 1989. "Antecedents of Companion Animal Bonding, Attitudes and Ownership: An Exploratory Analysis." *Abstracts of Presentations.* Delta Society Eighth Annual Conference, Parsippany, New Jersey.

Price, E. O. 1987. *The Veterinary Clinics of North America: Farm Animal Behavior.* Philadelphia: William B. Saunders.

Pritchard, William R. 1993. "Some Implications of Structural Changes in Veterinary Medicine and Its Impact on Veterinary Education." *Journal of the American Veterinary Medical Association* 203:361–64.

Quackenbush, Jamie. 1985. *When Your Pet Dies: How to Cope with Your Feelings.* New York: Pocket Books.

Quackenbush, J. E., and L. Glickman. 1984. "Helping People Adjust to the Death of a Pet." *Health and Social Work* 9:42–48.

Radnitz, C. L., K. A. Appelbaum, E. B. Blanchard, L. Elliott, and F. Andrasik. 1988. "The Effect of Self-Regulatory Treatment on Pain Behavior in Chronic Headache." *Behavior and Research Therapy* 26: 253–60.

Raloff, Janet. 1990. "Meaty Findings about Colon Cancer and Diets." *Science News* 138:374.

———. 1992. "Fighting Fat with Fat: Red Meat Redeemed." *Science News* 139: 22.

Rifkin, Jeremy. 1992. *Beyond Beef: The Rise and Fall of the Cattle Culture.* New York: NAL-Dutton.

Ritvo, Harriet. 1982. "Toward a More Peaceable Kingdom." *Technology Review* 95:54–62.

Rogers, Fred. 1988. *When a Pet Dies.* New York: Putnam.

Rollin, B. E. 1981. *Animal Rights and Human Morality.* Buffalo: Prometheus Books.

———. 1983. "The Concept of Illness in Veterinary Medicine." *Journal of the American Veterinary Medical Association* 182:122–25.

Rosch, Paul J. 1984. "Coping with Stress on the Job." *Nation's Business* 72: 65.

Ross, Elisabeth Kübler. 1966. "The Dying Patient as Teacher: An Experiment and an Experience." *Chicago Theological Seminary Register* 57:3.

Ruth, Rob. 1992. "Animals Are Helping Children Overcoming Physical and Emotional Challenges." *InterActions* 10:16–18.

Saint-Exupéry, Antoine de. [1943] 1971. *The Little Prince.* New York: Harcourt Brace Jovanovich.

Schaufl, Angelika, and Reinfhold Bergler. 1992. "Children and Dogs." *Abstracts of Presentations.* Sixth International Conference on Human-Animal Interactions, Montreal, Canada

Schleifer, S., E. Keller, M. Camerino, J. C. Thornton, and M. Stein. 1983. "Supression of Lymphocyte Stimulation Following Bereavement." *Journal of the American Medical Association* 250:374–77.

Schroefer, Lisa. 1991. "The Men's Health Job Stress Index." *Men's Health* 6:40–43.

Schwartz, Stephen G. 1991. "Holistic Health: Seeking a Link Between Medicine and Metaphysics." *Journal of the American Medical Association* 266:3064.

Seligman, Martin E. 1975. *Helplessness: On Depression, Development and Death.* San Francisco: W. H. Freeman and Company.

Self, Donnie, Dawn E. Schrader, DeWitt C. Baldwin, Jr., Susan Root, Frederic D. Wolinsky, John A. Shadduck. 1991. "Study of the Influence of Veterinary Medical Education on the Moral Development of Veterinary Students." *Journal of the American Veterinary Medical Association* 198:782–87.

Self, Donnie, Nancy S. Jecker, DeWitt C. Baldwin, Jr., John A. Shadduck. 1991. "Moral Orientations of Justice and Care among Veterinarians Entering Veterinary Practice." *Journal of the American Veterinary Medical Association* 199:569–73.

Serpell, J. A. 1990. "Evidence for Long Term Effects of Pet Ownership on Human Health." *Proceedings of the First Congress of the British Small Animal Veterinary Association,* 1–7.

Sheridan, Mary S. 1989. "Munchausen Syndrome by Proxy." *Health and Social Work* (February): 53–58.

Siegal, Bernard. 1986. *Love, Medicine, and Miracles.* New York: Harper and Row.

———. 1989. *Peace, Love, and Healing.* New York: Harper and Row.

Siegel, Judith M. 1990. "Stressful Life Events and Use of Physician Services among the Elderly: The Moderating Role of Pet Ownership." *Journal of Personality and Social Psychology* 58:1081–86.

Sinclair, Charles. 1993. "The Tough Job of Talking about Risk." *Journal of the American Veterinary Medical Association.* 202:884–86.

Singer, P. 1975. *Animal Liberation.* New York: Avon Books.

Smith, Brian R. 1991. *How to Become Successfully Self-Employed.* Holbrook, Mass.: Bob Adams, Inc.

Smith, Carin. 1992. "Acupuncture: An Ancient Treatment Modality under Scientific Scrutiny." *Journal of the American Veterinary Medical Association* 201:1321–25.

Spanos, N. P., et al. 1989. "Hypnosis, Suggestion, and Placebo in the Reduction of Experimental Pain." *Journal of Abnormal Psychology* 98:285–93.

Spencer, Lea. 1992a. "Pets Prove Therapeutic for People with AIDS." *Journal of the American Veterinary Medical Association* 201:1665–68

———. 1992b. "Study Explores Health Risks and the Human/Animal Bond." *Journal of the American Veterinary Medical Association* 201:1669

———. 1993. "*Escherichia coli* 0157:H7 Infection Forces Awareness of Food Production and Handling." *Journal of the American Veterinary Medical Association* 202:1043–47.

Spinelli, J. S., and H. Markowitz. 1987. "Clinical Recognition and Anticipation of Situations Likely to Induce Pain in Animals." *Journal of the American Veterinary Medical Association* 191:1216–18.

Stallones, Lorann. 1990. "Companion Animals and Health of the Elderly." *People, Animals, Environment* (Fall):18–19.

Stephenson, James. 1982. "Man's Best Friends: The Pleasures of Treating Animals." *Journal of the American Institute of Homeopathy* 75:4.

Stockner, Priscilla. 1986. "How to Handle a Client in Tears." *Trends* (January):61–63.

Stone, Elizabeth, Daniel A. Shugars, James D. Bader, and Edward H. O'Neill. 1992. "Attitudes of Veterinarians toward Emerging Competencies for Health Care Professionals."*Journal of the American Veterinary Medical Association* 201:1849–53.

Summers, Jim, and John New. 1985. "When Doing Good Can Help in Doing Well—A Case Study." *Journal of the American Veterinary Medical Association* 187:902–6.

Sussman, Vic. 1990. "A Fresh Attack on Red Meat: New Health Studies See More Perils." *U.S. News and World Report* 109:67.

Sykora, Jaroslav. 1992. "Stress Relieving Interactions Within a Complex of Animals and Humans in Experimental Isolation." *Abstracts of Presentations*. Sixth International Conference on Human-Animal Interactions, Montreal, Canada

Tannenbaum, Jerrold. 1986. "Animal Rights: Some Guideposts for the Veterinarian." *Journal of the American Veterinary Medical Association* 188: 1258–63.

———. 1989. *Veterinary Ethics*. Baltimore: Williams and Wilkins.

———. 1991. "Ethics and Animal Welfare: The Inextricable Connection." *Journal of the American Veterinary Medical Association* 198:1360–76.

"Tears: Medical Research Helps Explain Why You Cry." 1992. *Mayo Clinic Health Letter* 10:4 (2)

Telzak, Edward E., Lawrence D. Budnick, Michele S. Zweig Greenberg, Steve Blum, Mehdi Shayegani, Charles E. Berson, and Stephen Schultz. 1990. "A Nosocomial Outbreak of Salmonella Enteritidis Infection Due to the Consumption of Raw Eggs." *The New England Journal of Medicine* 323:394 (4).

Tevis, Cheryl. 1985. "There's More Help for Rural Stress." *Successful Farming* 83:15.

Thornburg, Larry. 1992. "Four Essential Components of Veterinary Education for the 21st Century." *Journal of the American Veterinary Medical Association* 201:1180–83.

Thornton, Gus. 1991. "Veterinarians as Members of the Humane Community." *Journal of the American Veterinary Medical Association* 198:1352–54.

Thomas, Lewis. 1974. *The Lives of a Cell: Notes of a Biology Watcher.* New York: Viking Press.

———. 1979. *The Medusa and the Snail.* New York: Viking Press.

———. 1983a. *Late Night Thoughts on Listening to Mahler's Ninth Symphony.* New York: Viking Press.

———. 1983b. *The Youngest Science.* New York: Viking Press.

———. 1992. *The Fragile Species.* New York: Charles Scribners Sons.

Toufexis, Anastasia. 1990. "Red Alert on Red Meat: The Link Between High-Fat Diets and Colon Cancer Gets Stronger." *Time* (December 24):70.

Turner, Dennis C., and Patrick Bateson. 1988. *The Domestic Cat: The Biology of Its Behavior.* Cambridge: Cambridge University Press.

Underwood, A. 1992. "Coping with On the Job Stress." *Black Enterprise* 23:86–88.

Viorst, Judith. 1971. *The Tenth Good Thing about Barney.* New York: Macmillan.

Wagner, William C. 1992. "Animal Research and Veterinary Medical Research Funding: A Vision of the Future." *Journal of the American Veterinary Medical Association* 200:1474–76.

Wallis, Claudia. 1991. "Why New Age Medicine Is Catching On." *Time* (November 4):68–76.

Wallis, Don, and Charles DeWolff. 1988. *Stress and Organization Problems in Hospitals.* New York: Routledge, Chapman and Hall.

Wexler, Scott. 1992a. *Living with a Passive-Aggressive Male.* New York: Simon & Schuster Trade.

———. 1992b. "Sugarcoated Hostility." *Newsweek* (October 12):14.

White, E. B. 1952. *Charlotte's Web.* New York: Harper and Row.

Wilkes, Darrell. 1993. "Assuring a Residue-free Food Supply: Beef." *Journal of the American Veterinary Medical Association* 202:1725–27.

Willensky, Diana. 1992. "Working Wonders (Health Benefits Enjoyed by Working Wives and Mothers)." *American Health* 11:104.

Willet, Walter C., Mair J. Stampfer, Graham A. Colditz, Bernard A. Rosner, and Frank E. Speizer. 1990. "Relation of Meat, Fat and Fiber Intake to the Risk of Colon Cancer in a Prospective Study of Among Women." *The New England Journal of Medicine* 323:1664–73.

Williams, Garth. 1991. "Flaming Out on the Job." *Modern Maturity* 34:26–29.

Wilson, Edward O. 1992. *The Diversity of Life.* New York: W. W. Norton.

Wilson, James F. 1988. *Law and Ethics of the Veterinary Profession.* Yardley, Pa.: Priority Press Ltd.

Ziegler, Jan. 1991. "Red Flags: Red Meat Doubles Risk of Colon Cancer." *American Health* 10:86.

Zitelli, Basil J., Mirian F. Seltman, and Rose Mary Shannon. 1987. "Munchausen's Syndrome by Proxy and Its Professional Participants." *American Journal of the Diseases of Childhood* 141:1099–1102.

Index

Abuse: client education and, 112–13; relative nature of, 113–14

Acceptance, client: chronic medical conditions and, 109–10; death of animal and, 215–16; dying animal and, 211–12; tolerance vs., 110

Acceptance, veterinarian: advantages of, 252–53; death of animal and, 233; different beliefs and, 30, 269–70; dying animal and, 231; unchangeable negative situations and, 251–57

Aggression, passive, 98–100; in clients, 98–99; in veterinarians, 100

Alternative therapies. See Therapies, alternative

Analgesics, behavioral vs. pharmacological, 189–91; use in terminally ill cases, 218, 219

Analogy: anthropomorphic owners and, 17; communication using, 66

Anger: death of animal and, 212–13, 214; dying animal and, 210, 228–29; euthanasia and, 212–13, 226; misbehaved animal and, 26–27, 93–94, 114

Anger, veterinarian: alternative therapies and, 171, 178–79; animal rights and, 183–84, death of animal and, 231–32; dying animal and, 227, 228–29; misbehaved animals and, 251–52; nonpaying clients and, 44; stressful client interactions and, 72–73; toward nonveterinary specialists, 94, 165

Animal rights. See Rights, animal

Animals, dominant: best friend clinicians and, 132–34; defined as loving, 110–11; god clinicians and, 118–20; handling of, 63–64; prepackaged best friend clinicians and, 133

Animals, submissive: best friend orientation and, 134; functioning as dominant, 119; god clinicians and, 118–19

Animals, terminally ill: home care of, 217–18; client acceptance of, 209–12; referring, 160–61; special considerations in treatment of, 216–18

Animals, territorial nature of. See Territoriality

Anorexia, behavioral vs. medical treatment of, 186–87

Anthropomorphically oriented owners. See Clients, anthropomorphically oriented

Anthropomorphically oriented veterinarians. See Veterinarians, relationships to animals

Antibiotics, as placebos, 173–74

Anxiety, separation, 79–80

Appetite, health and, 104–6

Appointments: educational, 94; end-of-day, 51–52; geriatric, 225–27; improper training of those making appointments, 97; making appointments with specialists, 166–67; variable length, 50–51

Balance, practitioner: achieving in patient-client orientation, 131, 153–55; at time of patient death, 223; problematic owner relationships and, 87; treating critically ill and injured animals and, 196, 207

Bargaining, death, dying and: client, 210–

This book has been set in Baskerville and Eras typefaces. Baskerville was designed by John Baskerville at his private press in Birmingham, England, in the eighteenth century. The first typeface to depart from oldstyle typeface design, Baskerville has more variation between thick and thin strokes. In an effort to insure that the thick and thin strokes of his typeface reproduced well on paper, John Baskerville developed the first wove paper, the surface of which was much smoother than the laid paper of the time. The development of wove paper was partly responsible for the introduction of typefaces classified as modern, which have even more contrast between thick and thin strokes.

Eras was designed in 1969 by Studio Hollenstein in Paris for the Wagner Typefoundry. A contemporary script-like version of a sans-serif typeface, the letters of Eras have a monotone stroke and are slightly inclined.

Printed on acid-free paper.